HUMAN
SECTIONAL
ANATOMY

Atlas of Body Sections, CT and MRI Images

SECOND EDITION

HAROLD ELLIS CBE MA DM MCh FRCS FRCOG
Clinical Anatomist
The Guy's, King's College and St.Thomas's Hospitals
Medical and Dental School
Guy's Campus
London SE1 9RT

BARI M LOGAN MA FMA Hon MBIE MAMAA
University Prosector
Department of Anatomy
University of Cambridge
Downing Street
Cambridge
CB2 3DY

ADRIAN K DIXON MD FRCP FRCR
Professor
Department of Radiology
University of Cambridge

Honorary Consultant Radiologist
Addenbrooke's Hospital
Hills Road
Cambridge
CB2 2QQ

Fellow, Peterhouse, Cambridge

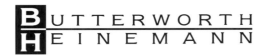

BUTTERWORTH
HEINEMANN

OXFORD • AUCKLAND • BOSTON • JOHANNESBURG • MELBOURNE • NEW DELHI

Butterworth-Heinemann
Linacre House, Jordan Hill, Oxford OX2 8DP
225 Wildwood Avenue, Woburn, MA 01801-2041
A division of Reed Educational and Professional Publishing Ltd

A member of the Reed Elsevier plc group

First published as Human Cross-sectional Anatomy 1991
Reprinted 1993
Second edition 1999
© Reed Educational and Professional Publishing Ltd, 1991, 1999

British Library Cataloguing in Publication Data
A catalogue record for this book is available from the British Library

Library of Congress Cataloguing in Publication Data
A catalogue record for this book is available from the Library of Congress

ISBN 0 7506 3367 0

Scanning and film origination by Graphic Ideas Studios, London

Printed in Great Britain By BAS Printers Ltd, Over Wallop, Hants

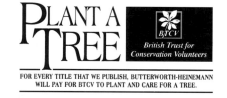

CONTENTS

PREFACE

The study of sectional anatomy of the human body goes back to the earliest days of systematic topographical anatomy. The beautiful drawings of the sagittal sections of the male and female trunk and of the pregnant uterus by Leonardo da Vinci (1452–1519) are well known. Among his figures, (which were based on some 30 dissections), are a number of transverse sections of the lower limb. These constitute the first known examples of the use of cross-sections for the study of gross anatomy and anticipate modern technique by several hundred years. In the absence of hardening reagents or methods of freezing it was only seldom used by Leonardo (O'Malley and Saunders 1952). Andreas Vesalius pictured transverse sections of the brain in his *Fabrica* published in 1543 and in the 17th century portrayals of sections of various parts of the body, including the brain, eye and the genitalia were made by Vidius, Bartholin, de Graaf and others. Drawings of sagittal section anatomy was used to illustrate surgical works in the 18th century, for example, those of Antonio Scarpa of Pavia and Peter Camper of Leyden. William Smellie, one of the fathers of British midwifery, published his magnificent *Anatomical Tables* in 1754, mostly drawn by Riemsdyk, which mainly comprised sagittal sections and William Hunter's illustrations of the human gravid uterus are also well known.

The obstacle to detailed sectional anatomical studies was, of course, the problem of fixation of tissues during the cutting process. De Riemer, a Dutch anatomist, published an atlas of human transverse sections in 1818 which were obtained by freezing the cadaver. The other technique which was developed during the early 19th century was the use of gypsum to envelope the parts and to retain the organs in their anatomical position – a method used by the Weber brothers in 1836.

Pirogoff, the well known Russian surgeon, produced his massive 5 volume cross-sectional anatomy between 1852 and 1859, which was illustrated with 213 plates. He used the freezing technique, which he claimed (falsely, as noted above), to have introduced as a novel method of fixation.

The second half of the 19th century saw the publication of a number of excellent sectional atlases, and photographic reproductions were used by Braun as early as 1875.

Perhaps the best known atlas of this era in the United Kingdom was that of Sir William Macewen, Professor of Surgery in Glasgow, and published in 1893. Entitled an *Atlas of Head Sections*, it comprised a series of coronal, sagittal and transverse sections of the head in the adult and child. This was the first atlas to show the skull and brain together in detail. Macewen intended his atlas to be of practical, clinical value and wrote in his preface 'the surgeon who is about to perform an operation on the brain has in these cephalic sections a means of refreshing his memory regarding the position of the various structures he is about to encounter'; this from the surgeon who first proved in his treatment of cerebral abscess, that clinical neurological localization could be correlated with accurate surgical exposure.

The use of formalin as a hardening and preserving fluid was introduced by Gerota in 1895 and it was soon found that thorough perfusion of the vascular system of the cadaver enabled satisfactory sections to be obtained of the formalin hardened material. The early years of the 20th century saw the publication of a number of atlases based on this technique. Perhaps the most comprehensive and beautifully executed of these was *A Cross-Section Anatomy* produced by Eycleshymer and Schoemaker of St Louis University, which was first published in 1911 and whose masterly historical introduction in the 1930 edition provides an extensive bibliography of sectional anatomy.

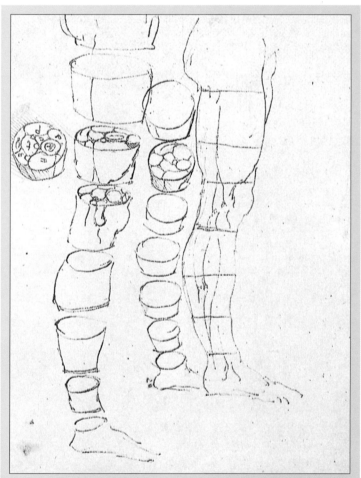

Leonardo da Vinci. The right leg of a man measured, then cut into sections (Source: Windsor Castle Royal Library © 1991 Her Majesty the Queen).

THE IMPORTANCE OF CROSS-SECTIONAL ANATOMY

Successive authors of atlases on sectional anatomy have emphasized the value to the anatomist and to the surgeon of being able to view the body in this dimension. It is always difficult to consider three dimensions in the mind's eye; to be able to view the relationships of the viscera and fascial planes in transverse and vertical section helps to clarify the conventional appearances of the body's structure as seen in the operating theatre, in the dissecting room and in the text-book.

The introduction of modern imaging techniques, especially Ultrasound, Computed Tomography (CT) and Magnetic Resonance Imaging (MRI) has enormously expanded the already considerable importance of sectional anatomy. The radiologist, neurologist, internist, chest physician and oncologist, as well as specialists in the various fields of surgery, have had to re-educate themselves in the appearances and relationships of anatomical structures in transverse and vertical section. Indeed, precise diagnosis, as well as the detailed planning of therapy (for example, the ablative surgery of extensive cancer) and of interventional radiology, often depends on the cross-sectional anatomical approach.

This atlas combines three presentations of cross-sectional anatomy, that of the dissecting room, Computed Tomography (CT) and Magnetic Resonance Imaging (MRI). The series are matched to each other as closely as possible on opposite pages. Students of anatomy, surgeons, clinicians and radiologists should find the illustrations of anatomical cross-sections (obtained by the most modern techniques of preparation and photographic reproduction) and the equivalent cuts on imaging (obtained on state-of-the-art apparatus) both interesting and rewarding.

PRESERVATION OF CADAVERS

Preservation of the cadavers used for the sections in this Atlas was by standard embalming technique, using two electric motor pumps set at a maximum pressure rate of 15 p.s.i. Preservative fluid was circulated through the arterial system via two cannulae inserted into the femoral artery of one leg. A partial flushing of blood was effected from the accompanying femoral vein by the insertion of a large bore drainage tube.

After the successful acceptance of 20 litres of preservative fluid, local injection by automatic syringe was carried out on those areas which remained unaffected.

On average, approximately 30 litres of preservative fluid was used to preserve each cadaver.

Following preservation, the cadavers were stored in thick-gauge polythene tubes and refrigerated to a temperature of 51°F (10.6°C) at 40% humidity, for a minimum 16 week period before sectioning.

This period allowed the preservative solution to saturate thoroughly the body tissues, resulting in a highly satisfactory state of preservation.

The chemical formula for the preservative solution (Logan et al 1989) is:

Methylated spirit 64 op	12.5 litres	
Phenol liquified 80%	2.5 litres	
Formaldehyde solution 38%	1.5 litres	
Glycerine BP	3.5 litres	= **20 litres**

The resultant working strengths of each constituent is:

Methylated spirit	55%
Glycerine	12%
Phenol	10%
Formaldehyde solution	3%

The advantages of this particular preservative solution are that (1) a state of soft preservation is achieved; (2) the low formaldehyde solution content obviates excessive noxious fumes during dissection; (3) a degree of natural tissue colour is maintained which benefits photography; and (4) mould growth does not occur on either whole cadavers thus preserved, or their subsequent prosected and stored parts.

SECTIONING

In order to produce the 117 cross-sections illustrated in this Atlas, five preserved cadavers, two male and three female were utilised, in addition to five upper and five lower separate limbs.

The parts to be sectioned were deep-frozen to a temperature of -40°C for a minimum three-day period immediately prior to sectioning.

Sectioning was carried out on a purpose-built AEW 600 stainless steel bandsaw (AEW Engineering Co Ltd, Gresham House, Pinetrees Business Park, Salhouse Road, Norwich, Norfolk, NR7 9BB, England). The machine is equipped with a 10 horse power, three phase electric motor which is capable of producing a constant blade speed of 6000 feet per minute.

A fine-toothed (four skip) stainless steel blade was used, 19 mm in depth and precisely 1 mm in thickness (including tooth set).

The design and precision manufacture of the machine results, during operation, in the loss of only 1 mm of material between each section.

Sections were taken from the cadavers to the following thickness of cut:

Head	1 cm serial
Neck	1.5 cm serial
Thorax	2 cm serial
Abdomen	2 cm serial
Pelvis male	2 cm serial
Pelvis female	2 cm serial
Lower limb	at selected levels
Upper limb	at selected levels

COMPUTED TOMOGRAPHY (CT)

Ever since the invention of CT by Hounsfield (1973) there has been renewed interest in sectional anatomy. Despite the high cost, CT systems are now widely used throughout the more affluent countries. Radiologists in particular have had to go through a rapid learning process. Several excellent sectional CT anatomy books have been produced. However, more modern CT technology allows a wider range of structures to be demonstrated with better image quality, mainly due to improved spatial resolution and shorter data acquisition times. Spiral CT techniques have lowered data acquisition time yet further, allowing a volume acquisition during a single breathold. Hence the justification for yet another atlas which correlates anatomical and CT images.

Most of the images in this volume have been obtained on a Siemens Somatom Plus CT system in Addenbrooke's Hospital, Cambridge. Imaging protocols have continued to evolve from the original descriptions (e.g. Dixon 1983a), particularly with the advent of spiral data acquisition. An Oral contrast medium is routinely given for abdominopelvic studies; thus the stomach and small bowel usually appear opaque. Contrast medium is often administered per rectum before a pelvic study. Intravenous contrast medium provides additional information and thus in some sections vessels appear opaque.

Precise correlation between the cadaveric sections and the clinical images is very difficult to obtain in practice. No two patients are quite the same shape! The distribution of fat, particularly in the abdomen, varies from patient to patient and between the sexes (Dixon, 1983b). Furthermore, there are the inevitable physiological discrepancies between cadaveric slices and images obtained in-vivo. These are especially noticeable in the juxta-diaphragmatic region. In particular, the vertebral levels do not quite correlate because of the effect of inspiration; all intrathoracic structures are better displayed on images obtained at suspended inspiration. Furthermore, in order to obtain as precise a correlation as possible, some CT images may not be quite of optimal quality. A further difficulty which is encountered when attempting to correlate the two sets of images is caused by the fact that CT involves ionising radiation. The radiation dose has to be kept to the minimum which answers the clinical problem. Thus it is not always possible to find photogenic examples of the anatomy shown in the cadavers for all parts of the body.

Some knowledge of the X-ray attenuation of normal structures is useful to assist interpretation of the images. The Hounsfield scale extends from air, which measures -1,000 HU (Hounsfield Units), through pure water at 0 HU to beyond +1,000 HU for dense cortical bone. Most soft tissues are in the range +35 to +70 HU (kidney, muscle, liver, etc). Fat provides useful negative contrast at around -100 HU. The displayed image can appear very different depending on the chosen window width (the spread of the grey scale) and the window level (the centre of the grey scale). These differences are especially apparent in the thorax where the images are displayed both at soft tissue settings (window 400, level +20 HU) and at lung settings (window c. 1250, level -850 HU). Such image manipulation merely requires alteration of the stored electronic data at the viewing console, where any parameters can be chosen. The 'hard copy' photographic record of the electronic data is always a rather poor representation. Indeed, in clinical practice, it may be difficult to display all structures and some lesions on hard copy film.

MAGNETIC RESONANCE IMAGING (MRI)

The evolution of Magnetic Resonance Imaging (MRI) to its present status from long established chemical magnetic resonance techniques has been gradual. A key milestone occured when Lauterbur (1973) first revealed the imaging potential of MRI. Clinical Images quickly followed, initially from Aberdeen and Nottingham (e.g. Hawkes et al 1980). Research by various manufacturers then led to a plethora of techniques, moving towards shorter and shorter acqusition times which are now approaching those of computed tomography (CT).

The physics of MRI is substantially more complex than CT, even though the principles of picture elements (pixels) derived from volume elements (voxels) within the body are similar, along with the partial volume artifacts that can occur. Much of the computing and viewing software is similar; indeed many manufacturers allow viewing of CT and MR images on the same viewing console.

Central to an MRI system is a very strong magnet, usually between 0.2 and 1.5 Tesla (T); (1T = 10,000 Gauss; the earth's magnetic field strength is approximately 0.5 Gauss). When the patient is in the magnet the protons within the body will align their spins according to the strength and direction of the magnetic field. The protons within the water of the body are particularly suitable for MR techniques. At 1.0 T protons within hydrogen nuclei will resonate at approximately 42.6 MHz. The protons can be excited so that the net magnetism of the spins is flipped by the application of a radiofrequency (RF) signal. Gradient magnetic fields are applied to vary the precessional frequency. The emitted radiofrequency signal is detected as an echo to provide spatial information and data about the chemical environment of the protons within the voxel, etc.

Some common imaging sequences are:

i) Proton density images. Conventionally acquired using a long repetition time (TR c. 2000 ms between signals) and a short echo time (TE c. 20 ms) before read out. These provide a map of the distribution of hydrogen protons (mainly within fat and water).

ii) T1 weighted images. These are conventionally acquired with short TR (c 700 ms) and short TE (c 20 ms). They are useful for demonstrating anatomy. The T1 time of the tissue refers to the time taken for the longitudinal magnetism to decay following the RF pulse and involves energy loss to the lattice in the chemical environment.

iii) T2 weighted images. These are conventionally acquired using long TR (e.g. 2000 ms) and long TE (80 plus ms). These images often show oedema and fluid most clearly and are good for demonstrating lesions. The T2 time of the tissue refers to the time taken for the transverse magnetism to decay following the RF pulse. It involves the way in which in the spin of one proton interacts with the spins of neighbouring protons.

iv) Fast imaging sequences. In order to complete acquisitions quickly (e.g. within a breath-hold) numerous techniques have been devised. These include gradient echo sequences whereby the magnetisation is never allowed to recover fully. Other techniques involve a rapid succession (train) of RF pulses and echoes, requiring advanced computer processing.

v) Tissue specific techniques. The different environments of protons (fat, water, flowing blood etc.) mean that protocols can be adapted to accentuate certain features. Fat can be suppressed by the application of a RF pulse at the resonant frequency of fat follwed by a gradient pulse to null the signal from fat. Images can also be generated to show either static fluid or flowing blood.

Because of the range of possible sequences, the appearance of the resulting images vary considerably. It is important to realise that the grey scale of the image reflects the intensity of the returning signal. There are no absolute values, such as in computed tomography (CT).

In general fat returns high signal and appears bright (white), unless fat suppression is used (see v. above). There is not sufficient water vapour in air to produce a signal. Therefore air always returns very little signal and appears dark (black). Dense cortical bone also appears black; cortical bone has very tightly bound protons within

its structure, the lack of mobility results in reduced signal. Medullary bone contains a lot of fatty marrow and thus usually appears bright. Sequences can be performed so that blood within the vessels will return high signal; this is the basis of MR angiography.

In the MR images presented here, the sequence(s) have been chosen to demonstrate certain anatomical features to best effect. Thus the precise parameters and the appearance vary extensively. On occasions T1 weighted image and corresponding T2 weighted image are displayed side by side for optimal demonstration of anatomical features.

ORIENTATION OF SECTIONS AND IMAGES

A concerted effort over recent years has meant that axial cross-sectional and coronal images are now viewed in a standard conventional manner. Hitherto there was wide variation which led to considerable confusion and even medico-legal complications.

ALL axial cross-sectional images in clinical practice are now viewed as shown in **Fig A**; that is from 'below' and 'looking up'. This is the logical method, in so far that the standard way in which a doctor approaches the examination of the supine patient is from the right hand, foot end of a couch. The image is thus in the correct orientation for his palpating right hand. For example, he has to 'reach across' the image to find the spleen, exactly as he would during the clinical examination of the abdomen. Similarly, for the head, the right eye is the one more accessible for right handed ophthalmoscopy. Thus, all axial sections should be considered, learned and even displayed with an orientation logo shown in **Fig B**. This is the same orientation as that used for other images (e.g. a chest X-ray). Here again, the right of the patient

is on the viewer's left, just as if the clinician was about to shake hands with the patient.

Happily there is now world-wide agreement over this matter with regard to axial imaging. Furthermore, many anatomy books have adopted this approach so that students learn this method from outset. Ideally, embryologists and members of all other disciplines concerned with anatomical orientation should ultimately conform to this method.

The orientation logo in **Fig B** is suitable for the head, neck, thorax, abdomen and pelvis. However in the limbs, when only one limb is displayed, further clarification is required. All depends on whether a right or left limb is being examined. To assist this quandary, a medial and a lateral marker is provided **Fig C**. In this volume a left limb has been used throughout. Again, viewing is as from 'below'.

The orientation of coronal images has also been standardised so that they are viewed with the patient's right on the left, exactly as for a chest X-ray or when talking to the patient face to face.

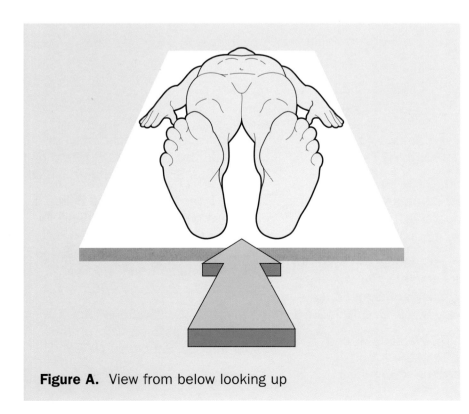

Figure A. View from below looking up

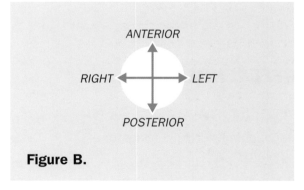

Figure B.

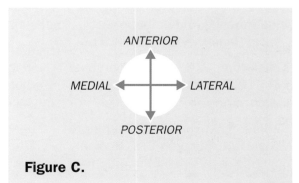

Figure C.

There is, as yet, no firm standardisation for viewing sagittal images. Various manufacturers display their images in different ways. Although there is a certain logic in viewing from the patient's right side, the visual approach for a clinician examining a patient on a couch, the majority of manufacturers display sagittal images viewed from the left. Thus in this volume most sagittal images are viewed from the left side of the patient.

Fig D Line A. The radiographic base line used for axial head sections and images in this atlas has been selected as that running from the inferior orbital margin to the external auditory meatus. This allows most of the brain to be demonstrated without excessive bony artefact.

Fig D Line B. For sections and images of the neck and the rest of the body a true axial plane has been used.

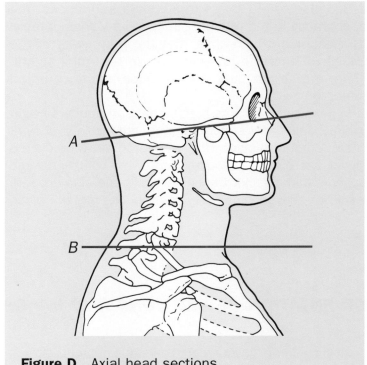

Figure D. Axial head sections

NOTES ON THE ATLAS

This Atlas presents various sections of the cadaver with corresponding radiological images. The logical sequence should enable the student to find the desired anatomical level with ease.

The numbers placed on the colour photographs and on the line drawings which accompany each radiological image match and the key to these numbers is given on the accompanying list on each page spread. Where numbers are highlighted in colour on the key, these refer to features which are apparent only on the radiological images.

Brief notes accompany each section and refer to important anatomical and radiological features.

In the majority of sections, bilateral structures have been labelled only on one side. This has been done in order to allow readers to have an unobscured view of structures and to put their own anatomical knowledge to the test.

A series of views of a minimally dissected brain is provided in order to clarify the orientation of cerebral topography in the series of head sections.

Several spreads of selected images (e.g. mediastinum) have been included in order to show features of important anatomical areas in more detail than can easily be demonstrated in cadavers and standard imaging.

REFERENCES

Dixon, A.K. (1983a) *Body* CT: *a handbook*. Churchill Livingstone, Edinburgh.

Dixon, A.K. (1983b) Abdominal fat assessed by computed tomography: sex difference in distribution. *Clinical Radiology* 34, 189–191.

Eycleshymer, A.C. and Schoemaker, D.M. (1930) *A Cross-Section Anatomy*. Appleton, New York.

Hawkes, R.C., Holland G.N., Moore W.S and Worthington B.S. Nuclear magnetic resonance tomography of the brain. *J. Comput. Assist. Tomogr.* 1980; 4: 577–80.

Hounsfield, G.N. (1973) Computerized transverse axial scanning (tomography). *British Journal of Radiology*, 46, 1016–102.

Lauterbur. P.C. Image formation by induced local interaction: examples employing nuclear magnetic resonance. *Nature*. 1973; 242: 190–1.

Logan, B.M., Watson, M. and Tattersall, R. (1989) A basic synopsis of the 'Cambridge'

procedure for the preservation of whole human cadavers. *Institute of Anatomical Sciences Journal*, 3, 25.

Logan, B.M., Liles, R.P. and Bolton, I. (1990) A photographic technique for teaching topographical anatomy from whole body transverse sections. *The Journal of Audio Visual Media in Medicine* 13 (No 2), 45–48.

O'Malley, C.D. and Saunders, J.B. (1952) *Leonardo da Vinci on the human body*. Schuman, New York.

ACKNOWLEDGEMENTS

DISSECTING ROOM STAFF

'for skilled technical assistance in the preservation and sectioning of the cadavers'

Mr M Watson, Senior Technician
Mr R Tattersall, Technician
Mrs C Bester, Technician
Mr M O'Hannan, Porter

Department of Anatomy, University of Cambridge

AUDIO VISUAL UNIT

'for photographic expertise'

Mr J Bashford
Mr R Liles, LMPA
Mr I Bolton
Mr A Newman

Department of Anatomy, University of Cambridge

'for all the excellent art work and graphics'

Mrs Rachel Chesterton

PRINTING OF COLOUR PHOTOGRAPHS

Streamline Colour Labs, Cambridge

SECRETARIAL

'for typing of manuscript'

Miss J McLachlan, Miss A J J Burton,
Miss S Clark and Mrs K Frans

Departments of Anatomy and Radiology,
University of Cambridge

ANNOTATION OF CENTRAL NERVOUS SYSTEM (BRAIN & HEAD SECTIONS)

Professor Roger Lemon
The Sobell Department of Neurophysiology,
Institute of Neurology,
Queen's Square, London

Dr Catherine Horner, Lecturer in Neurobiology,
Department of Anatomy,
University of Cambridge

ANNOTATION OF HEAD AND LIMB SECTIONS.

Dr Ian Parkin, Clinical Anatomist,
Department of Anatomy,
University of Cambridge

COMPUTED TOMOGRAPHY AND MAGNETIC RESONANCE IMAGING

'for performing many of the procedures'

Mrs B Housden, DCR
Miss H Szutowicz, HDCR
Mrs C Sims DCR
Mrs L Clements, DCR

and many other Radiographers at Addenbrooke's Hospital, Cambridge.

Many radiological colleagues provided useful advice and some kindly provided images (e.g. Dr David J Lomas, Lead Consultant, MRI).

PRODUCTION OF THE ATLAS

The authors would also like to thank the staff at Butterworth-Heinemann for their help and advice in the production of this Atlas.

DESIGN, LAYOUT AND REPROGRAPHICS

A very special thanks from the authors to Lee Smith, Paul Wilkinson and Andrew Wallis of Graphic Ideas Studios, London, for all their advice and care with the design and final layout of the book to press.

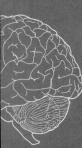
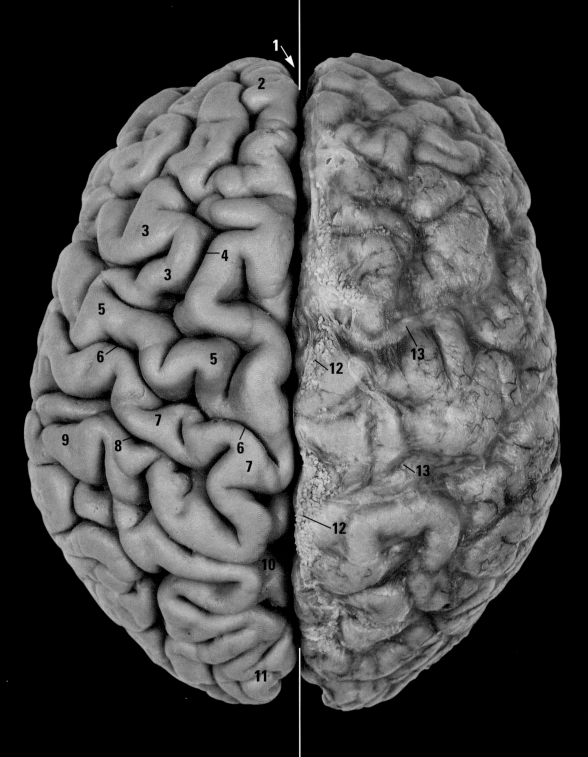

A Left cerebral hemisphere. From
   above with the arachnoid mater
   and blood vessels removed

B Right cerebral hemisphere. From
   above with the arachnoid mater
   and blood vessels intact

1 Longitudinal cerebral
   fissure (arrowed)
2 Frontal pole
3 Middle frontal gyrus
4 Superior frontal sulcus
5 Precentral gyrus
6 Central sulcus
7 Postcentral gyrus
8 Postcentral sulcus
9 Inferior parietal lobe
10 Parieto-occipital fissure
11 Occipital gyri

12 Arachnoid granulations
13 Superior cerebral veins

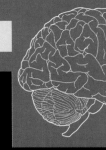

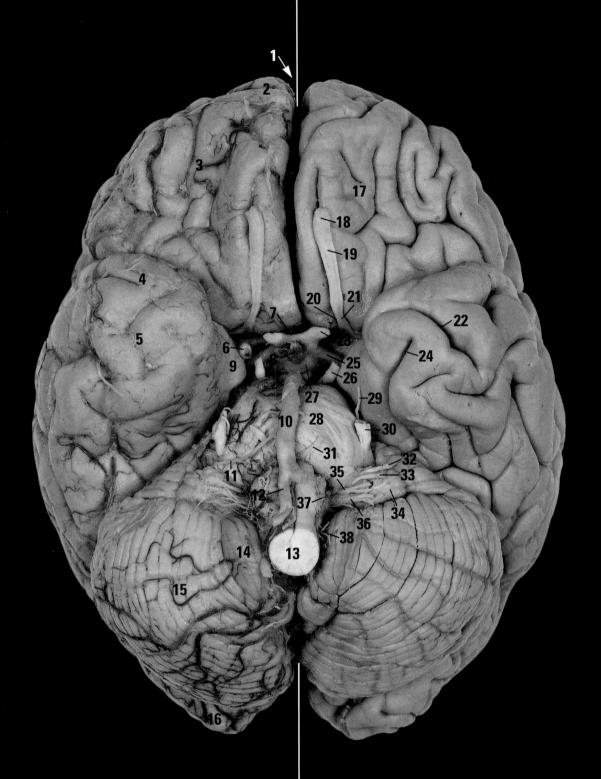

C Right cerebral hemisphere, cerebellum and brain stem. From below with the arachnoid mater and blood vessels intact

D Left cerebral hemisphere, cerebellum and brain stem. From below with the arachnoid mater and blood vessels removed

1 Longitudinal cerebral fissure (arrowed)
2 Frontal pole
3 Inferior surface of frontal pole
4 Temporal pole
5 Inferior surface of temporal pole
6 Internal carotid artery
7 Optic chiasma
8 Infundibulum
9 Parahippocampal gyrus
10 Basilar artery
11 Labyrinthine artery
12 Right vertebral artery
13 Medulla oblongata
14 Tonsil of cerebellum
15 Cerebellar hemisphere
16 Occipital pole

17 Orbital gyri
18 Olfactory bulb
19 Olfactory tract (I)
20 Medial olfactory stria
21 Lateral olfactory stria
22 Inferior temporal sulcus
23 Optic nerve (II)
24 Collateral sulcus
25 Optic tract
26 Oculomotor nerve (III)
27 Mamillary body
28 Pons

29 Trochlear nerve (IV)
30 Trigeminal nerve (V)
31 Abducent nerve (VI)
32 Facial nerve (VII)
33 Vestibulocochlear nerve (VIII)
34 Flocculus
35 Glossopharyngeal nerve (IX)
36 Vagus nerve (X)
37 Hypoglossal nerve (XII)
38 Accessory nerve (XI)

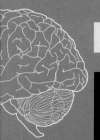

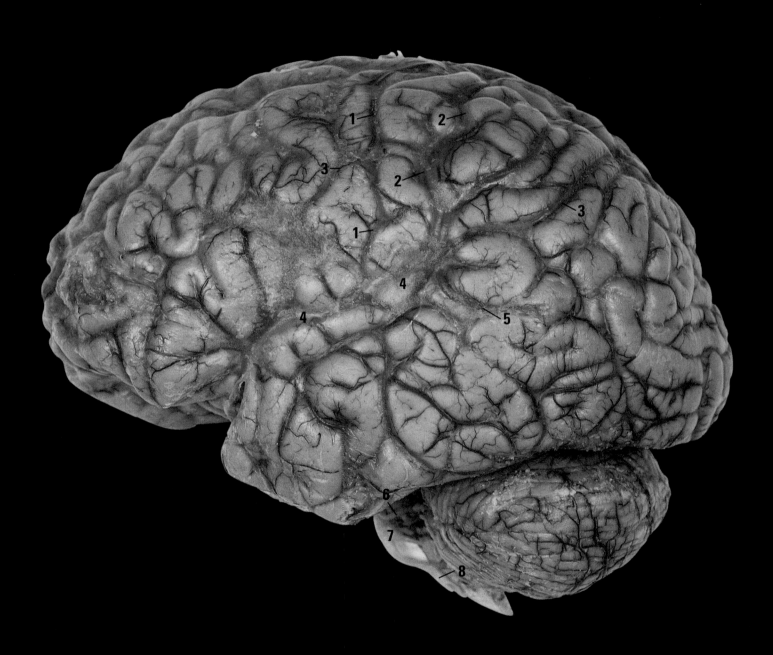

E From the left with the arachnoid mater and blood vessels intact

1 Rolandic artery (in central sulcus)
2 Superior anastomotic vein (Troland)
3 Superior cerebral veins
4 Lateral fissure
5 Inferior anastomotic vein (Labbé)
6 Superior cerebellar artery
7 Basilar artery
8 Vertebral artery

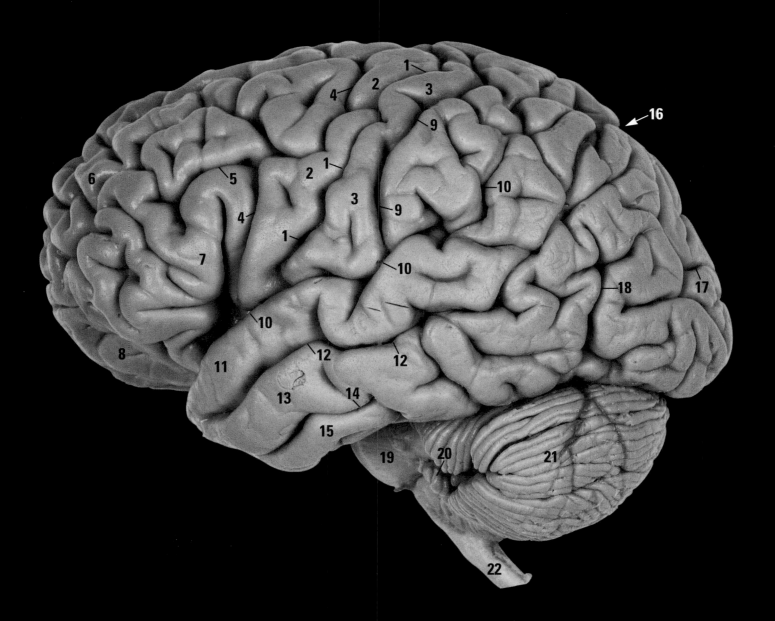

F From the left with the arachnoid mater and blood vessels removed

1 Central sulcus
2 Precentral gyrus
3 Postcentral gyrus
4 Precentral sulcus
5 Inferior frontal sulcus
6 Superior frontal gyrus
7 Inferior frontal gyrus
8 Orbital gyri
9 Postcentral sulcus
10 Lateral fissure
11 Superior temporal gyrus
12 Superior temporal sulcus

13 Middle temporal gyrus
14 Inferior temporal sulcus
15 Inferior temporal gyrus
16 Parieto-occipital fissure
    (arrowed)
17 Lunate sulcus
18 Anterior occipital sulcus
19 Pons
20 Flocculus
21 Cerebellar hemisphere
22 Medulla oblongata

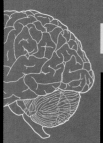

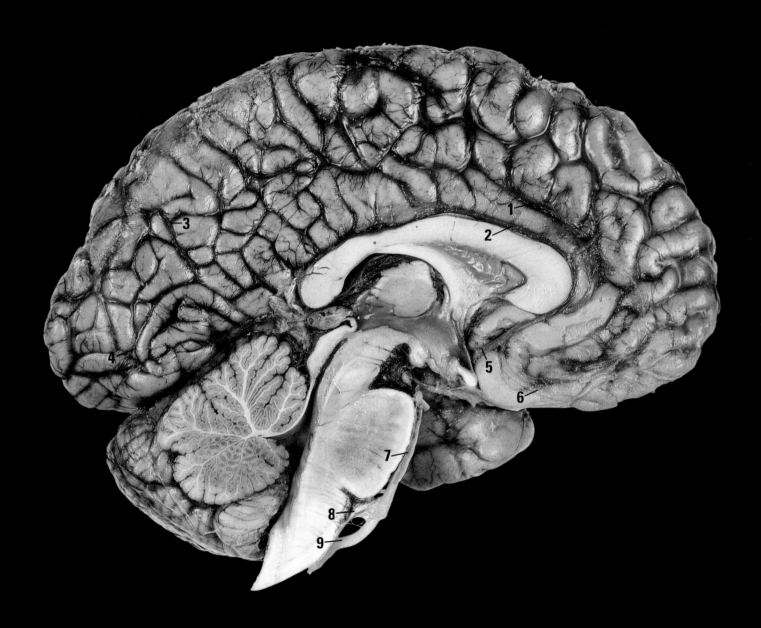

G A median sagittal section. The left half, from the right, with the arachnoid mater and blood vessels intact

1 Callosomarginal artery
2 Pericallosal artery
3 Calcarine artery
4 Posterior cerebral artery
5 Anterior cerebral artery
6 Orbital artery
7 Basiliar artery
8 Anterior inferior cerebellar artery
9 Left vertebral artery

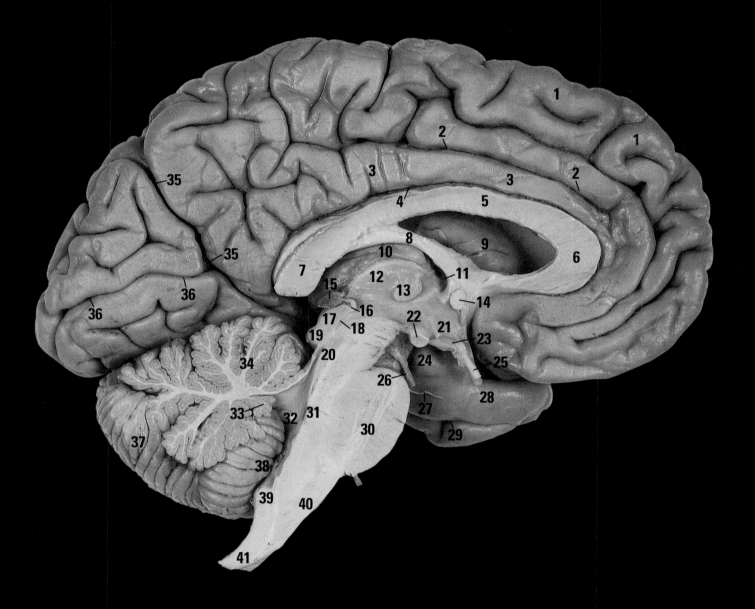

H A median sagittal section. The left half, from the right, with the arachnoid mater and blood vessels removed

1 Superior frontal gyrus
2 Cingulate sulcus
3 Cingulate gyrus
4 Callosal sulcus
5 Corpus callosum – body
6 Corpus callosum – genu
7 Corpus collosum – splenium
8 Fornix
9 Caudate nucleus (head) in
   wall of lateral ventricle
10 Choroid plexus, third vetricle
11 Interventricular foramen
   (Monro)
12 Thalamus
13 Massa intermedia

14 Anterior commissure
15 Pineal body
16 Posterior commissure
17 Superior colliculus
18 Aqueduct (of Sylvius)
19 Inferior colliculus
20 Mesencephalon
21 Hypothalamus
22 Mamillary body
23 Infundibulum
24 Uncus
25 Optic nerve (II)
26 Oculomotor nerve (III)
27 Trochlear nerve (IV)
28 Parahippocampal gyrus

29 Rhinal sulcus
30 Pons
31 Pontine tegmentum
32 Fourth ventricle
33 Nodulus
34 Anterior lobe of cerebellum
35 Parieto-occipital fissure
36 Calcarine sulcus
37 Cerebellar hemisphere
38 Tonsil of cerebellum
39 Inferior cerebellar peduncle
40 Pyramid
41 Medulla oblongata

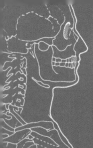

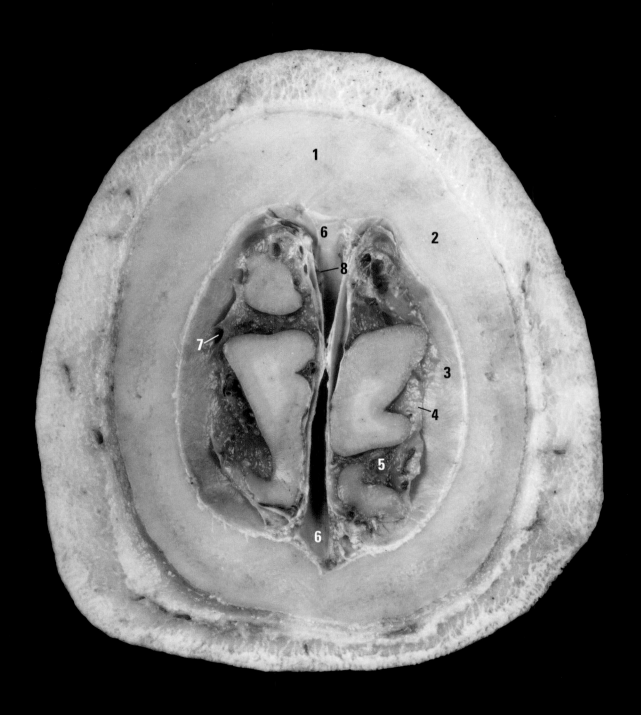

1 Frontal bone
2 Parietal bone
3 Dura mater
4 Arachnoid mater
5 Pia mater
6 Superior sagittal sinus
7 Superior cerebral vein
8 Arachnoid granulation

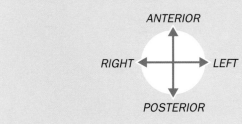

Section level

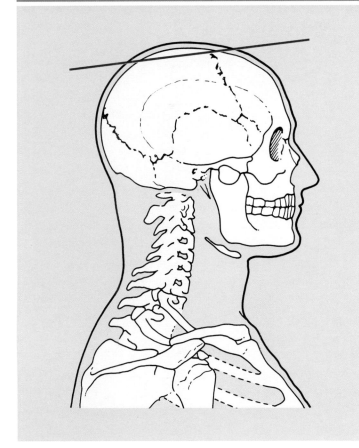

Orientation guide

ANTERIOR

RIGHT ← → LEFT

POSTERIOR

Notes

This section passes through the apex of the skull vault and traverses the parietal bones (**2**) and the superior portion of the frontal bone (**1**).

The dura mater which lines the inner aspect of the skull comprises an outer, or endosteal, layer, or endocranium (**3**) (which is, in fact, the periosteum which lines the inner aspect of the skull) and an inner, or meningeal, layer (**4**). Most of the intracranial venous sinuses are formed as clefts between these two layers, as demonstrated in this section by the superior sagittal sinus (**6**). The exceptions to this rule are the inferior sagittal sinus and the straight sinus, which are clefts within the meningeal layer.

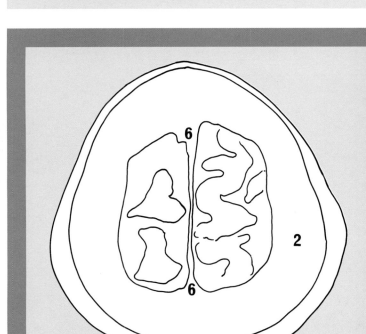

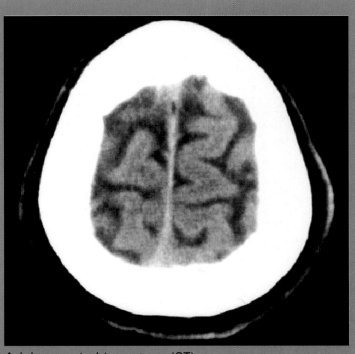

Axial computed tomogram (CT)

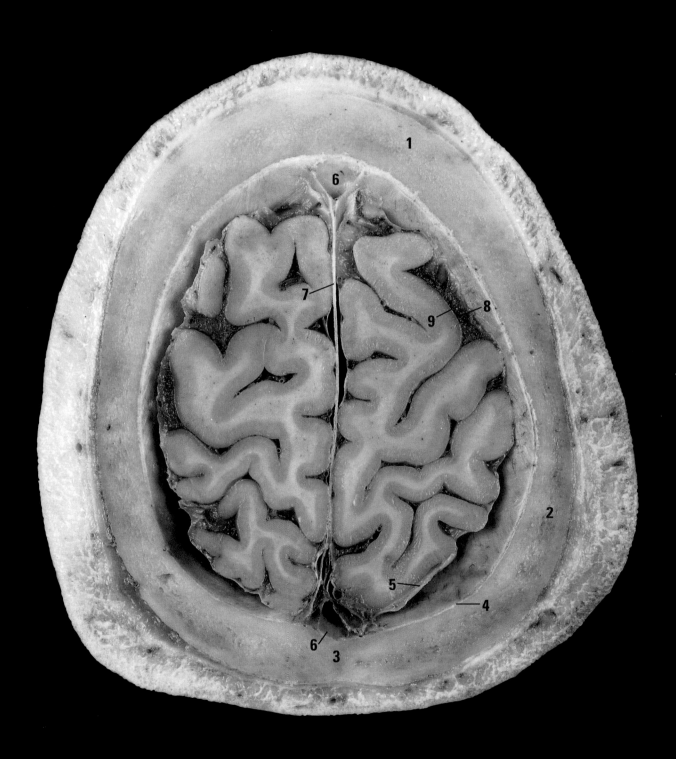

1 Frontal bone
2 Parietal bone
3 Sagittal suture
4 Dura mater
5 Arachnoid mater
6 Superior sagittal sinus
7 Falx cerebri
8 Subarachnoid space
9 Pia mater

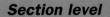

Section level

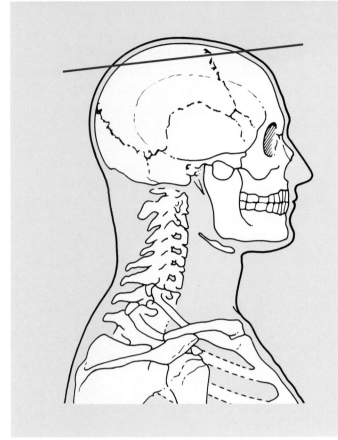

Orientation guide

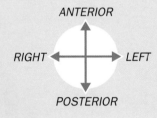

ANTERIOR

RIGHT   LEFT

POSTERIOR

Notes

This section, at a deeper plane through the skull vault, demonstrates the falx cerebri (**7**), which is formed as a double fold of the inner, meningeal, layer of the dura mater (**5**) and which forms the dural septum between the cerebral hemispheres.

The inner layer of the dura is lined by the delicate arachnoid mater. The pia mater (**9**) is vascular and invests the brain, spinal cord, cranial nerves and the spinal nerve roots. It remains in close contact with the surface of the brain, including the depths of the cerebral sulci and fissures.

Over the convexities of the brain, the pia and arachnoid are in close contact. Over the cerebral sulci and the cisterns of the brain base, the pia and arachnoid are separated by the subarachnoid space (**8**), which contains cerebrospinal fluid. This space is traversed by a fine spider's web of fibres (*arachnoid*: pertaining to the spider).

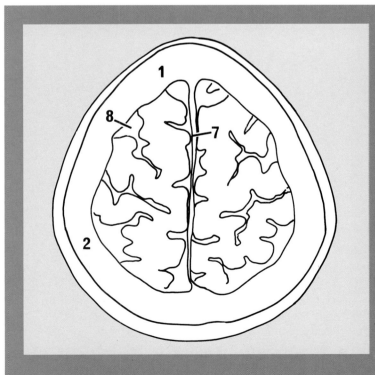

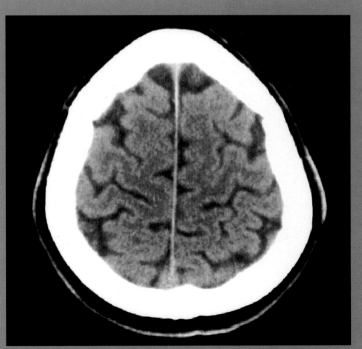

Axial computed tomogram (CT)

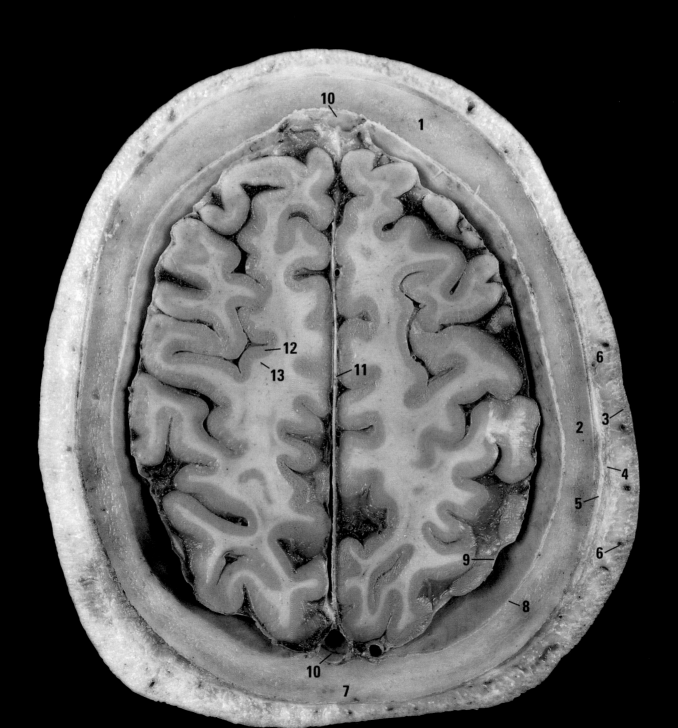

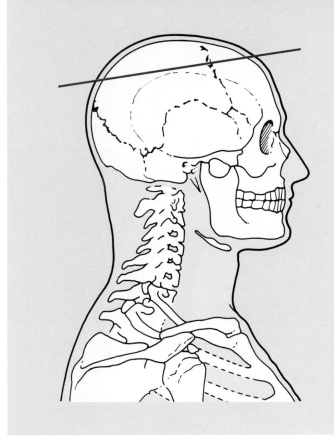

Section level

Orientation guide

ANTERIOR

RIGHT ← → LEFT

POSTERIOR

Notes

This section, through the upper parts of the cerebral hemispheres, gives a clear picture of the distinction between the outer grey matter (**12**), which contains nerve cells, and the inner white matter (**13**), made up of nerve fibres. This is in contradistinction to the arrangement of the spinal cord, with the central grey and surrounding white matter.

Note the five layers of the scalp – skin, underlying dense connective tissue (**3**), the dense epicranial aponeurosis, or galea aponeurotica (**4**), which is separated by a film of loose areolar connective tissue from the outer periosteum of the skull – the pericranium (**5**). The pericranium is densely adherent to the surface of the skull and passes through the various foramina, where it becomes continuous with the outer endosteal layer of the dura (**8**) and is also continuous with the sutural ligaments which occupy the cranial sutures.

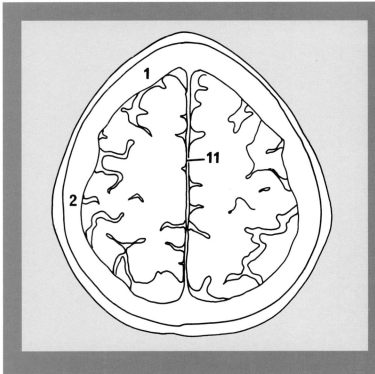

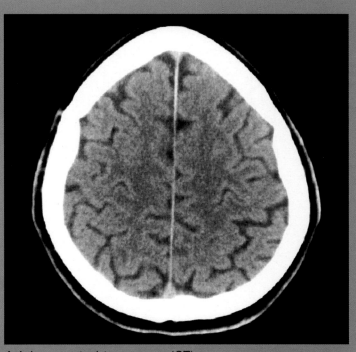

Axial computed tomogram (CT)

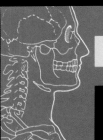

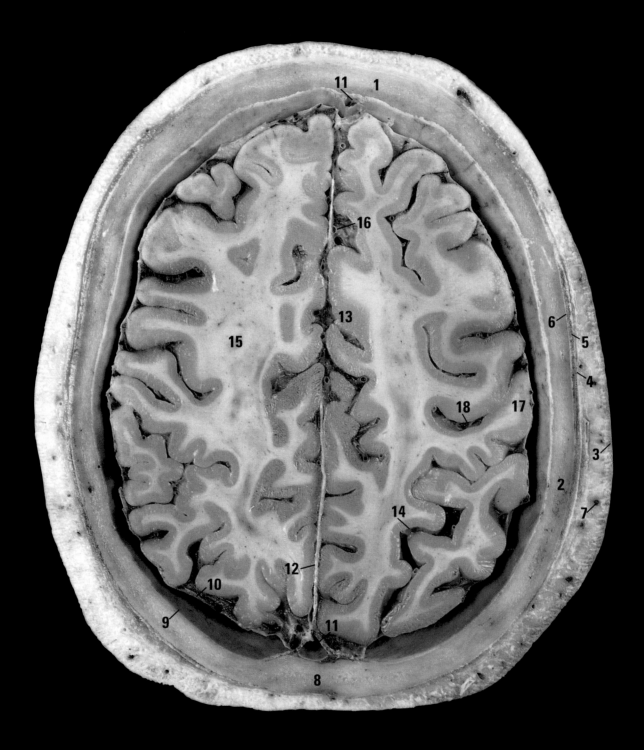

1	Frontal bone	**9**	Dura mater
2	Parietal bone	**10**	Arachnoid mater
3	Skin and dense	**11**	Superior sagittal sinus
	subcutaneous tissue	**12**	Falx cerebri
4	Epicranial aponeurosis	**13**	Cingulate gyrus
	(galea aponeurotica)	**14**	Parieto-occipital sulcus
5	Temporalis	**15**	Corona radiata
6	Pericranium	**16**	Anterior cerebral artery
7	Branch of superficial		(branches)
	temporal artery	**17**	Postcentral gyrus
8	Sagittal suture	**18**	Central sulcus

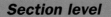

Section level

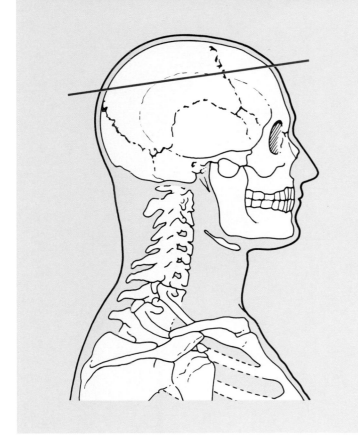

Orientation guide

ANTERIOR

RIGHT — LEFT

POSTERIOR

Notes

This section allows some of the main gyri and sulci of the cerebrum to be identified. Cross-reference should be made to the photographs of the external aspects and sagittal sections of the brain for orientation (see pages 1–6).

The corona radiata (**15**) comprises a fan-shaped arrangement of afferent and efferent projection fibres which join the grey matter to lower centres. On the CT image it appears as a curved linear area of low attenuation termed the *centrum semiovale*.

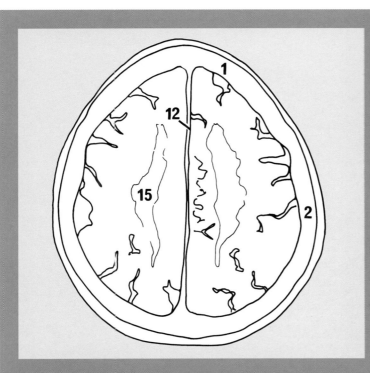

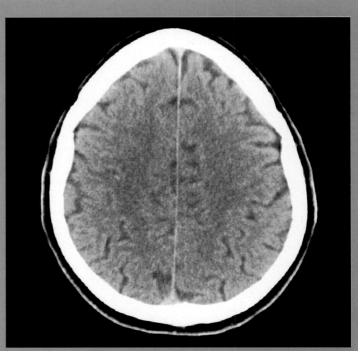

Axial computed tomogram (CT)

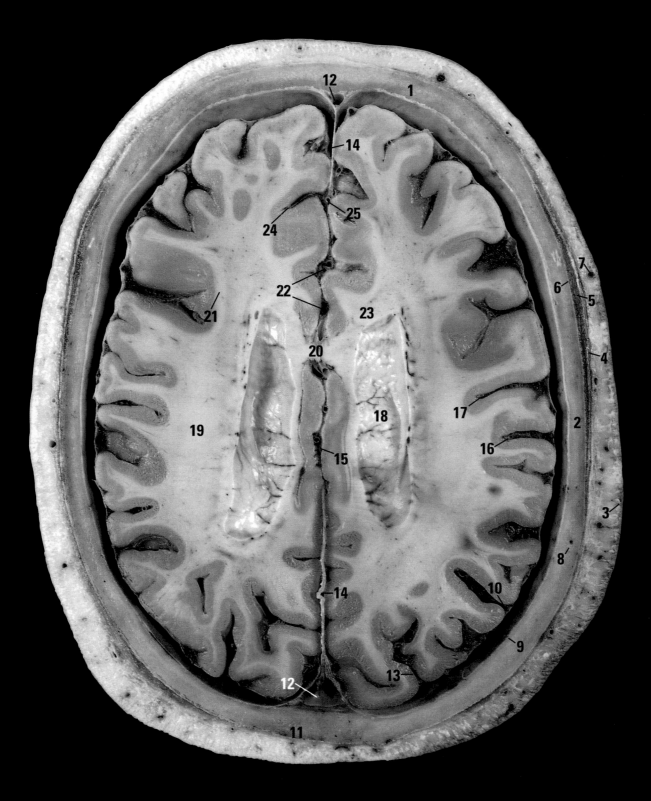

1 Frontal bone	**9** Dura mater	**19** Corona radiata
2 Parietal bone	**10** Arachnoid mater	**20** Corpus callosum
3 Skin and dense	**11** Sagittal suture	**21** Longitudinal fasciculus
subcutaneous tissue	**12** Superior sagittal sinus	(cortico cortical fibres)
4 Epicranial aponeurosis	**13** Lunate sulcus	**22** Anterior cerebral artery
(galea aponeurotica)	**14** Falx cerebri	(branches)
5 Temporalis	**15** Cingulate gyrus	**23** Forceps minor
6 Pericranium	**16** Postcentral sulcus	**24** Cingulate sulcus
7 Branches of superficial	**17** Central sulcus	**25** Inferior sagittal sinus
temporal artery	**18** Roof of body of lateral	
8 Diploic vein	ventricle	

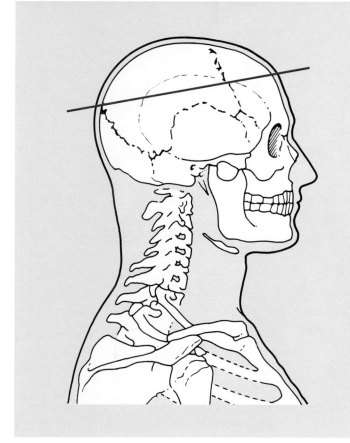

Section level

Orientation guide

ANTERIOR

RIGHT ← → LEFT

POSTERIOR

Notes

This section passes through the roof of the lateral ventricle (**18**).

The central sulcus, or fissure of Rolando (**17**), is the most important of the sulcal landmarks, since it separates the precentral (motor) gyrus from the post-central (sensory) gyrus. It also helps demarcate the frontal and parietal lobes of the cerebrum.

Again the corona radiata (**19**), or centrum semi-ovale, is well seen in both the section and CT image.

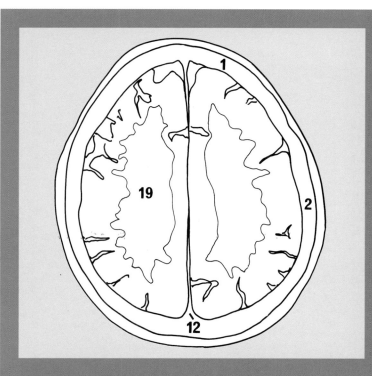

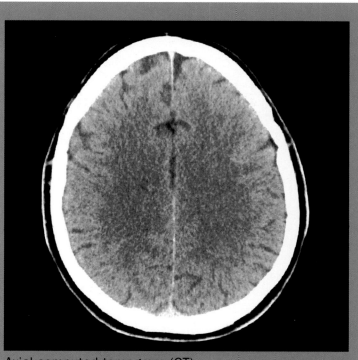

Axial computed tomogram (CT)

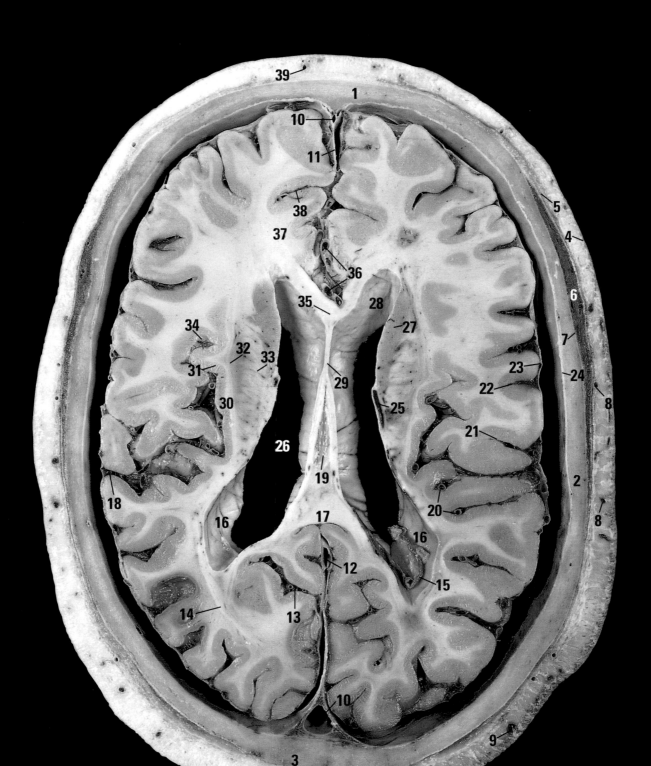

1 Frontal bone	**13** Parieto-occipital sulcus	**27** Body of caudate nucleus
2 Parietal bone	**14** Optic radiation	**28** Frontal horn of lateral
3 Sutural bone	**15** Choroid plexus	ventricle
4 Skin and dense	**16** Posterior horn lateral ventricle	**29** Septum pellucidum
subcutaneous tissue	**17** Splenium of corpus callosum	**30** Insula
5 Epicranial aponeurosis	**18** Lateral sulcus (Sylvian fissure)	**31** Claustrum
(galea aponeurotica)	**19** Third ventricle	**32** Putamen
6 Temporalis	**20** Middle cerebral artery	**33** Internal capsule
7 Pericranium	(branches)	**34** Circular sulcus
8 Branches of superficial	**21** Postcentral sulcus	**35** Genu of corpus callosum
temporal artery	**22** Central sulcus	**36** Anterior cerebral artery
9 Occipital vein	**23** Arachnoid mater	(branches)
10 Superior sagittal sinus	**24** Dura mater	**37** Forceps minor
11 Falx cerebri	**25** Thalamostriate vein	**38** Cingulate sulcus
12 Straight sinus	**26** Body of lateral ventricle	**39** Supra-orbital artery

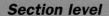

Section level

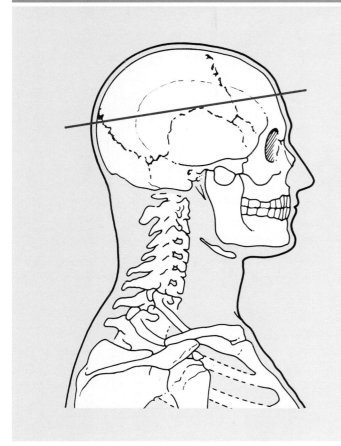

Orientation guide

ANTERIOR

RIGHT ← → LEFT

POSTERIOR

Notes

This section passes through the bodies of the lateral ventricles (**26**) and the third ventricle (**19**).

The lateral ventricles comprise a frontal horn (**28**) and body (**26**), which continues with the posterior or occipital horn (**16**), which, in turn, enters the inferior horn within the temporal lobe. This will be seen in later sections. The lateral ventricles are almost completely separated from each other by the septum pellucidum (**29**) but communicate indirectly via the third ventricle (**19**), a narrow slit-like cavity.

The choroid plexuses of the lateral ventricles (**15**), which are responsible for the production of most of the cerebrospinal fluid (CSF), extend from the inferior horn, through the body to the interventricular foramen, where they become continuous with the plexus of the third ventricle.

In addition to the centres of ossification of the named bones of the skull, other centres may occcur in the course of the sutures which give rise to irregular sutural (Wormian) bones (**3**). They occur most frequently in the region of the lambdoid suture as here, but may sometimes be seen at the anterior, or more especially the posterior fontanelle. They are usually limited to two or three in number, but may occur in greater numbers in congenital hydrocephalic skulls and other developmental disorders.

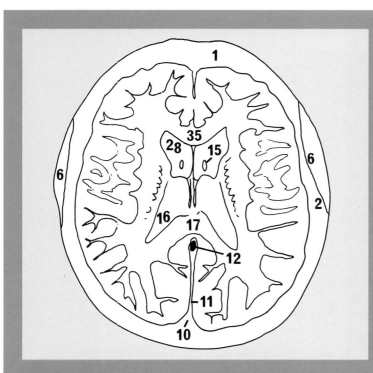

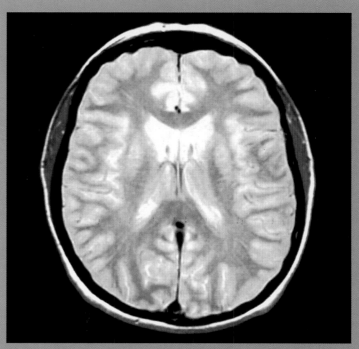

Axial magnetic resonance image (MRI)

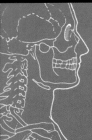

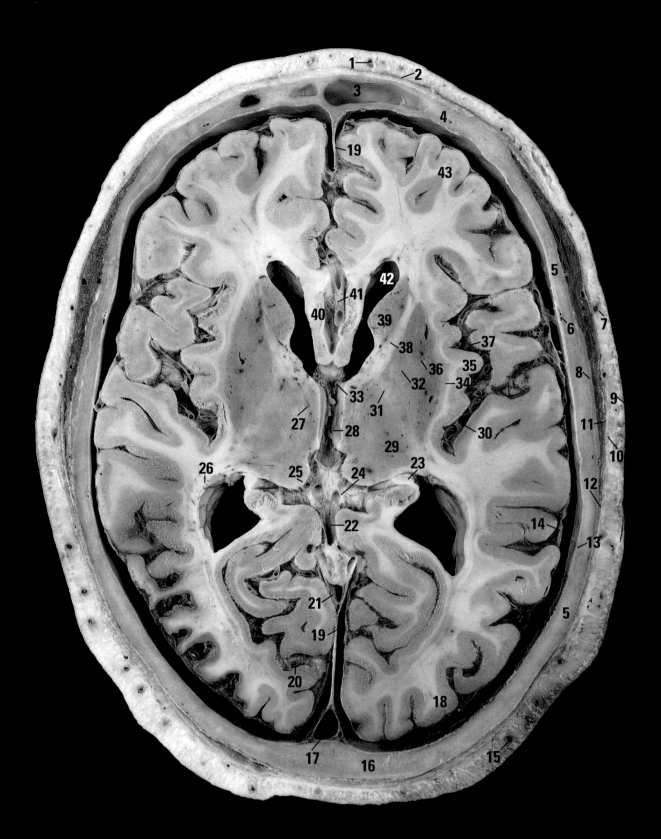

1 Supra orbital artery
2 Frontal belly of occipitofrontalis
3 Frontal sinus
4 Frontal bone
5 Parietal bone
6 Middle meningeal artery
   and vein
7 Branch of temporal artery
8 Sliver of squamous
   part of temporal bone
9 Skin and dense
   subcutaneous tissue
10 Epicranial aponeurosis
   (galea aponeurotica)
11 Temporalis
12 Pericranium
13 Dura mater

14 Arachnoid mater
15 Occipital artery
16 Squamous part of occipital bone
17 Superior sagittal sinus
18 Occipital lobe
19 Falx cerebri
20 Calcarine sulcus
21 Straight sinus
22 Great cerebral vein
23 Fornix
24 Internal cerebral vein (branches)
25 Pulvinar of thalamus
26 Optic radiation
27 Medial nucleus of thalamus
28 Third ventricle
29 Ventroposterior thalamic
   nucleus

30 Circular sulcus
31 Globus pallidus – internal
   segment
32 Globus pallidus – external
   segment
33 Choroid plexus in interventricular
   foramen (Monro)
34 Claustrum
35 Insula
36 Putamen
37 Middle cerebral artery (branches)
38 Anterior limb of internal capsule
39 Caudate nucleus – head
40 Corpus callosum
41 Anterior cerebral artery
42 Frontal horn of lateral ventricle
43 Frontal lobe

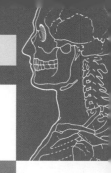

Section level

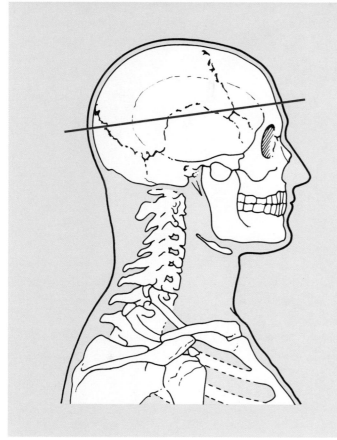

Notes

This section passes through the apex of the squamous part of the occipital bone (**16**) and the frontal sinus (**3**). The latter varies greatly in size from subject to subject, as may be appreciated by the inspection a number of skull radiographs.

The interventricular foramen of Monro (**33**) is well demonstrated and drains the lateral ventricle on both sides into the third ventricle (**28**), thus providing a link between the ventricular systems within the two cerebral hemispheres.

This section also demonstrates the components of the basal ganglia; the claustrum (**34**), the lentiform nucleus, made up of the globus pallidus (**31**, **32**) and putamen (**36**). The latter is largely separated from the head of the caudate nucleus (**39**) by the anterior limb of the internal capsule (**38**).

Orientation guide

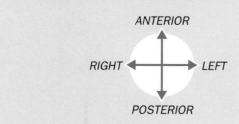

ANTERIOR

RIGHT   LEFT

POSTERIOR

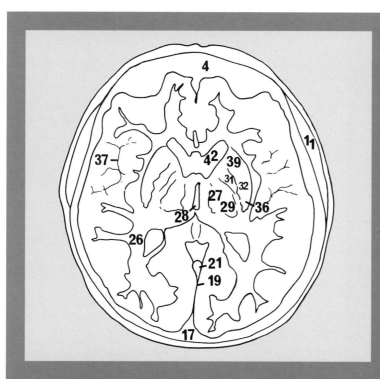

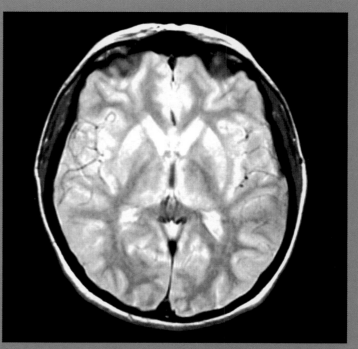

Axial magnetic resonance image (MRI)

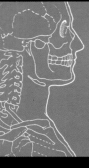

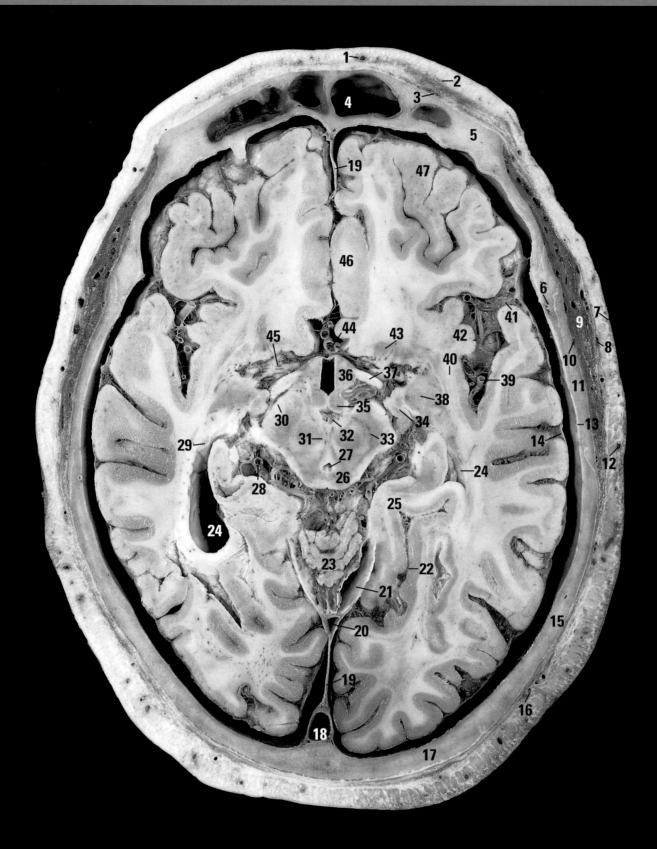

1 Supra orbital artery	**12** Superficial temporal artery	**26** Superior colliculus	**40** Claustrum
2 Orbital part of occipitofrontalis	**13** Dura mater	**27** Aqueduct of Sylvius	**41** Lateral sulcus (Sylvius)
3 Frontal belly of occipitofrontalis	**14** Arachnoid mater	**28** Posterior cerebral artery	**42** Insula
4 Frontal sinus	**15** Parietal bone	**29** Tail of caudate nucleus	**43** Nucleus accumbens septi
5 Frontal bone	**16** Occipital artery	**30** Cerebral peduncle	**44** Anterior cerebral artery
6 Middle meningeal artery and vein	**17** Squamous part of occipital bone	**31** Red nucleus	**45** Anterior perforated substance
7 Skin and dense subcutaneous tissue	**18** Superior sagittal sinus	**32** Third ventricle	**46** Cingulate gyrus
8 Epicranial aponeurosis (galea aponeurotica)	**19** Falx cerebri	**33** Substantia nigra	**47** Orbitofrontal cortex
9 Temporalis	**20** Straight sinus	**34** Cornu ammonis (hippocampus)	**48** Cisterna ambiens
10 Pericranium	**21** Tentorium cerebelli	**35** Mamillary body	**49** Temporal lobe
11 Squamous part of temporal bone	**22** Collateral sulcus	**36** Hypothalamus	**50** Interpeduncular cistern
	23 Anterior lobe of cerebellum	**37** Optic tract	
	24 Lateral ventricle	**38** Amygdala	
	25 Parahippocampal gyrus	**39** Middle cerebral artery (branches)	

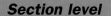

Section level

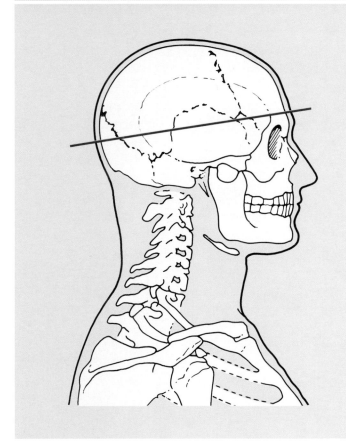

Notes

This section passes through the upper part of the squamous temporal bone (**11**) and traverses the mid brain at the level of the cerebral peduncle (**30**) and the red nucleus (**31**).

The aqueduct of Sylvius (**27**) is the communication between the third ventricle (see section 7, page 19) and the fourth ventricle (see section 10, page 25).

The colliculi, two superior (**26**) and two inferior, blend to form the tectum over the aqueduct (**27**). This is sometimes termed the quadrigeminal plate, hence an alternative name for the cisterna ambiens (**48**) is the quadrigeminal cistern. Other names for this include: superior cistern and cistern of the great cerebral vein. As this cistern contains the great cerebral vein and the pineal body, it is an important anatomical landmark.

Orientation guide

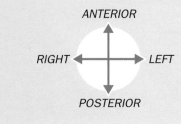

ANTERIOR

RIGHT   LEFT

POSTERIOR

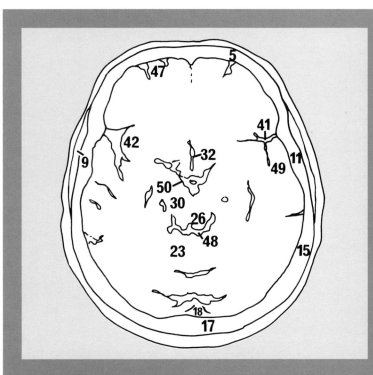

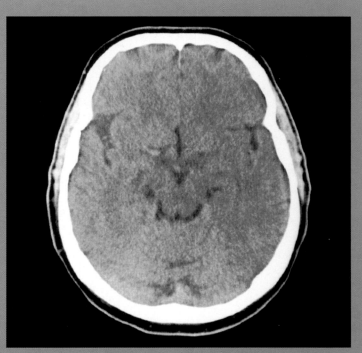

Axial computed tomogram (CT)

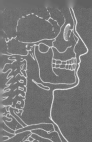

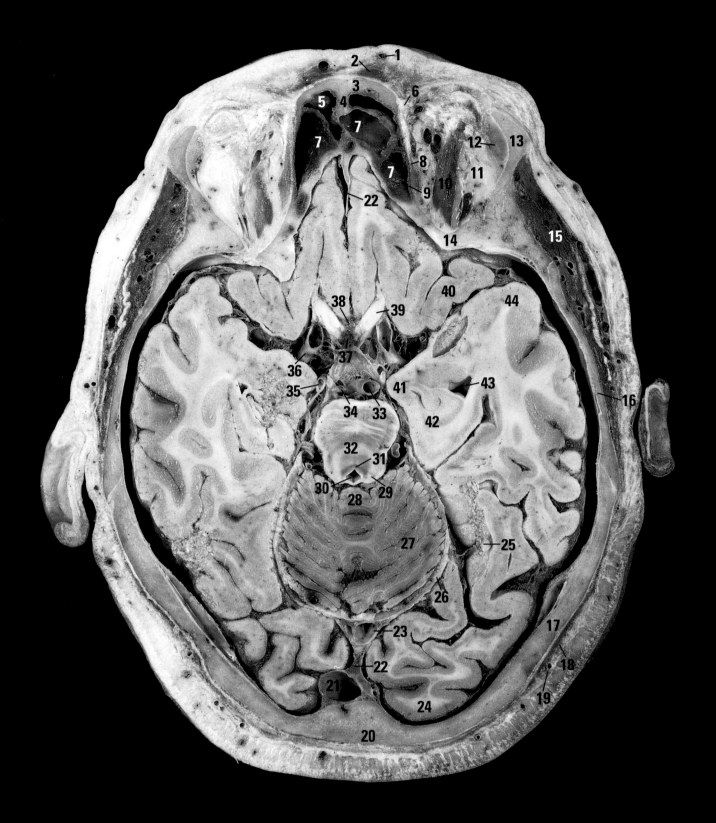

1 Supraorbital artery	**13** Zygomatic process of frontal bone	**25** Floor of lateral ventricle (occipital horn)	**36** Internal carotid artery
2 Frontal belly of occipitofrontalis	**14** Lesser wing of sphenoid bone	**26** Tentorium cerebelli (outer edge)	**37** Pituitary infundibulum
3 Frontal bone	**15** Temporalis	**27** Anterior lobe of cerebellum	**38** Optic chiasma
4 Frontal crest	**16** Temporal bone	**28** Cerebellar vermis	**39** Optic nerve (II)
5 Frontal sinus	**17** Parietal bone	**29** Inferior colliculus	**40** Orbitofrontal cortex
6 Trochlea	**18** Posterior belly of occipitofrontalis	**30** Aqueduct of Sylvius	**41** Uncus of parahippocampal gyrus
7 Ethmoid air sinuses	**19** Occipital artery	**31** Locus coeruleus	**42** Hippocampus
8 Superior oblique	**20** Occipital bone	**32** Decussation of superior cerebellar peduncle	**43** Temporal horn of lateral ventricle
9 Orbital plate of ethmoid bone	**21** Superior sagittal sinus	**33** Basilar artery	**44** Temporal pole
10 Superior rectus underlying levator palpebri superioris	**22** Falx cerebri	**34** Superior cerebellar artery	**45** Vitreous humour
11 Orbital fat	**23** Straight sinus	**35** Posterior cerebral artery	**46** Lens
12 Lacrimal gland	**24** Occipital pole		**47** Middle cerebral artery

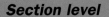

Section level

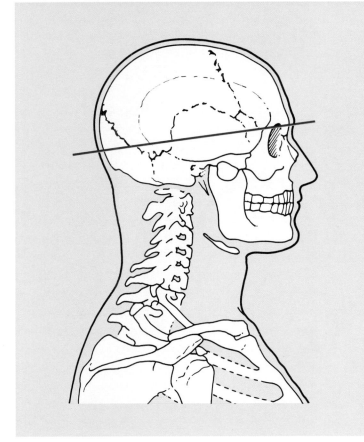

Notes

This section traverses the upper part of the orbits, the mid brain at the level of the inferior colliculus (**29**) and the anterior lobe of the cerebellum (**27**).

The straight sinus (**23**) lies in the sagittal plane of the tentorium cerebelli (**26**) at its attachment to the falx cerebri (**22**). It receives both the inferior sagittal sinus and the great cerebral vein, and drains posteriorly, usually into the left but occasionally into the right, transverse sinus.

Orientation guide

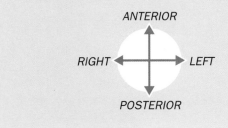

ANTERIOR

RIGHT ⟷ LEFT

POSTERIOR

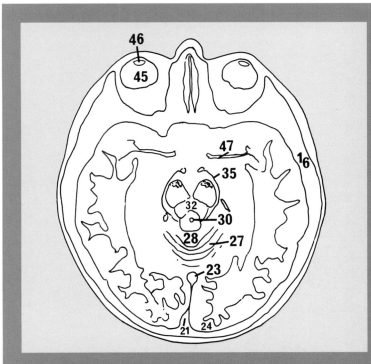

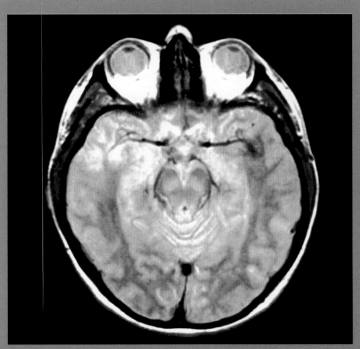

Axial magnetic resonance image (MRI)

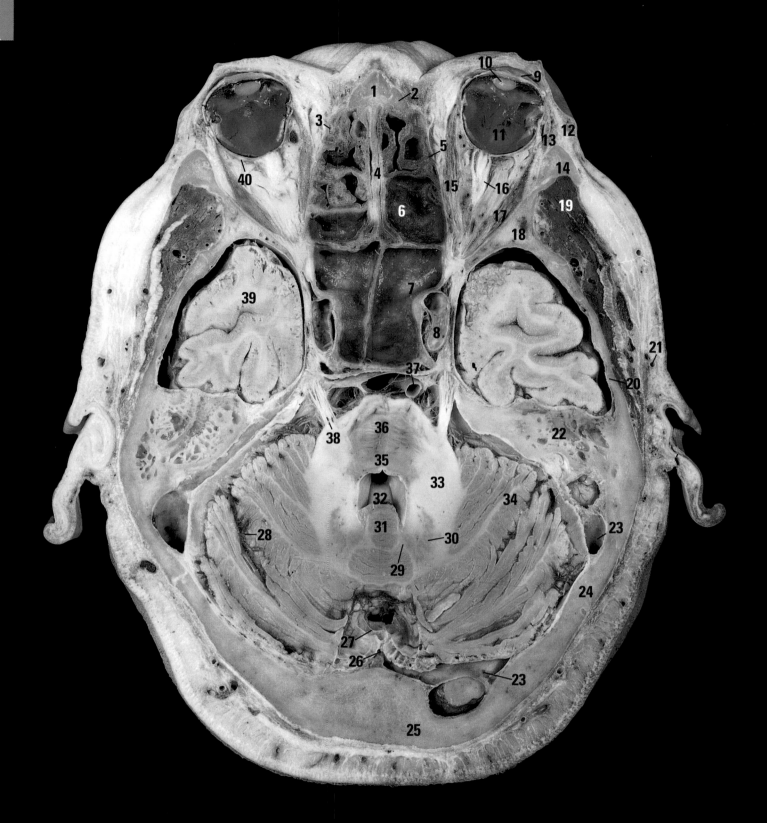

1 Nasal bone	**11** Vitreous humour
2 Frontal process of maxilla	**12** Orbicularis oculi – orbital part
3 Nasolacrimal duct	**13** Orbicularis oculi – palpebral part
4 Perpendicular plate of ethmoid bone	**14** Frontal process of zygomatic bone
5 Orbital plate of ethmoid bone	**15** Medial rectus
6 Posterior ethmoidal air cells	**16** Optic nerve (II)
7 Sphenoidal sinus	**17** Lateral rectus
8 Internal carotid artery within cavernous sinus	**18** Greater wing of sphenoid bone
9 Cornea	**19** Temporalis
10 Lens	**20** Squamous part of temporal bone

21 Superficial temporal artery and vein	**33** Middle cerebellar peduncle
22 Mastoid air cells	**34** Hemisphere of cerebellum
23 Transverse sinus	**35** Pontine tegmentum
24 Parietal bone	**36** Pontine nuclei
25 Squamous part of occipital bone	**37** Basilar artery
26 Falx cerebelli	**38** Trigeminal nerve (V)
27 Superior sagittal sinus	**39** Temporal lobe
28 Posterolateral fissure	**40** Sclera
29 Emboliform (interposed) nucleus	**41** Crista galli of ethmoid
30 Dentate nucleus	**42** Petrous part of temporal bone
31 Vermis of cerebellum	**43** Internal auditory meatus
32 Fourth ventricle	

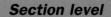

Section level

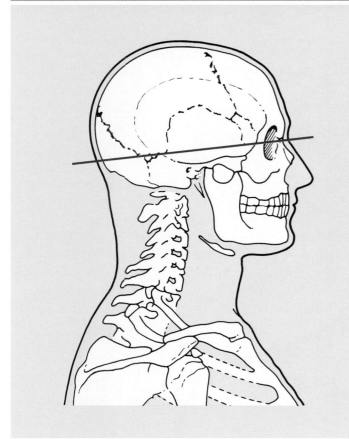

Notes

This section transects the eyeballs, the sphenoid sinus (**7**) and the pons (**36**) at the level of the middle cerebellar peduncles (**33**).

The structure of the orbit in horizontal section can be appreciated in this section. The eyeball with its cornea (**9**), lens (**10**) and vitreous humour (**11**) contained within the tough sclera (**40**), and the optic nerve (**16**) lie surrounded by the extrinsic muscles (**15**, **17**). The slit like naso-lacrimal duct (**3**) drains downwards into the inferior meatus.

The fourth ventricle (**32**) lies above the tegmentum of the pons (**35**) and below the vermis of the cerebellum (**31**).

Orientation guide

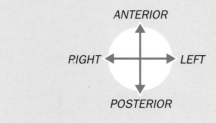

ANTERIOR

RIGHT   LEFT

POSTERIOR

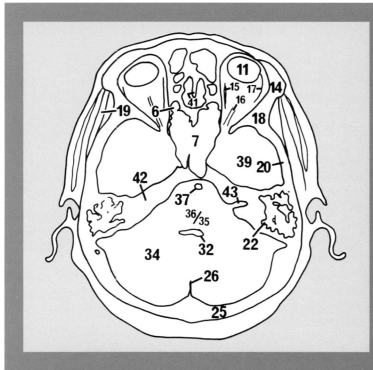

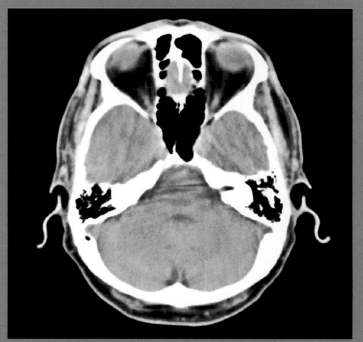

Axial computed tomogram (CT)

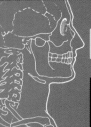

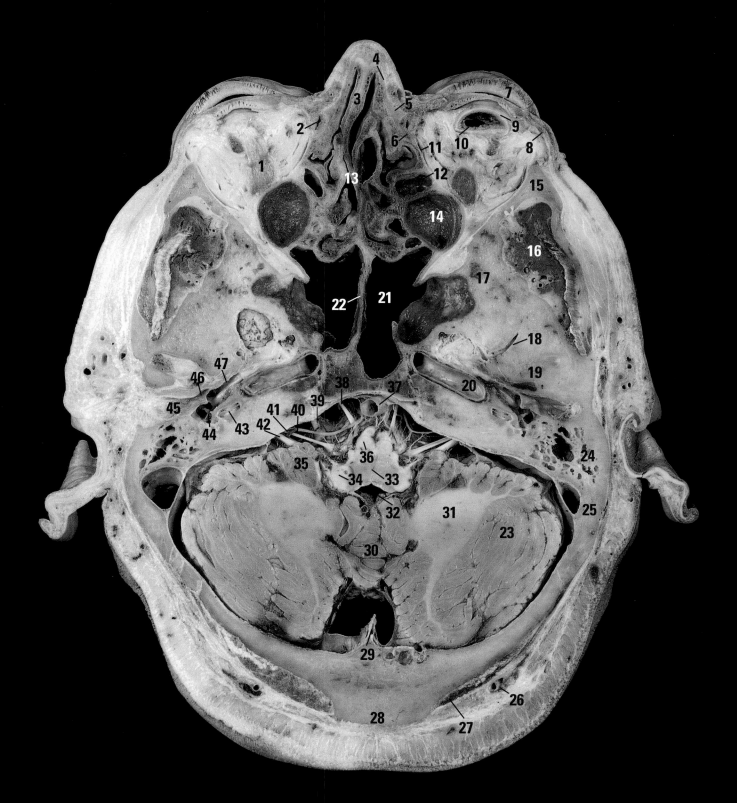

1 Inferior rectus	**15** Frontal process of	**28** External occipital	**42** Vestibulocochlear
2 Nasolacrimal duct	zygomatic bone	protruberance	(auditory) nerve (VIII)
3 Cartilage of nasal septum	**16** Temporalis	**29** Falx cerebelli	**43** Cochlea
4 Nasal bone	**17** Greater wing of	**30** Vermis	**44** Stapes
5 Frontal process of	sphenoid bone	**31** Middle cerebellar	**45** External auditory
maxilla	**18** Middle meningeal	peduncle	meatus
6 Lacrimal bone	artery	**32** Fourth ventricle with	**46** Tympanic membrane
7 Upper eyelid	**19** Petrous part of	choroid plexus	and handle of malleus
8 Orbicularis oculi	temporal bone	**33** Medulla oblongata	**47** Auditory tube
9 Sclera	**20** Internal carotid artery	**34** Inferior cerebellar	(eustachian)
10 Vitreous humour	**21** Sphenoidal sinus	peduncle	
11 Orbital plate of ethmoid	**22** Septum of sphenoidal	**35** Flocculus	**48** Lens
bone	sinus	**36** Pyramidal tract	**49** Medial rectus
12 Ethmoid air cells	**23** Cerebellar hemisphere	**37** Basilar artery	**50** Lateral rectus
13 Perpendicular plate of	**24** Mastoid air cells	**38** Abducent nerve (VI)	**51** Foramen rotundum
ethmoid bone	**25** Transverse sinus	**39** Trigeminal nerve (V)	
14 Apex of maxillary	**26** Occipital artery and vein	**40** Labyrinthine artery	
antrum	**27** Trapezius	**41** Facial nerve (VII)	

Section level

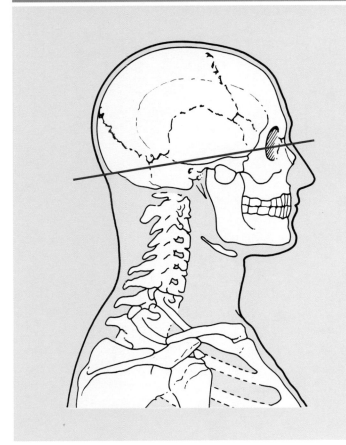

Orientation guide

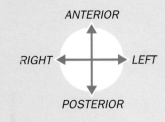

ANTERIOR

RIGHT ←→ LEFT

POSTERIOR

Notes

This section passes through the upper part of the nasal cavity, the medulla oblongata (**33**) and, posteriorly, through the external occipital protruberance (**28**).

The sphenoidal sinus (**21**) is unusually large in this specimen. It is divided by a median septum (**22**) and drains anteriorly into the nasal cavity at the spheno-ethmoidal recess.

Note the relations of the labyrinthine artery (**40**), a branch of the basilar artery (**37**), the facial nerve (**41**) and the vestibulocochlear (or auditory) nerve (**42**) as they enter the internal auditory meatus of the temporal bone.

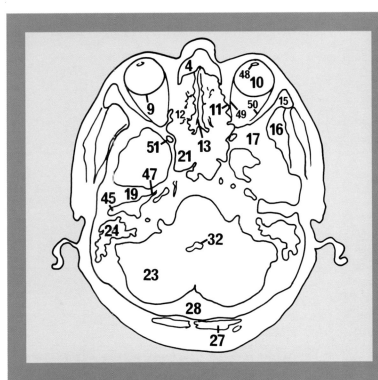

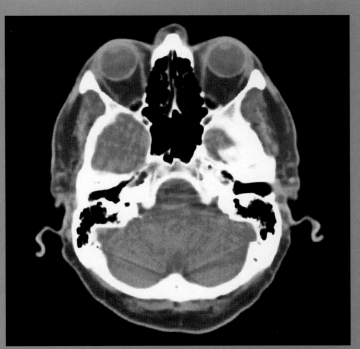

Axial computed tomogram (CT)

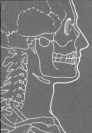

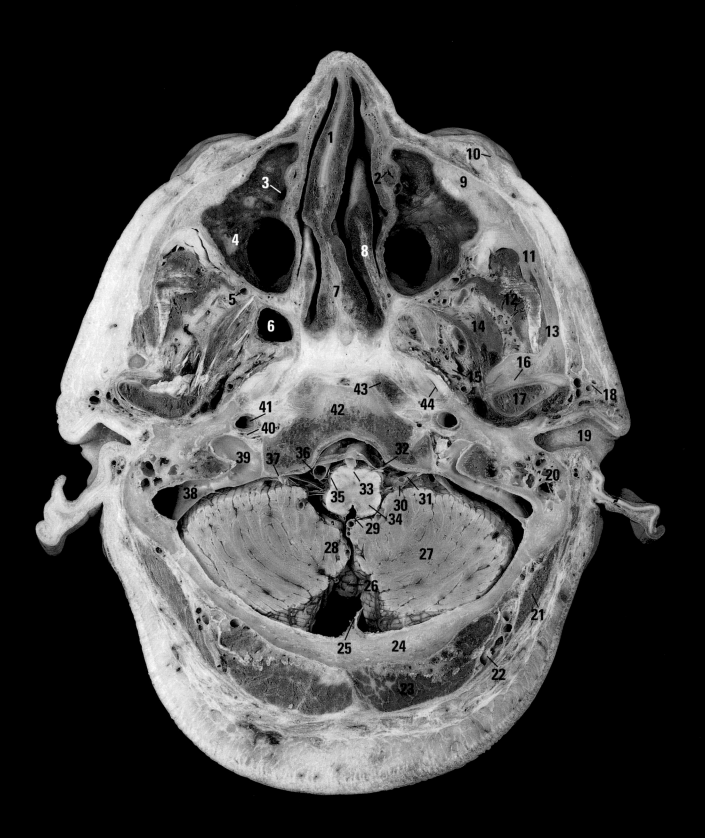

1 Cartilage of nasal septum	**15** Trigeminal nerve (V)	**26** Vermis	**39** Bulb of internal jugular vein
2 Nasolacrimal duct	**16** Articular disc of temporo mandibular joint	**27** Cerebellar hemisphere	**40** Glossopharyngeal nerve, vagus nerve, and accessory nerve (IX, X and XI)
3 Orifice of maxillary sinus		**28** Tonsil of cerebellum	
4 Maxillary sinus	**17** Head of mandible	**29** Fourth ventricle (median aperture of roof)	**41** Internal carotid artery
5 Maxillary artery	**18** Superficial temporal artery and vein		**42** Basi-occiput
6 Sphenoidal sinus	**19** External auditory meatus	**30** Anterior inferior cerebellar artery	**43** Longus capitis
7 Vomer		**31** Glossopharyngeal nerve (IX)	**44** Auditory (Eustachian) tube
8 Middle nasal concha	**20** Mastoid air cells		
9 Maxilla	**21** Sternocleidomastoid	**32** Hypoglossal nerve (XII)	
10 Orbicularis oculi	**22** Occipital artery and vein	**33** Pyramidal tract	**45** Pterygopalatine fossa (apex)
11 Zygomatic bone	**23** Trapezius	**34** Medulla	**46** Foramen ovale
12 Temporalis and tendon	**24** Occipital bone – squamous part	**35** Inferior olive	
13 Zygomatic process of temporal bone	**25** Falx cerebelli	**36** Vertebral artery	
14 Lateral pterygoid		**37** Vagus nerve (X)	
		38 Sigmoid sinus	

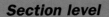

Section level

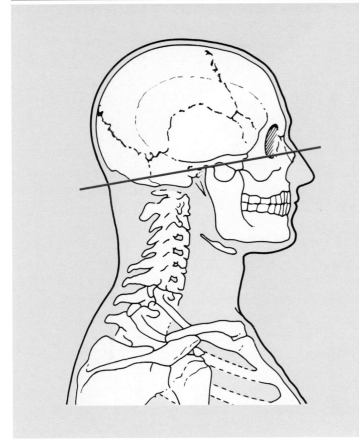

Orientation guide

ANTERIOR

RIGHT ←→ LEFT

POSTERIOR

Notes

This section transects the maxillary sinus (**4**) and the basiocciput (**42**) and passes through the external auditory meatus (**19**).

At this level the vertebral arteries (**36**) are running cranially from their entry into the skull at the foramen magnum to form the basilar artery.

The sigmoid sinus (**38**) runs forward to emerge from the skull at the jugular foramen, at which it becomes the bulb of the internal jugular vein (**39**). Exiting through the jugular foramen anterior to the vein lie, from anterior to posterior, the glossopharyngeal, vagus and accessory cranial nerves (**40**).

The maxillary nerve (V^{ii}) passes into the pterygopalatine fossa (**45** on this CT image) having traversed the foramen rotundum (see (**51**) CT image, section 11, page 28). The mandibular nerve (V^{iii}) leaves the skull via the foramen ovale (**46**).

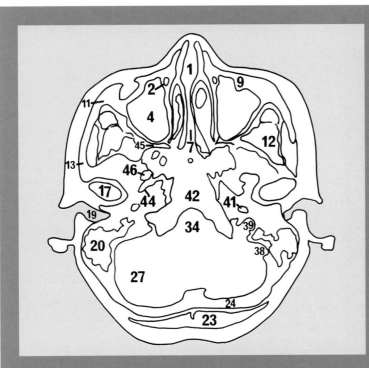

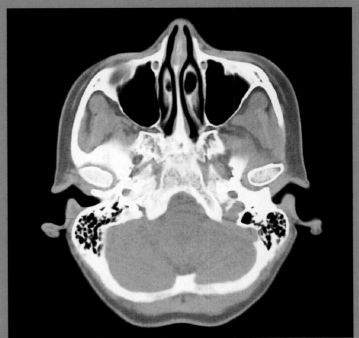

Axial computed tomogram (CT)

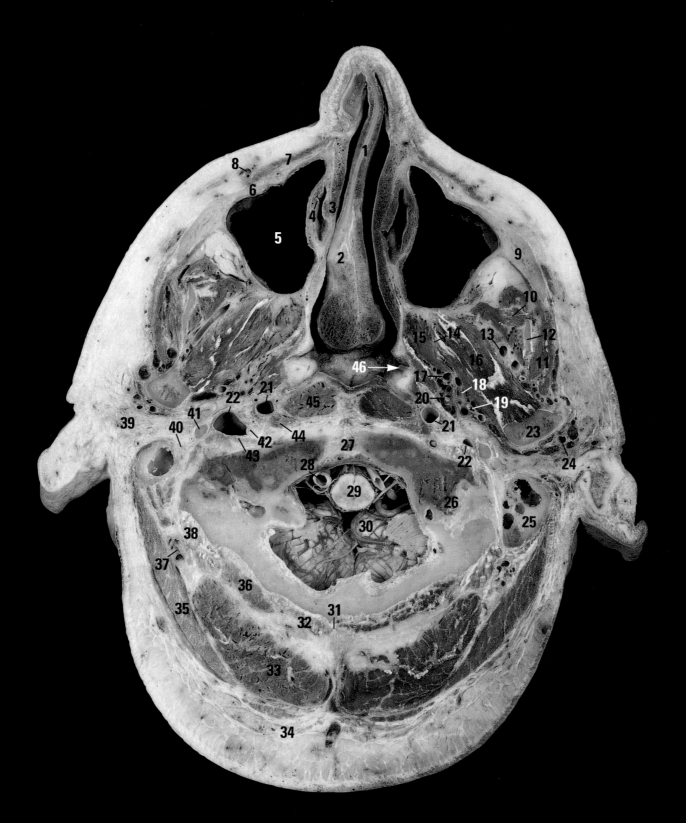

1 Cartilage of nasal septum	**14** Lateral pterygoid plate of sphenoid	**26** Base of occipital condyle	**38** Obliquus capitis superior
2 Vomer	**15** Medial pterygoid	**27** Basilar part of occipital bone	**39** Parotid gland
3 Inferior nasal concha	**16** Lateral pterygoid	**28** Vertebral artery	**40** Facial nerve (VII)
4 Orifice of nasolacrimal duct	**17** Pterygoid artery and pterygoid venous plexus	**29** Spinal cord	**41** Styloid process
5 Maxillary sinus	**18** Lingual nerve (V^{iii})	**30** Tonsil of cerebellum	**42** Glossopharyngeal nerve (IX), vagus nerve (X) and accessory nerve (XI)
6 Maxilla	**19** Inferior alveolar nerve (V^{iii})	**31** External occipital crest	**43** Hypoglossal nerve (XII)
7 Levator labii superioris	**20** Chorda tympani	**32** Rectus capitis posterior minor	**44** Rectus capitis anterior
8 Facial vein	**21** Internal carotid artery	**33** Semispinalis capitis	**45** Longus capitis
9 Zygomatic bone	**22** Internal jugular vein	**34** Trapezius	**46** Opening of auditory (Eustachian) tube (arrowed)
10 Tendon of temporalis	**23** Head of mandible	**35** Sternocleidomastoid	
11 Masseter	**24** Superficial temporal artery	**36** Rectus capitis posterior major	
12 Coronoid process of mandible	**25** Mastoid air cells	**37** Occipital artery and vein	**47** Nasopharynx
13 Maxillary artery and vein			**48** Parapharyngeal space
			49 Pharyngeal recess

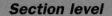

Section level

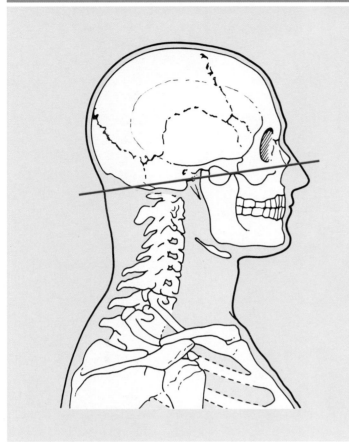

Orientation guide

ANTERIOR

RIGHT ←→ LEFT

POSTERIOR

Notes

This section traverses the nasal septum (**1**) at the level of the inferior nasal concha (**3**), beneath which opens the nasolacrimal duct (**4**). Posteriorly the plane passes through the uppermost part of the spinal cord (**29**) and the cerebellar tonsil (**30**).

The internal jugular vein (**22**) in this specimen is small, especially on the left side. The chorda tympani (**20**) is seen here as it emerges from the petrotympanic fissure to join the lingual nerve (**18**) about 2 cm below the base of the skull. It subserves taste sensation to the anterior two-thirds of the tongue as well as supplying secretomotor fibres to the submandibular and sublingual salivary glands.

The tonsil of the cerebellum (**30**), on the inferior aspect of the cerebellar hemisphere, lies immediately above the foramen magnum. Withdrawal of CSF at lumbar puncture in a patient with raised intracranial pressure is dangerous as it may result in potentially lethal herniation of the tonsils through this bony ring.

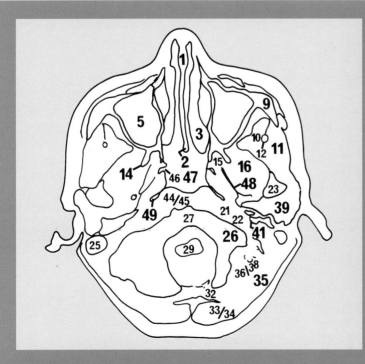

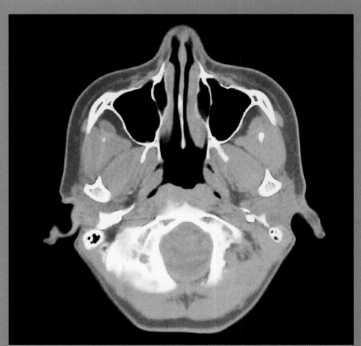

Axial computed tomogram (CT)

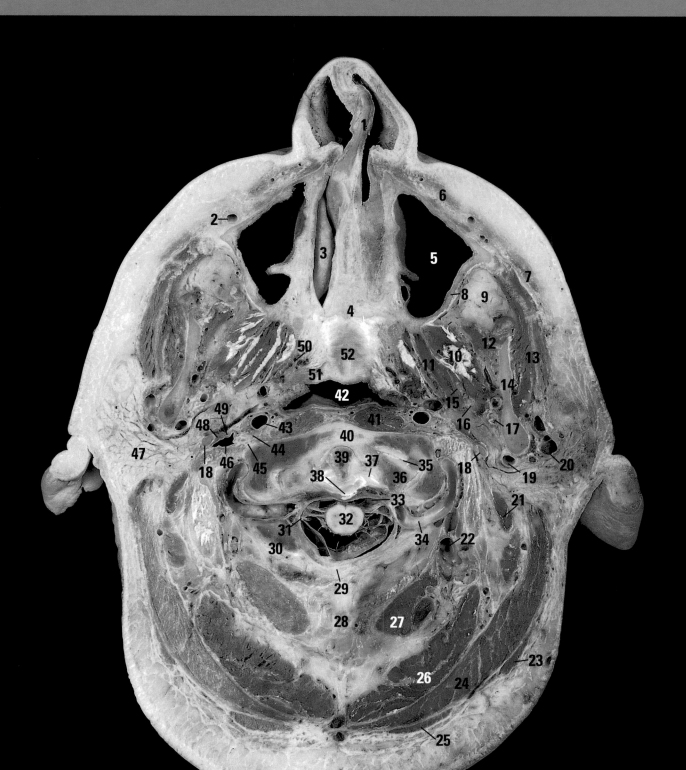

1 Cartilage of nasal septum
2 Facial vein
3 Inferior nasal concha
4 Horizontal plate of palatine bone
5 Maxillary sinus
6 Levator labii superioris
7 Zygomaticus major
8 Maxilla
9 Buccal pad of fat
10 Lateral pterygoid
11 Medial pterygoid
12 Temporalis
13 Masseter
14 Ramus of mandible
15 Lingual nerve (V^{iii})
16 Inferior alveolar artery vein and nerve (V^{iii})

17 Maxillary artery
18 Styloid process
19 External carotid artery
20 Retromandibular vein
21 Posterior belly of digastric
22 Vertebral vein
23 Sternocleidomastoid
24 Splenius
25 Trapezius
26 Semispinalis capitis
27 Rectus capitis posterior major
28 Ligamentum nuchae
29 Posterior atlanto-occipital membrane
30 Posterior arch of atlas
31 Spinal root of accessory nerve (XI)

32 Spinal cord within dural sheath
33 Membrana tectoria
34 Vertebral artery
35 Atlanto-occipital joint
36 Condyle of occipital bone
37 Alar ligament
38 Transverse ligament of atlas (first cervical vertebra)
39 Dens of axis (odontoid process of second cervical vertebra)
40 Anterior arch of atlas (first cervical vertebra)
41 Longus capitis
42 Nasopharynx
43 Internal carotid artery

44 Glossopharyngeal nerve (IX), vagus nerve (X)
45 Sympathetic chain
46 Internal jugular vein
47 Parotid gland
48 Stylopharyngeus
49 Accessory nerve (XI)
50 Pterygoid venous plexus
51 Tensor veli palatini
52 Soft palate

53 Pharyngeal recess
54 Parapharyngeal space

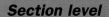

Section level

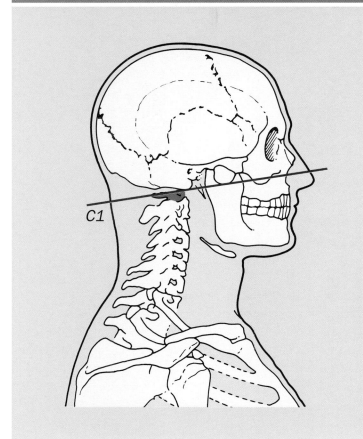

C1

Orientation guide

ANTERIOR

RIGHT ←→ LEFT

POSTERIOR

Notes

This section traverses the nasal cavity through its inferior meatus below the inferior concha (**3**), the hard palate at the horizontal plate of the palatine bone (**4**) and the tip of the dens of the axis, the second cervical vertebra (**39**).

The external carotid artery (**19**) divides at the neck of the mandible into the superficial temporal artery and the maxillary artery (**17**).

Note that the outer endosteal layer of the dura mater of the skull blends with the pericranium at the foramen magnum. The dural sheath surrounding the spinal cord (**32**) represents the continuation of the inner meningeal layer of the cerebral dura (see section 1, page 7).

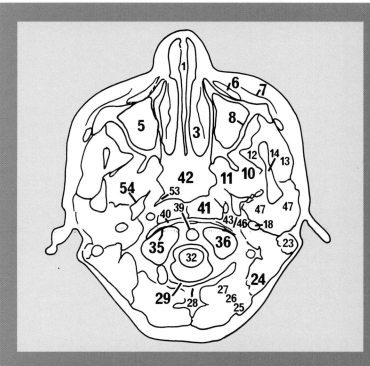

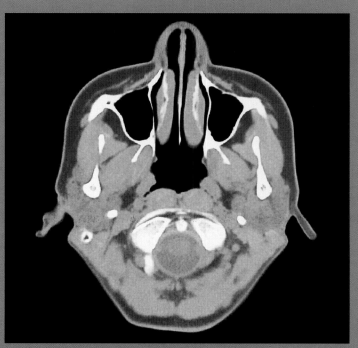

Axial computed tomogram (CT)

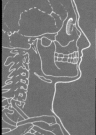

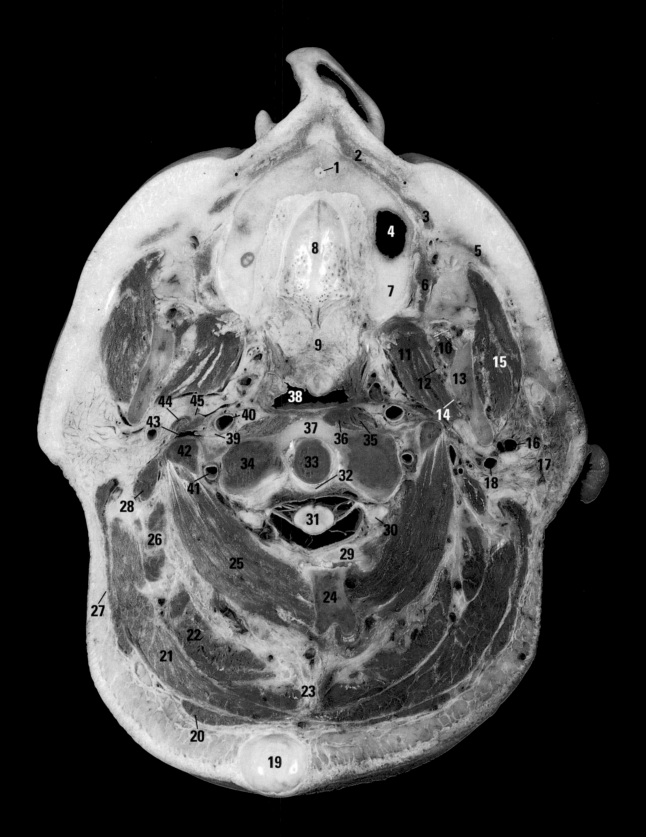

1 Nasopalatine nerve (V^{ii}) within incisive canal
2 Orbicularis oris
3 Levator anguli oris
4 Maxillary antrum
5 Zygomaticus major
6 Buccinator
7 Alveolar process of maxilla
8 Hard palate
9 Soft palate
10 Temporalis
11 Medial pterygoid
12 Lingual nerve (V^{iii})
13 Ramus of mandible
14 Inferior alveolar artery vein and nerve
15 Masseter

16 Retromandibular vein
17 Parotid gland
18 External carotid artery
19 Dermoid cyst of scalp
20 Trapezius
21 Splenius capitis
22 Semispinalis capitis
23 Ligamentum nuchae
24 Spine of axis
25 Obliquus capitis inferior
26 Longissimus capitis
27 Sternocleidomastoid
28 Posterior belly of digastric
29 Posterior arch of atlas (first cervical vertebra)
30 Dorsal root ganglion of second cervical nerve

31 Spinal cord within dural sheath
32 Transverse ligament of atlas
33 Dens of axis (odontoid process of second cervical vertebra)
34 Lateral mass of atlas (first cervical vertebra)
35 Longus capitis
36 Longus colli
37 Anterior arch of atlas (first cervical vertebra)
38 Nasopharynx
39 Vagus nerve (X), and hypoglossal nerve (XII)
40 Internal carotid artery
41 Vertebral artery

42 Transverse process of atlas (first cervical vertebra)
43 Internal jugular vein
44 Styloid process with origins of styloglossus and stylohyoid and glossopharyngeal nerve (IX)
45 Stylopharyngeus

46 Levator and tensor veli palatini
47 Parapharyngeal space
48 Inferior nasal concha
49 Cartilage of nasal septum

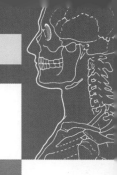

Section level

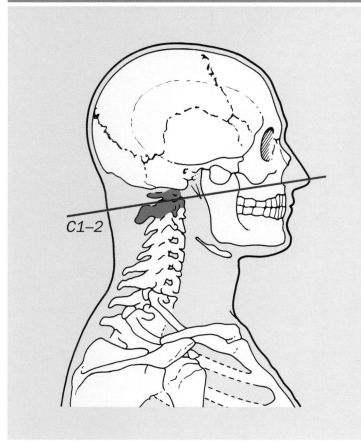

C1–2

Orientation guide

ANTERIOR

RIGHT ←→ LEFT

POSTERIOR

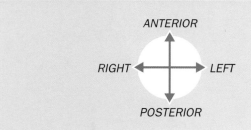

Notes

This section traverses the hard and soft palate (**8** and **9**), the nasopharynx (**38**), the dens (**33**) and the spine of the axis (**24**). The CT image is rather more cranial.

Flexion and extension of the skull (nodding movements of the head) take place at the atlanto-occipital joint between the upper facet of the lateral mass of the atlas (**34**) and the corresponding facet on the occipital bone. Rotation of the skull (looking to the left and right) takes place at the atlanto-axial articulation between the dens (**33**) and the facet on the anterior arch of the atlas (**37**). Additional gliding movements take place at the intervertebral joints between the lower cervical vertebrae. The transverse ligament of the atlas (**32**) is dense and is the principal structure in preventing posterior dislocation of the dens.

Obliquus capitis inferior (**25**) forms the lower outer limb of the sub-occipital triangle. The vertebral artery (**41**), on emerging from the foramen transversarium of the atlas, enters this triangle on its ascending course to the foramen magnum.

Note that this subject has a large dermoid cyst of the scalp (**19**).

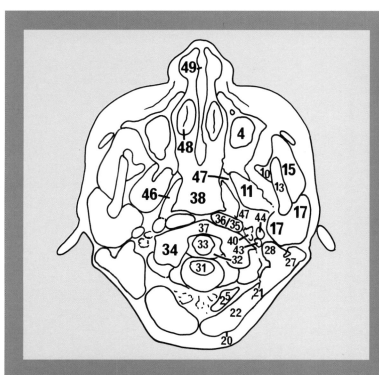

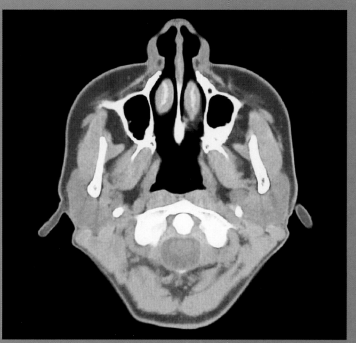

Axial computed tomogram (CT)

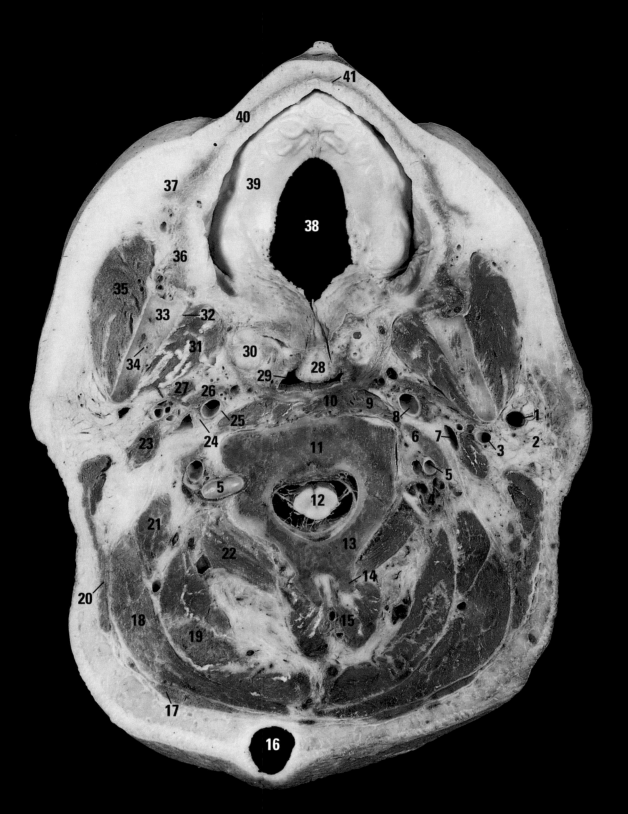

1	Retromandibular vein	**15**	Semispinalis cervicis	**28**	Base of uvula
2	Parotid gland	**16**	Dermoid cyst of scalp	**29**	Nasopharynx
3	External carotid artery	**17**	Trapezius	**30**	Palatine tonsil
4	Vertebral vein	**18**	Splenius	**31**	Medial pterygoid
5	Vertebral artery	**19**	Semispinalis capitis	**32**	Lingual nerve (V^{iii})
6	Scalenus medius	**20**	Sternocleidomastoid	**33**	Ramus of mandible
7	Internal jugular vein	**21**	Longissimus capitis	**34**	Inferior alveolar artery,
8	Internal carotid artery	**22**	Obliquus capitis inferior		vein and nerve (V^{iii})
9	Longus capitis	**23**	Posterior belly of		within mandibular
10	Longus colli		digastric		canal
11	Body of axis (second	**24**	Vagus nerve (X) and	**35**	Masseter
	cervical vertebra)		hypoglossal nerve (XII)	**36**	Buccinator
12	Spinal cord within	**25**	Sympathetic chain	**37**	Levator anguli oris
	dural sheath	**26**	Stylopharyngeus , and	**38**	Mouth
13	Lamina of axis (second		glossopharyngeal	**39**	Alveolar margin
	cervical vertebra)		nerve (IX)	**40**	Orbicularis oris
14	Spine of axis (second	**27**	Styloglossus and stylo-	**41**	Mucous gland of lip
	cervical vertebra)		hyoid (posteriorly)		

42	Hard palate
43	Soft palate
44	Styloid process
45	Parapharyngeal space
46	Anterior arch of atlas
47	Dens of axis (odontoid process of second cervical vertebra)
48	Posterior arch of atlas (first cervical vertebra)
49	Foramen transversarium

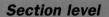

Section level

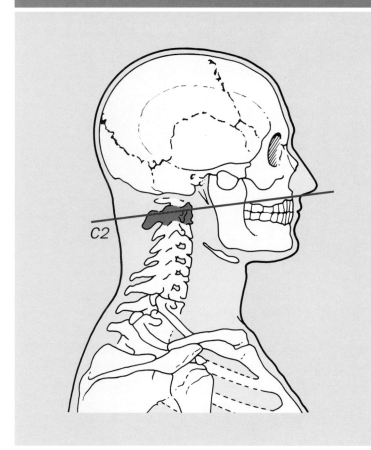

C2

Orientation guide

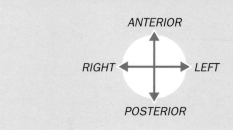

ANTERIOR

RIGHT ← → LEFT

POSTERIOR

Notes

This section passes through the alveolar margin (**39**) of the upper jaw and through the body of the axis (**11**). The CT image is at a more cranial level.

The vertebral artery (**5**) on the right side of this specimen is tortuous and bulges laterally between the transverse processes of the atlas and axis, a not uncommon feature in arteriosclerotic subjects. Each cervical vertebra bears its characteristic foramen transversarium (**49**) within its transverse process. The vertebral artery, with its accompanying vein, ascends through the foramina of C6 to C1 to gain access to the foramen magnum.

The lips are lined by mucous membrane enclosing orbicularis oris (**40**), the labial vessels and nerves, fibrofatty connective tissue and the labial mucous glands (**41**). These lie between the mucosa and underlying muscle, are about 0.5 cm in diameter and resemble mucous salivary glands. Their ducts drain into the vestibule of the mouth. These glands, like those studded over the oral aspect of the palate, are occasional sites of pleiomorphic adenomas, which are similar to those more commonly seen in the parotid gland.

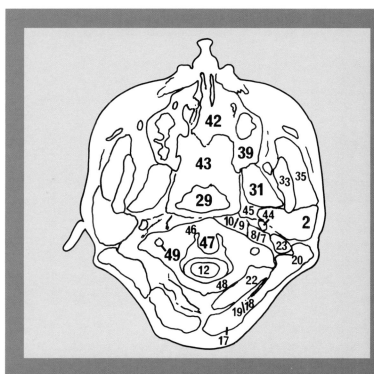

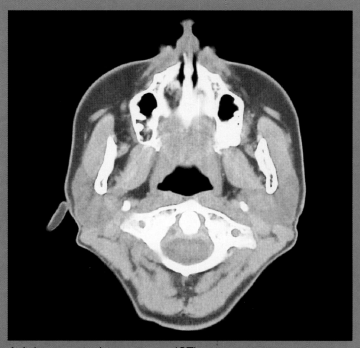

Axial computed tomogram (CT)

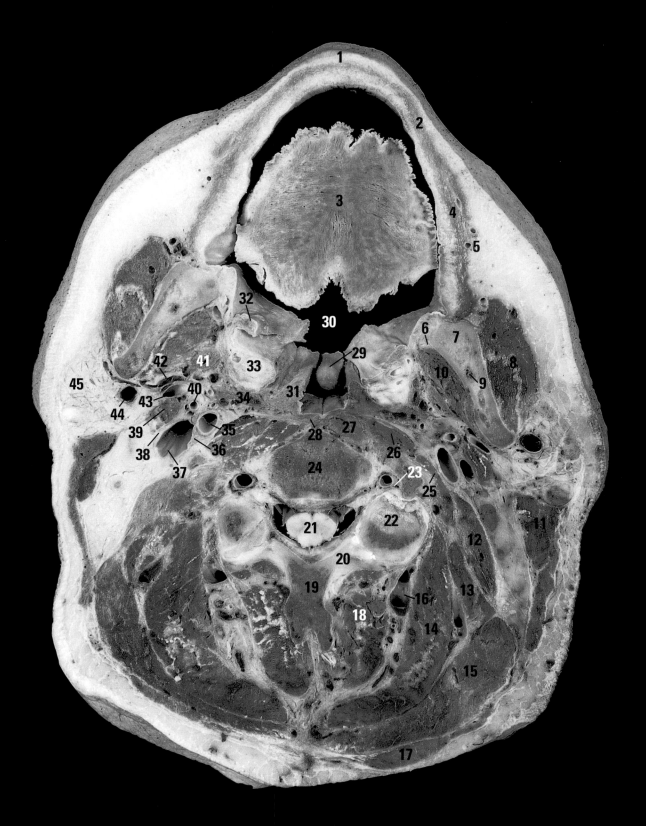

1 Upper lip
2 Orbicularis oris
3 Tongue
4 Buccinator
5 Facial artery and vein
6 Lingual nerve (V^{iii})
7 Ramus of mandible
8 Masseter
9 Inferior alveolar artery vein and nerve (V^{iii}) within mandibular canal
10 Medial pterygoid
11 Sternocleidomastoid
12 Levator scapulae
13 Longissimus capitis

14 Semispinalis capitis
15 Splenius
16 Deep cervical vein
17 Trapezius
18 Semispinalis cervicis
19 Spine of axis (second cervical vertebra)
20 Lamina of axis (second cervical vertebra)
21 Spinal cord within dural sheath
22 Superior articular process of axis (second cervical vertebra)
23 Vertebral artery and vein

24 Body of axis (second cervical vertebra)
25 Scalenus medius
26 Longus capitis
27 Longus colli
28 Constrictor of pharynx
29 Uvula
30 Oropharynx
31 Palatopharyngeal arch with palatopharyngeal
32 Palatoglossal arch with palatoglossus
33 Palatine tonsil
34 Stylopharyngeus
35 Internal carotid artery
36 Vagus nerve (X)

37 Internal jugular vein
38 Accessory nerve (XI)
39 Digastric (posterior belly)
40 External carotid artery
41 Styloglossus
42 Stylohyoid
43 Posterior auricular artery
44 Retromandibular vein
45 Parotid gland

46 Nasopharynx
47 Parapharyngeal space
48 Alveolar process of maxilla

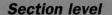

Section level

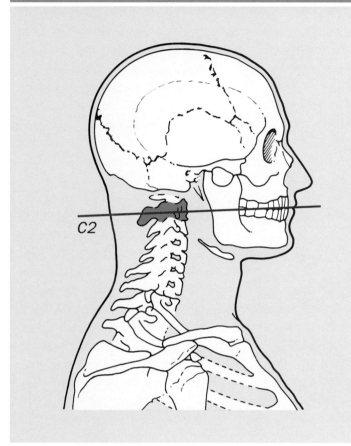

C2

Orientation guide

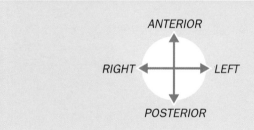

ANTERIOR

RIGHT ←→ LEFT

POSTERIOR

Notes

This section traverses the upper lip (**1**), the tongue (**3**), the uvula (**29**) and the axis (**19, 20, 22, 24**). The plane of the CT image is slightly more cranial.

The palatine tonsil (**33**) lies in the tonsillar fossa between the anterior and posterior pillars of the fauces. The anterior pillar, or palatoglossal arch, (**32**) forms the boundary between the buccal cavity and the oropharynx (**30**); it fuses with the lateral wall of the tongue and contains the palatoglossus muscle. The posterior pillar, or palatopharyngeal arch (**31**), blends with the wall of the pharynx and contains the palatopharyngeus muscle.

The tonsil consists of a collection of lymphoid tissue covered by a squamous epithelium; a unique histological combination which makes it easy to identify under the microscope. From late puberty onwards the lymphoid tissue undergoes progressive atrophy.

The prominent deep cervical vein (**16**) is a useful landmark in separating the deeply placed semispinalis cervicis muscle (**18**) from the more superficially placed semispinalis capitis (**14**); this is seen again in section 18, page 41.

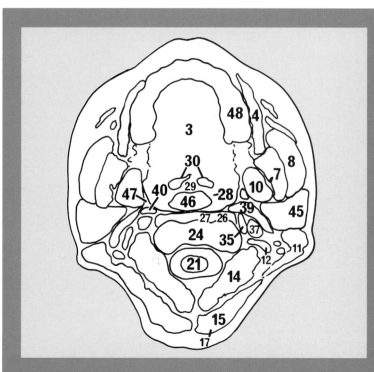

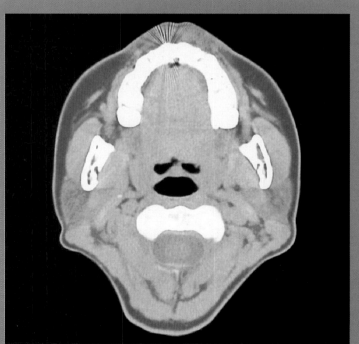

Axial computed tomogram (CT)

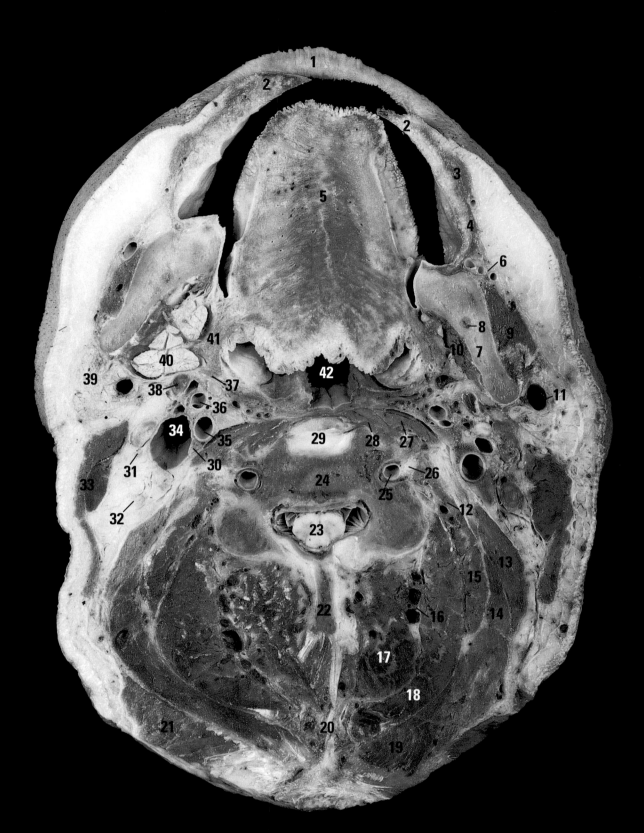

1 Upper lip
2 Lower lip
3 Orbicularis oris
4 Buccinator
5 Transverse intrinsic
   muscle of tongue
6 Facial artery and vein
7 Ramus of mandible
8 Inferior alveolar artery
   vein and nerve (V^{iii})
   within mandibular
   canal
9 Masseter
10 Medial pterygoid
11 Retromandibular vein
12 Scalenus medius
13 Levator scapulae

14 Splenius cervicis
15 Longissimus capitis
16 Deep cervical vein
17 Semispinalis cervicis
18 Semispinalis capitis
19 Splenius capitis
20 Ligamentum nuchae
21 Trapezius
22 Spine of third cervical
   vertebra
23 Spinal cord within
   dural sheath
24 Body of third cervical
   vertebra
25 Vertebral artery and
   vein within foramen
   transversarium

26 Anterior primary ramus
   of third cervical nerve
27 Longus capitis
28 Longus colli
29 Part of intervertebral
   disc between second
   and third cervical
   vertebrae
30 Vagus nerve (X)
31 Accessory nerve (XI)
32 Deep cervical lymph
   node
33 Sternocleidomastoid
34 Internal jugular vein
35 Internal carotid artery
36 External carotid artery
37 Stylohyoid

38 Tendon of digastric
39 Parotid gland
40 Submandibular salivary
   gland
41 Styloglossus entering
   tongue
42 Oropharynx

43 Genioglossus
44 Constrictor of pharynx
45 Base of tongue
46 Mylohyoid
47 Hyoglossus
48 External jugular vein

Section level

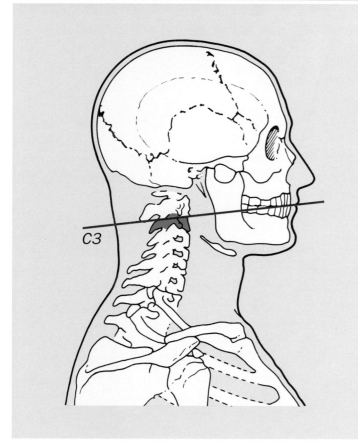

C3

Orientation guide

ANTERIOR

RIGHT ← → LEFT

POSTERIOR

Notes

This section passes between the lips (**1** and **2**), the body of the third cervical vertebra (**24**) and its spine (**22**). The CT image, is from a different subject and comes from the series which traverses the neck. This is because few cranial CT runs extend as caudal as this level. Moreover, artefacts from the amalgam of dental fillings often obscure this region. Bolus enhancement with intravenous iodinated contrast medium has opacified the major vessels (**34–36**) and assists in their identification.

The submandibular salivary gland (**40**) lies against the ramus of the mandible (**7**) at its angle, separated by the medial pterygoid muscle (**10**). Its close relationship to the parotid gland (**39**) is well demonstrated; it is separated from the latter only by the fascial sheet of the sphenomandibular ligament.

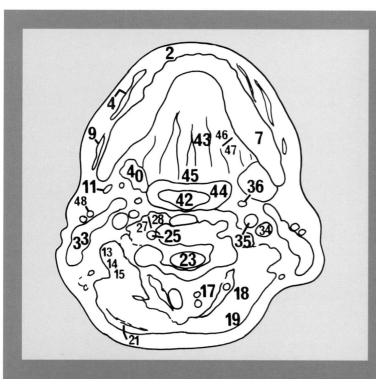

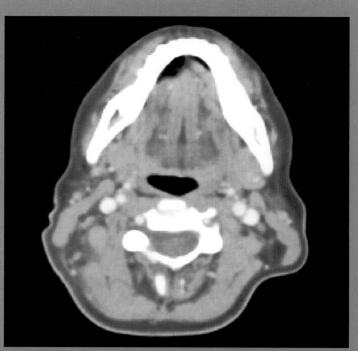

Axial computed tomogram (CT)

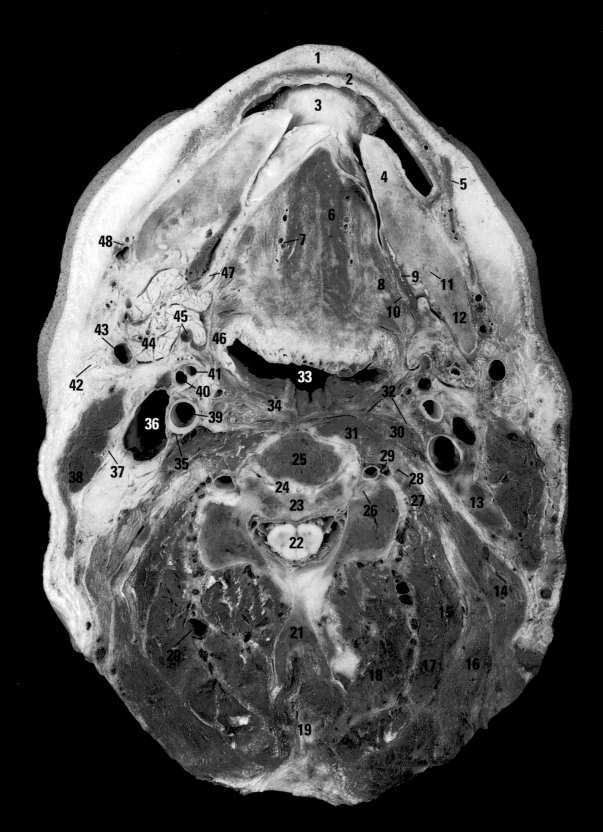

1 Lower lip	**16** Splenius capitis	**27** Scalenus medius	**41** Origin of facial artery
2 Orbicularis oris	**17** Semispinalis capitis	**28** Scalenus anterior	**42** Parotid gland
3 Under surface of	**18** Semispinalis cervicis	origin	**43** Retromandibular vein
tongue	**19** Ligamentum nuchae	**29** Vertebral artery and	**44** Submandibular salivary
4 Body of mandible	**20** Deep cervical vein	vein within foramen	gland – superficial lobe
5 Depressor anguli oris	**21** Spine of fourth cervical	transversarium	**45** Tendon of digastric
6 Genioglossus	vertebra	**30** Longus capitis	**46** Styloglossus
7 Lingual artery and vein	**22** Spinal cord within	**31** Longus colli	**47** Deep lobe of
8 Hyoglossus	dural sheath	**32** Prevertebral fascia	submandibular salivary
9 Mylohyoid	**23** Part of body of fourth	**33** Oropharynx	gland
10 Lingual nerve (V^{iii})	cervical vertebra	**34** Constrictor muscles of	**48** Facial artery and vein
11 Inferior alveolar nerve	**24** Part of intervertebral	pharynx	
(V^{iii}) within mandibular	disc between third and	**35** Vagus nerve (X)	**49** Platysma
canal	fourth cervical vertebrae	**36** Internal jugular vein	**50** Hyoid bone
12 Ramus of mandible	**25** Part of body of third	**37** Accessory nerve (XI)	**51** External jugular vein
13 Cervical lymph nodes	cervical vertebra	**38** Sternocleidomastoid	
14 Levator scapulae	**26** Dorsal root ganglion of	**39** Internal carotid artery	
15 Splenius cervicis	fourth cervical nerve	**40** External carotid artery	

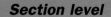

Section level

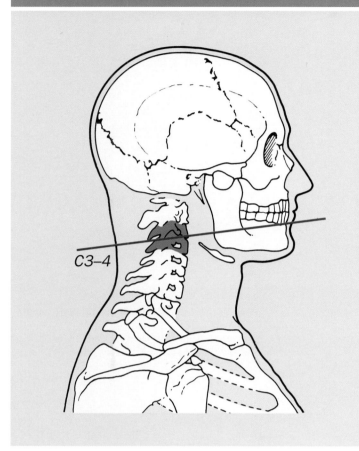

C3–4

Notes

This section passes through the upper border of the lower lip (**1**), genioglossus at the base of the tongue (**6**) and the cartilaginous disc between the third and fourth cervical vertebrae (**24**).

The prevertebral fascia (**32**) invests the front of the bodies of the cervical vertebrae, the prevertebral muscles (**30, 31**) and the scalene muscles (**27, 28**). It forms an almost avascular transverse plane behind the pharynx (**33**) and the great vessels (**36, 39**).

The facial artery at its origin from the external carotid artery (**40**) is seen at (**41**). It arches over the submandibular salivary gland (**44**) to cross the lower border of the mandible (**4**) where its pulse is palpable (**48**).

Orientation guide

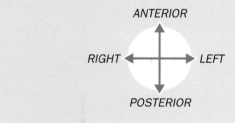

ANTERIOR

RIGHT — LEFT

POSTERIOR

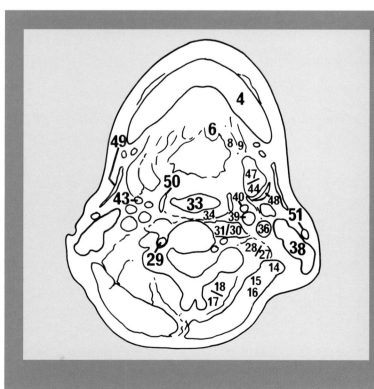

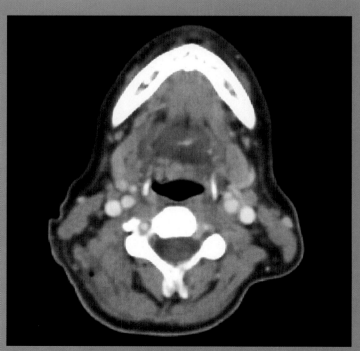

Axial computed tomogram (CT)

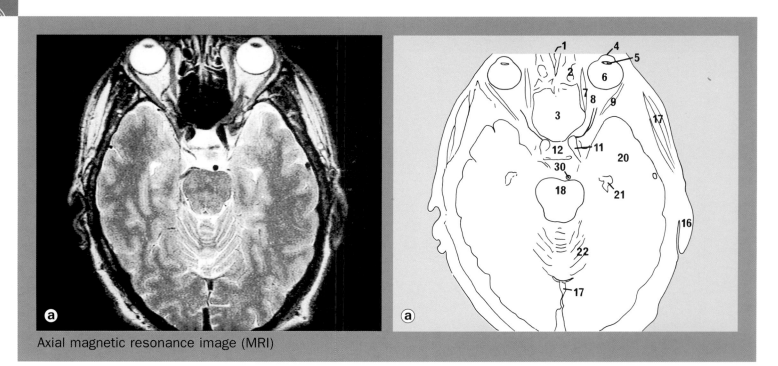

Axial magnetic resonance image (MRI)

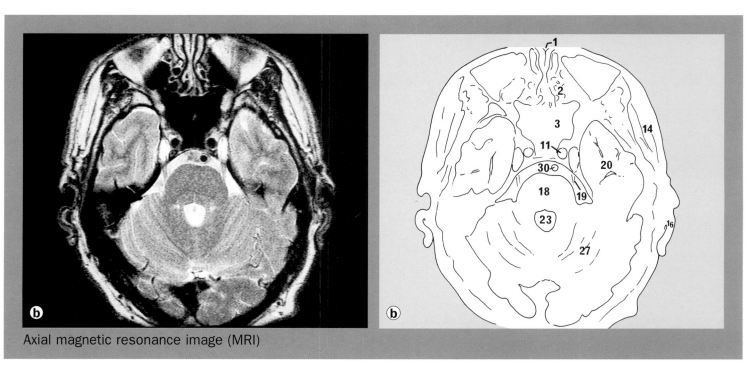

Axial magnetic resonance image (MRI)

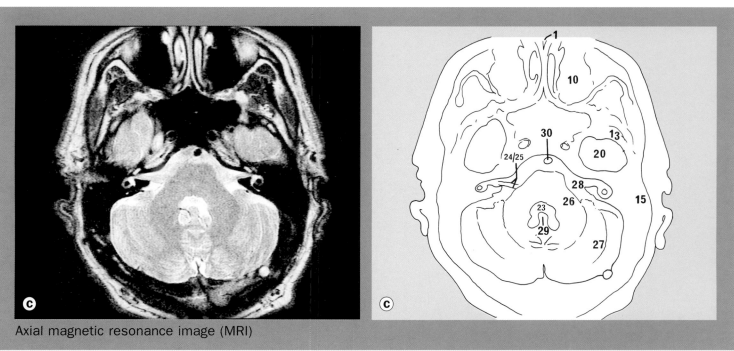

Axial magnetic resonance image (MRI)

Section level

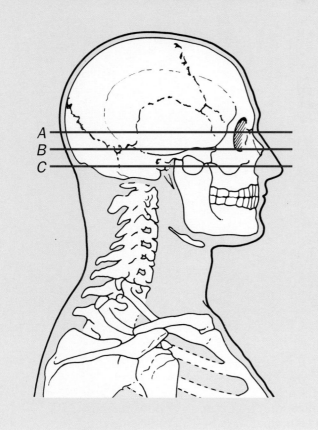

Notes

These three axial T2 weighted images show many important structures at the base of the brain, along with the orbits and sinuses. The water content of the globe provides good contrast with the lens. On this sequence the fluid in the globe and cerebrospinal spaces yields similar signal intensity to the fat within the orbit. The T2 weighting also demonstrates the emerging nerves within the CSF to good effect. Demonstration of a normal VIIIth (vestibulocochlear) nerve and fluid entering the internal auditory canal (meatus) effectively excludes a neuroma here. Possible lesions at this site (the cerebello-pontine angle) provide one of the commonest referrals for MRI. On the spin-echo sequence used here, flowing arterial blood returns no signal and thus appears black; in this way the internal carotid and basilar arteries are well visualised. Air containing structures, such as the sphenoid sinus, also appear black.

Orientation guide

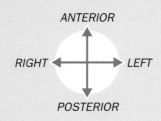

1	Nasal bone
2	Ethmoid sinus
3	Sphenoid sinus
4	Cornea
5	Lens
6	Vitreous humour
7	Medial rectus
8	Optic nerve (II)
9	Lateral rectus
10	Maxillary sinus
11	Internal carotid artery – within cavernous sinus (image b)
12	Pituitary fossa
13	Greater wing of sphenoid bone
14	Temporalis
15	Mastoid
16	Pinna
17	Straight sinus
18	Pons
19	Trigeminal nerve (V)
20	Temporal lobe of brain
21	Temporal horn of lateral ventricle
22	Anterior lobe of cerebellum
23	Fourth ventricle
24	Facial nerve (VII)
25	Vestibulocochlear (auditory) nerve (VIII)
26	Middle cerebral peduncle
27	Cerebellar hemisphere
28	Internal auditory meatus
29	Vermis of cerebellum
30	Basilar artery

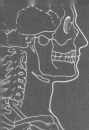

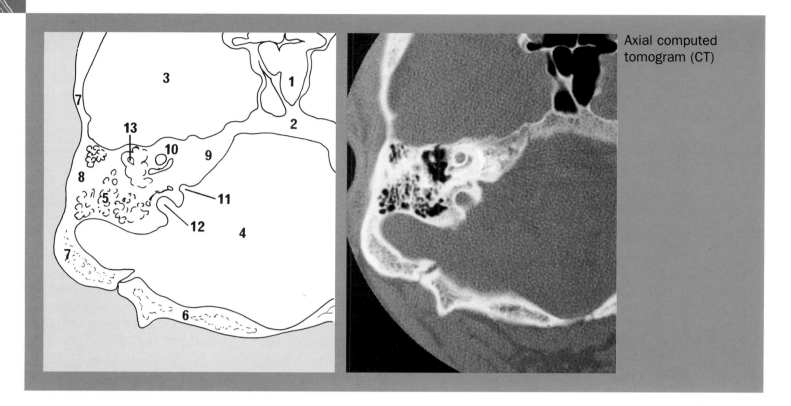

Axial computed tomogram (CT)

1 Sphenoidal sinus
2 Basi-sphenoid joining basi-occiput (forming clivus)
3 Temporal lobe of brain (in middle cranial fossa)
4 Posterior cranial fossa
5 Mastoid air cells (within temporal bone)
6 Occipital bone

7 Temporal bone (squamous part)
8 Temporal bone (mastoid part)
9 Temporal bone (apex of petrous part)
10 Cochlea
11 Internal auditory meatus
12 Superior aspect of jugular bulb
13 Malleus

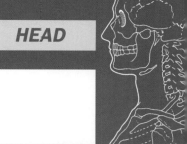

Section level

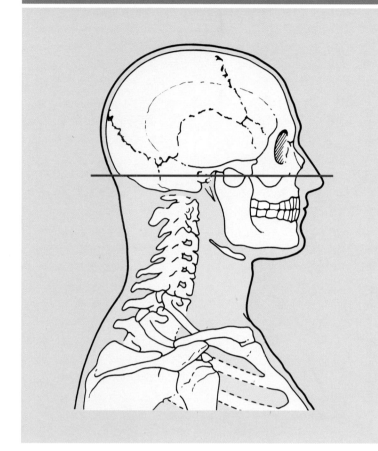

Orientation guide

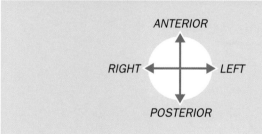

ANTERIOR

RIGHT — LEFT

POSTERIOR

Notes

This thin section CT image has been reconstructed using a bony algorithm and displayed at settings to demonstrate the bony structures. Hence the bone texture is well seen (and the detail of cerebral tissue absent). Such high resolution images are essential to study the anatomy of the inner ear before complex surgery.

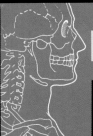

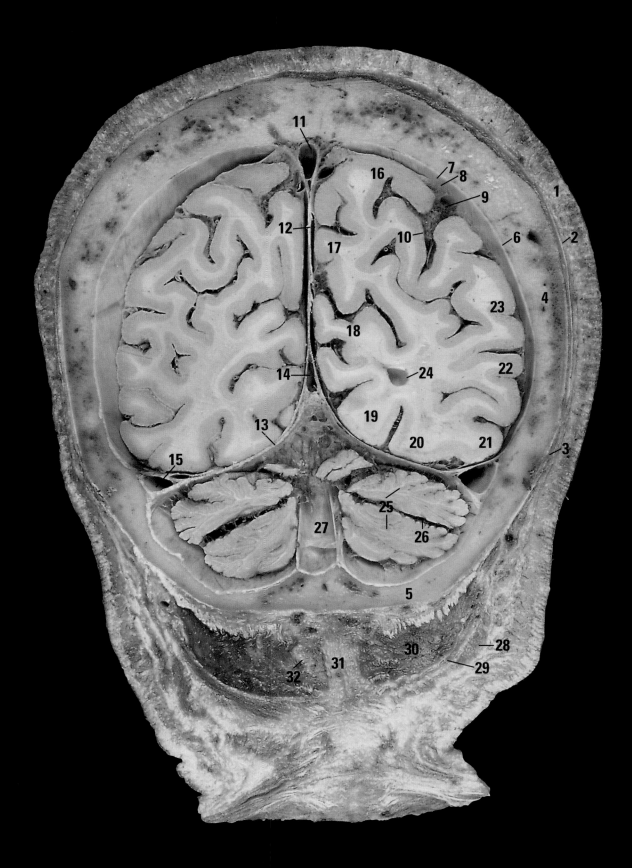

1 Skin and dense subcutaneous tissue	**10** Pia mater	**22** Middle temporal gyrus
2 Epicranial aponeurosis (galea aponeurotica)	**11** Superior sagittal sinus	**23** Inferior parietal lobule
	12 Falx cerebri	**24** Posterior horn of lateral ventricle
3 Occipital belly of occipitofrontalis	**13** Tentorium cerebelli	**25** Cerebellar hemisphere
	14 Straight sinus	**26** Horizontal fissure of cerebellum
4 Parietal bone	**15** Transverse sinus	**27** Internal occipital crest
5 Occipital bone	**16** Superior parietal lobule	**28** Trapezius
6 Dura mater	**17** Precuneus	**29** Splenius capitis
7 Subdural space	**18** Cuneus	**30** Semispinalis capitis
8 Arachnoid mater	**19** Lingual gyrus	**31** Ligamentum nuchae
9 Subarachnoid space	**20** Medial occipitotemporal gyrus	**32** Greater occipital nerve
	21 Lateral occipitotemporal gyrus	

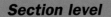

Section level

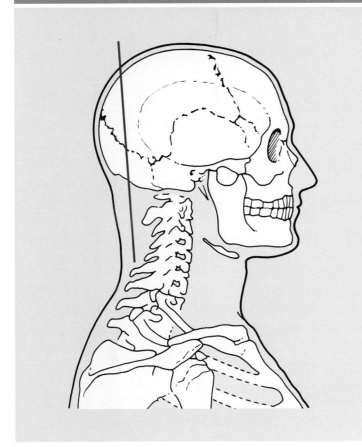

Notes

This coronal section passes through the posterior part of the occipital bone (**5**) immediately anterior to the external occipital protuberance. It passes through the posterior extremity of the posterior, or occipital, horn of the lateral ventricle (**24**).

In this, as in all subsequent sections, cross-reference should be made between a coronal section with the photographs of the external aspects and sagittal sections of the brain for orientation of the positions of the main sulci and gyri (see pages 1–6).

On this proton density MR image flowing blood in the venous sinuses appears black (low signal intensity) because the protons which were excited have moved out of the slice before measurement (creating a flow void).

Orientation guide

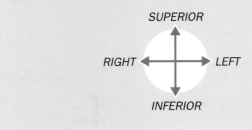

SUPERIOR

RIGHT   LEFT

INFERIOR

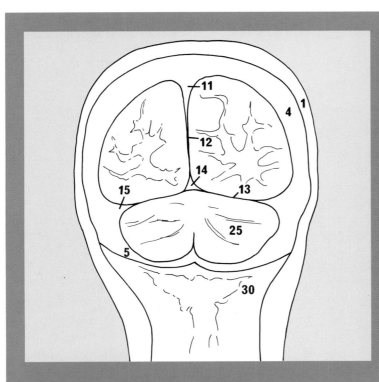

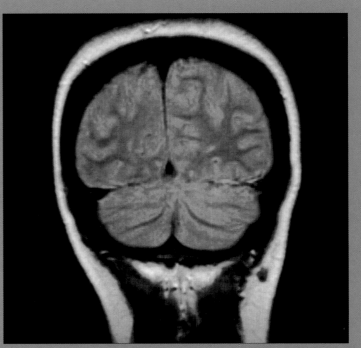

Coronal magnetic resonance image (MRI)

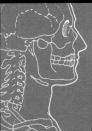

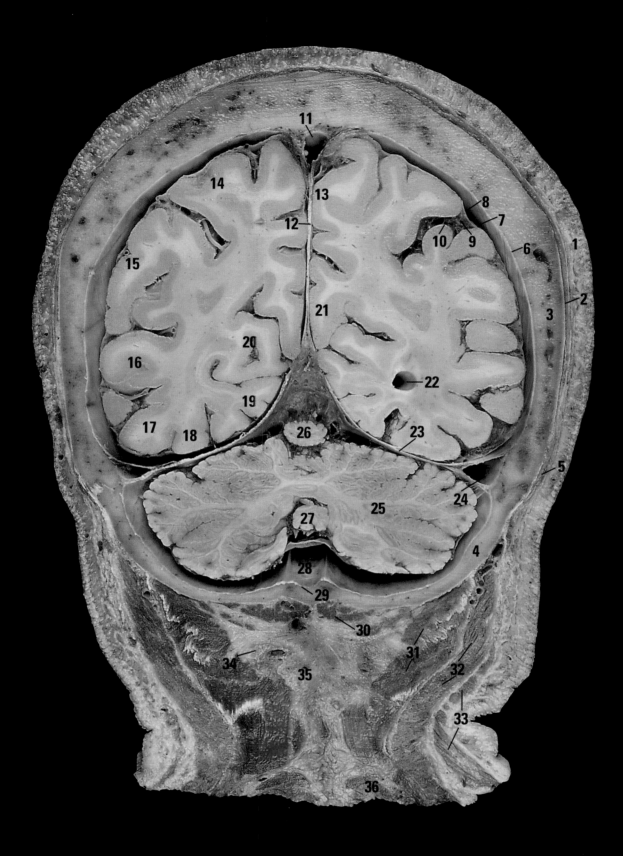

1 Skin and dense subcutaneous tissue	**11** Superior sagittal sinus	**24** Transverse sinus
2 Epicranial aponeurosis (galea aponeurotica)	**12** Falx cerebri	**25** Cerebellar hemisphere
3 Parietal bone	**13** Precuneus	**26** Superior vermis
4 Occipital bone	**14** Superior parietal lobule	**27** Inferior vermis
5 Occipital belly of occipitofrontalis	**15** Inferior parietal lobule	**28** Falx cerebelli
6 Dura mater	**16** Middle temporal gyrus	**29** Internal occipital crest
7 Subdural space	**17** Lateral occipitotemporal gyrus	**30** Rectus capitis posterior minor
8 Arachnoid mater	**18** Medial occipitotemporal gyrus	**31** Semispinalis capitis
9 Subarachnoid space	**19** Lingual gyrus	**32** Splenius capitis
10 Pia mater	**20** Cuneus	**33** Trapezius
	21 Cingulate gyrus	**34** Greater occipital nerve
	22 Posterior horn of lateral ventricle	**35** Ligamentum nuchae
	23 Tentorium cerebelli	**36** Semispinalis cervicis

Section level

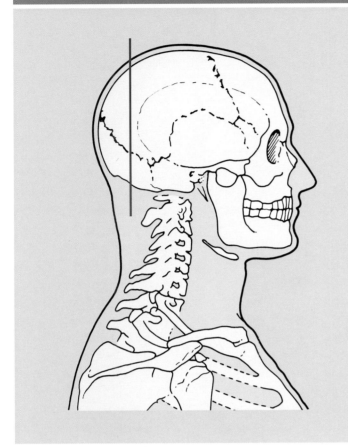

Orientation guide

SUPERIOR

RIGHT ← → LEFT

INFERIOR

Notes

The make up of the layers of the scalp can be appreciated in this and subsequent sections. It comprises hair-bearing skin, lying on dense, highly vascular connective tissue (**1**); note the large vessels seen in many of the sections. This, in turn, is adherent to a tough aponeurosis (**2**), which is the aponeurotic sheet joining the occipital belly of occipitofrontalis (**5**) to the frontalis muscle. The former arises from the superior nuchal line, while the latter inserts into the fascia above the eyebrows. The occipital part is supplied by the auricular, the frontal part by the temporal, branch of the facial nerve (VII). Paralysis of the facial nerve is followed by inability to wrinkle the forehead on the affected side. Beneath the aponeurosis lies a layer of loose areolar tissue, which again can be appreciated in these sections. It is in this plane that avulsion of the scalp can take place in tearing injuries and in which a flap of scalp can be turned down during surgical exposure of the skull. The final layer, the periosteum, is closely adherent to the skull.

This T2 weighted image is through the same position as MRI image, section 1, page 50. The cerebrospinal fluid in the subarachnoid space (**9**) now yields high signal intensity (white), providing contrast with the gyri.

The various layers of the meninges are well demonstrated (**6**, **8**, **10**). Haemorrhage around these layers is a serious event. An extradural haematoma develops between bone (**3**) and the dura mater (**6**) and usually arises soon after trauma which ruptures a meningeal vessel. A subdural haematoma collects in the subdural space (**7**), usually due to venous bleeding following minor trauma in the elderly. Subarachnoid haemorrage develops suddenly in the subarachnoid space (**9**), usually following the spontaneous rupture of a cerebral artery, or berry aneurysm.

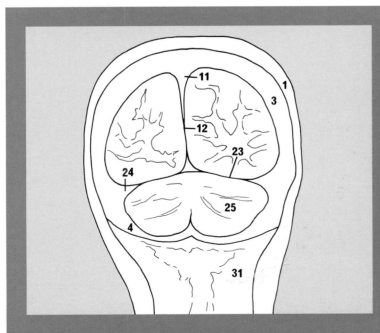

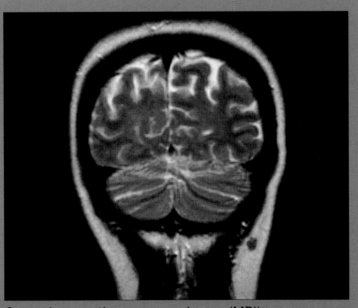

Coronal magnetic resonance image (MRI)

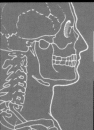

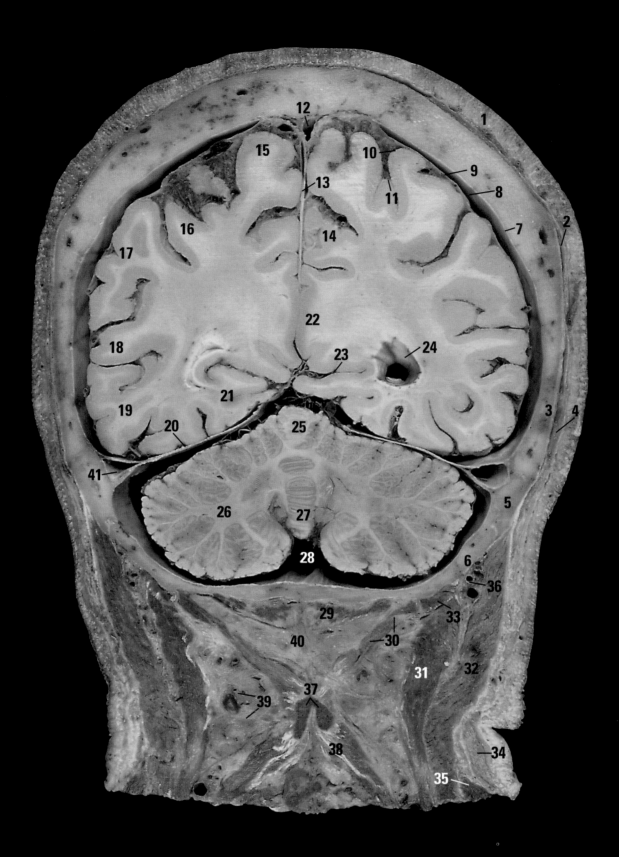

1 Skin and dense subcutaneous tissue	**13** Falx cerebri	**29** Rectus capitis posterior minor
2 Epicranial aponeurosis (galea aponeurotica)	**14** Precuneus	**30** Rectus capitis posterior major
3 Parietal bone	**15** Superior parietal lobule	**31** Semispinalis capitis
4 Occipital belly of occipitofrontalis	**16** Inferior parietal lobule	**32** Splenius capitis
5 Occipital margin of temporal bone	**17** Superior temporal gyrus	**33** Superior oblique
	18 Middle temporal gyrus	**34** Trapezius
	19 Inferior temporal gyrus	**35** Levator scapulae
6 Occipital bone	**20** Tentorium cerebelli	**36** Occipital artery and vein
7 Dura mater	**21** Lingual gyrus	**37** Bifid spine of axis
8 Subdural space	**22** Cingulate gyrus	**38** Semispinalis cervicis
9 Arachnoid mater	**23** Calcarine sulcus	**39** Occipital lymph nodes
10 Subarachnoid space	**24** Posterior horn of lateral ventricle	**40** Ligamentum nuchae
11 Pia mater	**25** Superior vermis	**41** Transverse sinus
12 Superior sagittal sinus	**26** Cerebellar hemisphere	
	27 Inferior vermis	**42** Small infarct (see notes)
	28 Cerebello-medullary cistern	

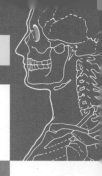

Section level

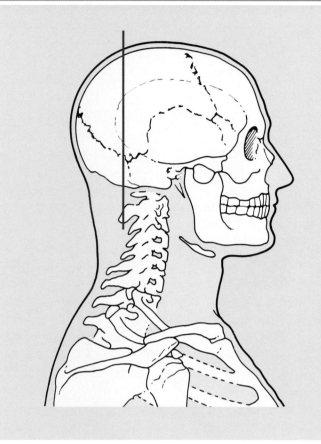

Notes

This and neighbouring sections give clear views of the structure of the superior sagittal sinus (**12**) and the transverse sinus (**11**), which are formed as clefts between the outer (endosteal) and inner (meningeal) layer of the dura mater.

The bifid spine of the axis (**37**) gives attachment to semispinalis cervicis (**38**), rectus capitis posterior major (**30**) and the ligamentum nuchae (**40**), as well as the inferior oblique, which can be seen in the next section.

The small occipital lymph nodes (**39**) are of clinical significance in that they are classically enlarged in rubella (German Measles) and some forms of cancer.

This T2 weighted MR image shows cerebrospinal fluid (white) in the subarachnoid space (**10**) surrounding the gyri and within the posterior horn of the left lateral ventricle (**24**).

This MR image shows a small area of abnormal high signal intensity (**42**) medially in the occipital lobe. The clinical features and radiological features were those of a small infarct.

Orientation guide

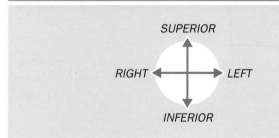

SUPERIOR

RIGHT ← → LEFT

INFERIOR

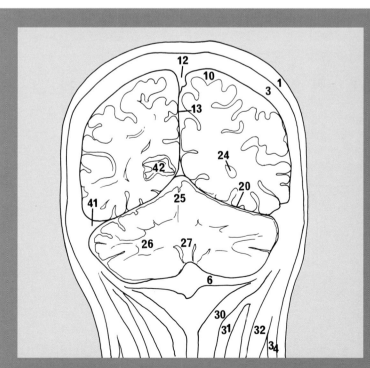

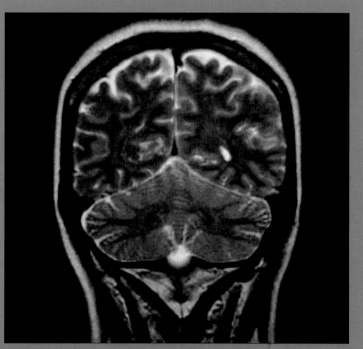

Coronal magnetic resonance image (MRI)

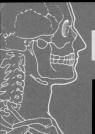

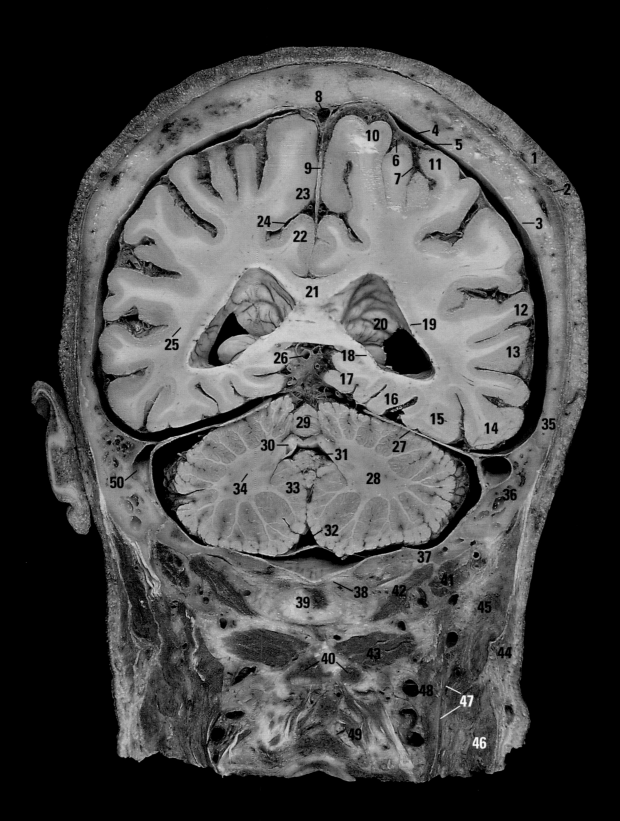

1 Skin and dense subcutaneous tissue	**15** Lateral occipitotemporal gyrus	**27** Tentorium cerebelli	**39** Posterior tubercle of atlas
2 Epicranial aponeurosis (galea aponeurotica)	**16** Medial occipitotemporal gyrus	**28** Cerebellar hemisphere	**40** Bifid spinous process of axis
3 Dura mater	**17** Parahippocampal gyrus	**29** Superior vermis	**41** Superior oblique
4 Subdural space	**18** Fimbria of hippocampus	**30** Superior medullary vellum	**42** Rectus capitis posterior major
5 Arachnoid mater	**19** Tapetum	**31** Fourth ventricle	**43** Inferior oblique
6 Subarachnoid space	**20** Posterior horn of lateral ventricle	**32** Cerebello-medullary cistern	**44** Sternocleidomastoid
7 Pia mater	**21** Splenium of corpus callosum	**33** Tonsil of cerebellum	**45** Splenius capitis
8 Superior sagittal sinus	**22** Cingulate gyrus	**34** Dentate nucleus	**46** Levator scapulae
9 Falx cerebri	**23** Paracentral lobule	**35** Parietal bone	**47** Longissimus capitis
10 Postcentral gyrus	**24** Cingulate sulcus	**36** Mastoid air cells within petrous part of temporal bone	**48** Semispinalis capitis
11 Inferior parietal lobule	**25** Optic radiation	**37** Occipital bone	**49** Semispinalis cervicis
12 Superior temporal gyrus	**26** Great cerebral vein	**38** Posterior atlanto-occipital membrane	**50** Transverse sinus
13 Middle temporal gyrus			**51** Small infarct (see notes)
14 Inferior temporal gyrus			

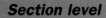

Section level

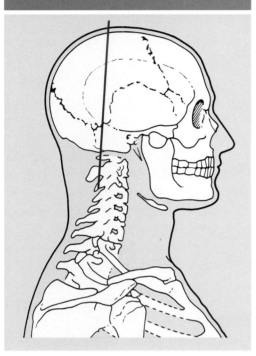

Notes

This section passes through the posterior part of the opening in the tentorium cerebelli (**27**). Note the great cerebral vein (**26**), a short median vessel formed by the union of the two internal cerebral veins. It passes backwards to open into the anterior end of the straight sinus, which lies at the junction of the falx cerebri (**9**) with the tentorium cerebelli.

On the two T2 weighted images (a & b) shown here, the extent of the cerebrospinal fluid is well demonstrated in image (a) especially in the subarachnoid space (**6**) around the gyri, but also in the cisterns around the base of the brain (**32**).

Also to be seen in image (a) is the small infarct (**51**), this is an area where there has been damage caused by interruption to the blood supply, most commonly due to a small embolus.

Orientation guide

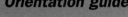

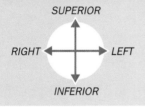

SUPERIOR

RIGHT — LEFT

INFERIOR

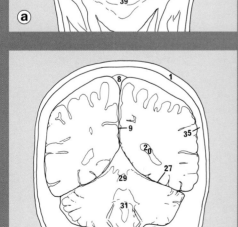

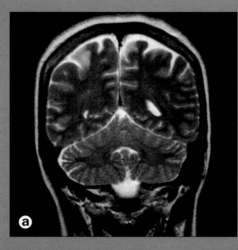

Coronal magnetic resonance image (MRI)

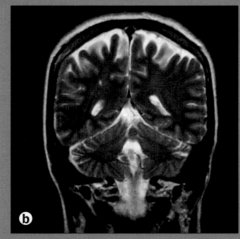

Coronal magnetic resonance image (MRI)

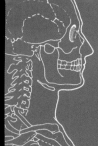

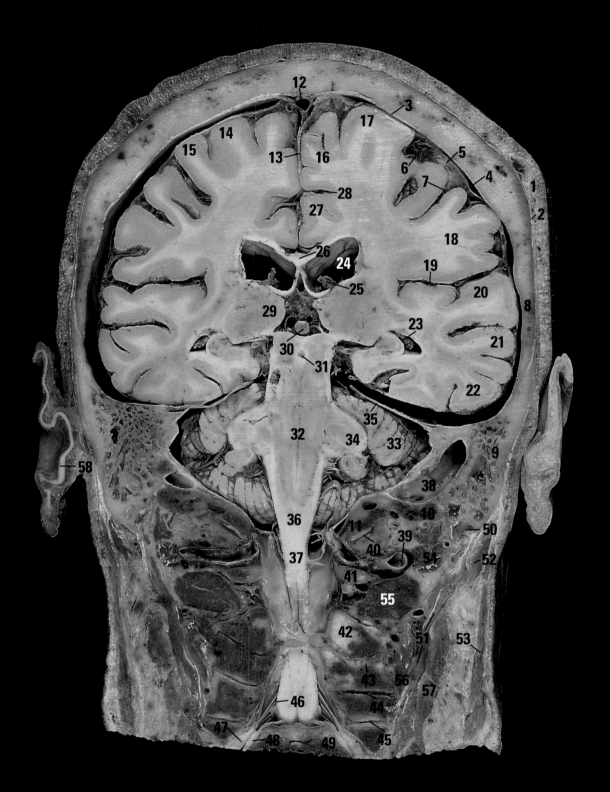

1 Skin and dense subcutaneous tissue	**17** Precentral gyrus	**33** Cerebellar hemisphere
2 Epicranial aponeurosis (galea aponeurotica)	**18** Supramarginal gyrus	**34** Middle cerebellar peduncle
3 Dura mater	**19** Lateral sulcus	**35** Tentorium cerebelli
4 Subdural space	**20** Superior temporal gyrus	**36** Termination of medulla oblongata
5 Arachnoid mater	**21** Middle temporal gyrus	**37** Commencement of spinal cord
6 Subarachnoid space	**22** Inferior temporal gyrus	**38** Sigmoid sinus
7 Pia mater	**23** Choroid plexus within posterior horn of lateral ventricle (see 25)	**39** Vertebral artery entering foramen magnum
8 Parietal bone	**24** Body of lateral ventricle	**40** Atlanto-occipital joint
9 Mastoid air cells within petrous part of temporal bone	**25** Choroid plexus within body of lateral ventricle (see 23)	**41** Posterior arch of atlas
10 Occipital bone	**26** Corpus callosum	**42** Lamina of axis
11 Margin of foramen magnum	**27** Cingulate gyrus	**43** Facet joint between C2/3 vertebrae
12 Superior sagittal sinus	**28** Cingulate sulcus	**44** Facet joint between C3/4 vertebrae
13 Falx cerebri	**29** Thalamus	**45** Facet joint between C4/5 vertebrae
14 Precentral gyrus	**30** Pineal gland	**46** Dorsal nerve root C5
15 Postcentral gyrus	**31** Aqueduct (of Sylvius)	
16 Para central lobule	**32** Pons	

47 Dorsal root ganglion C5	
48 Ventral nerve root C5	
49 Body of fifth cervical vertebra	
50 Posterior belly of digastric	
51 Longissimus capitis	
52 Splenius capitis	
53 Sternocleidomastoid	
54 Superior oblique	
55 Inferior oblique	
56 Semispinalis capitis	
57 Levator scapulae	
58 Auricular cartilage of ear	

59 Occipital condyle
60 Dens of axis (odontoid peg of second cervical vertebra)

Section level

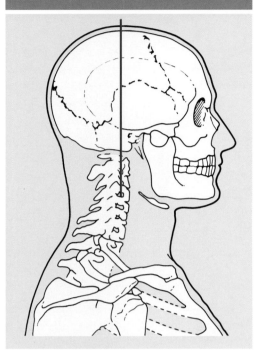

Orientation guide

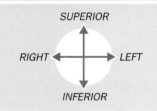

SUPERIOR

RIGHT ← → LEFT

INFERIOR

Notes

This section provides an excellent view of the foramen magnum (**11**) in the coronal section. It can be appreciated that the medulla oblongata (**36**) terminates at its superior margin and the spinal cord (**37**) commences at its inferior margin.

The vertebral artery (**39**) passes over the posterior arch of the atlas (**41**) to enter the skull through the foramen magnum. The first cervical dorsal spinal ramus lies between the artery and posterior arch. Muscular branches of the artery supply the deep muscles of this region and anastomose with the occipital, ascending and deep cervical arteries.

Formation of the fifth cervical spinal nerve from its dorsal (**46**) and ventral (**48**) root is clearly seen. Note that the dorsal root ganglion (**47**) lies within the intervertebral foramen between the fourth and fifth (**49**) cervical vertebrae.

The nerve roots in the cervical spine emerge cranial to their numbered vertebra (ie C5 roots emerge between C4 and C5 but C8 emerges between C7 and T1). In the thoracic, lumbar and sacral spine, roots emerge caudal to their numbered vertebra (ie L5 emerges between L5 and S1).

Note the close relationship between the pons (**32**), medulla oblongata (**36**) and the atlanto-occipital joints (**40**) and dens of the axis (odontoid peg) (**60**). This explains why injuries at the C1/C2 level are so serious and diseases which affect this region (eg. rheumatoid arthritis eroding the dens of the axis (odontoid peg) and weakening ligaments) can be so disabling.

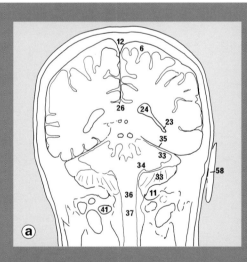

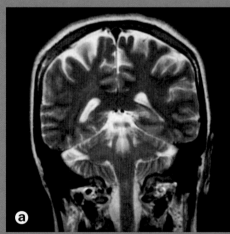

Coronal magnetic resonance image (MRI)

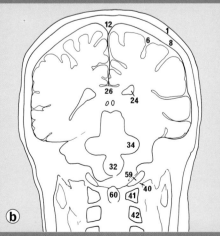

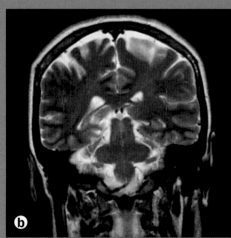

Coronal magnetic resonance image (MRI)

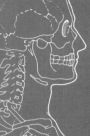

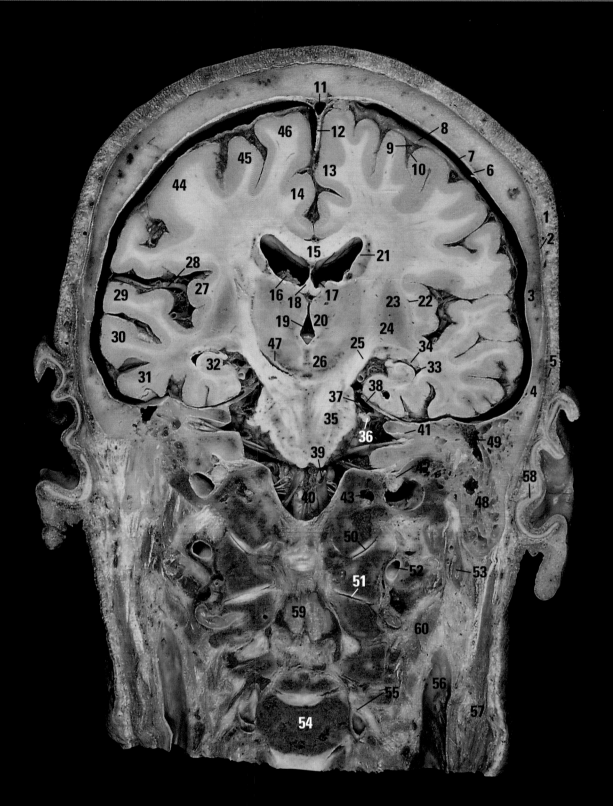

1	Skin and dense subcutaneous tissue	**21**	Caudate nucleus	
2	Epicranial aponeurosis (galea aponeurotica)	**22**	Claustrum	
3	Parietal bone	**23**	Putamen	
4	Temporal bone	**24**	Globus pallidus	
5	Temporalis	**25**	Posterior limb of internal capsule	
6	Dura mater	**26**	Mamillary body	
7	Subdural space	**27**	Insula	
8	Arachnoid mater	**28**	Lateral cerebral fissure and branches of middle cerebral artery	
9	Subarachnoid space	**29**	Superior temporal gyrus	
10	Pia mater	**30**	Middle temporal gyrus	
11	Superior sagittal sinus	**31**	Inferior temporal gyrus	
12	Falx cerebri	**32**	Hippocampus	
13	Medial frontal gyrus	**33**	Inferior horn of lateral ventricle	
14	Cingulate gyrus	**34**	Tail of caudate nucleus	
15	Body of corpus callosum	**35**	Pons	
16	Choroid plexus within lateral ventricle	**36**	Trigeminal nerve (V)	
17	Septum pellucidum	**37**	Trochlear nerve (IV)	
18	Fornix	**38**	Free margin of tentorium cerebelli	
19	Third ventricle			
20	Thalamus			

39 Vertebral artery (see 52)
40 Medulla oblongata
41 Facial nerve (VII) and Vestibulocochlear nerve (VIII) entering internal auditory meatus within petrous part of temporal bone
42 Glossopharyngeal nerve (IX), vagus nerve (X) and cranial part of accessory nerve (XI) entering jugular foramen within petrous part of temporal bone
43 Hypoglossal nerve (XII) entering hypoglossal canal within petrous part of temporal bone
44 Post central gyrus
45 Precentral gyrus
46 Superior frontal gyrus
47 Substantia nigra
48 Mastoid air cells within mastoid process of the

petrous part of temporal bone
49 Mastoid antrum within petrous part of temporal bone
50 Atlanto-occipital joint
51 Atlanto-axial joint
52 Vertebral artery within foramen transversarium of axis (see 39)
53 Posterior belly of digastric
54 Body of C4 vertebra
55 C4 dorsal root ganglion
56 Internal jugular vein
57 Sternocleidomastoid
58 Auricular cartilage of ear
59 Dura of spinal canal
60 Levator scapulae

61 Lateral ventricle
62 Basilar artery
63 Body of second cervical vertebra

Section level

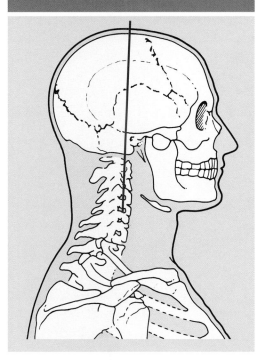

Orientation guide

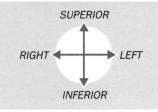

SUPERIOR

RIGHT ← → LEFT

INFERIOR

Notes

The posterior limb of the internal capsule is transected in this section (**25**) and can be seen descending into the pons (**35**). Medial to the internal capsule can be seen the tail of the caudate nucleus (**21**) and the thalamus (**20**), while laterally lies the lentiform nucleus, made up of the putamen (**23**) and, more medially, the globus pallidus (**24**). Lateral to the lentiform nucleus lies the claustrum (**22**), sandwiching the narrow external capsule between the two.

The internal auditory meatus is cut along its length and demonstrates the facial nerve (VII) and vestibulocochlear, or auditory, nerve (VIII) lying within it (**41**).

MRI is an excellent method of demonstrating small acoustic neurinomata which develop close to the internal auditory meatus. It is now possible to diagnose these benign tumours long before the bony meatus becomes enlarged.

These two MR images, obtained at the same anatomical plane, graphically demonstrate the different information which can be obtained using different MR parameters:

(a) – is the proton density image whereas
(b) – is the T2 weighted image from a dual echo acquisition.

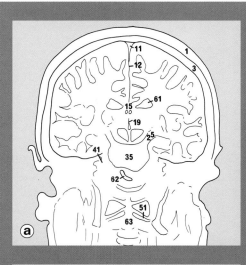

(a)

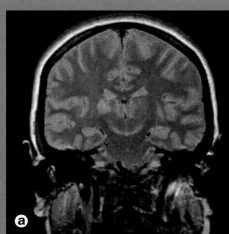

Coronal magnetic resonance image (MRI)

(a)

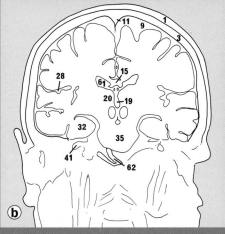

(b)

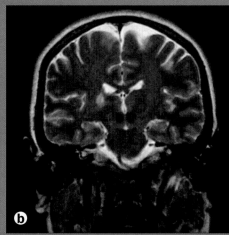

Coronal magnetic resonance image (MRI)

(b)

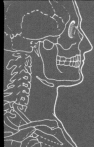
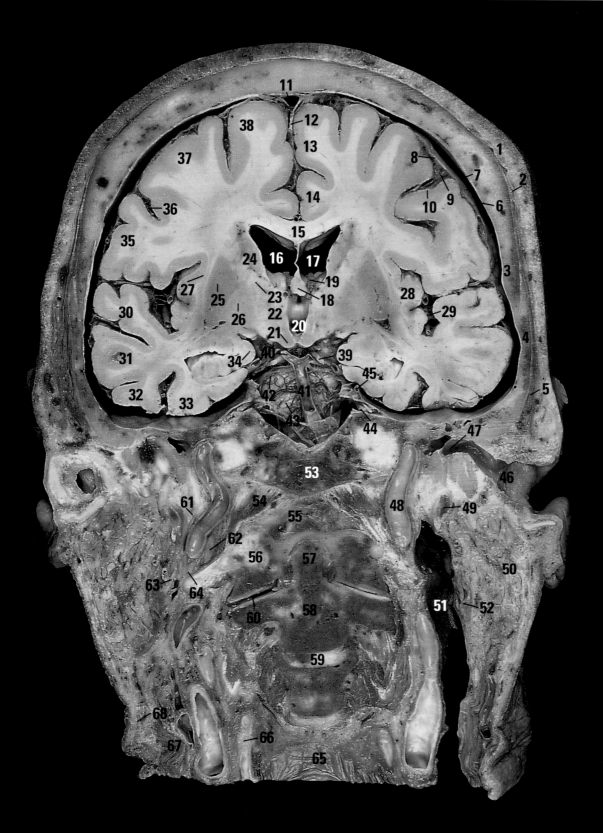

1 Skin and dense
   subcutaneous tissue
2 Epicranial aponeurosis
   (galea aponeurotica)
3 Parietal bone
4 Squamous part of
   temporal bone
5 Temporalis
6 Dura mater
7 Subdural space
8 Arachnoid mater
9 Subarachnoid space
10 Pia mater
11 Superior sagittal sinus
12 Falx cerebri
13 Medial frontal gyrus
14 Cingulate gyrus
15 Body of corpus callosum
16 Body of lateral ventricle
17 Septum pellucidum
18 Fornix

19 Choroid plexus with
   floor of lateral ventricle
20 Third ventricle
21 Mamillary body
22 Thalamus
23 Anterior limb of internal
   capsule
24 Caudate nucleus
25 Putamen
26 Globus pallidus
27 Claustrum
28 Insula
29 Lateral cerebral fissure
   and branches of middle
   cerebral artery
30 Superior temporal gyrus
31 Middle temporal gyrus
32 Inferior temporal gyrus
33 Lateral occipitotemporal
   gyrus
34 Parahippocampal gyrus

   adjacent (lateral) to
   hippocampus
35 Post central gyrus
36 Central sulcus
37 Pre central gyrus
38 Superior frontal gyrus
39 Oculomotor nerve (III)
40 Posterior cerebral artery
41 Basilar artery
42 Superior cerebral artery
43 Pons
44 Trigeminal nerve (V)
45 Free margin of tentorium
   cerebelli
46 External auditory meatus
47 Tympanic membrane
48 Internal carotid artery
49 Styloid process
50 Parotid gland
51 Internal jugular vein
52 Digastric

53 Base of occipital
   bone (clivus)
54 Rectus capitis anterior
55 Anterior atlanto-occipital
   membrane
56 Anterior arch of atlas
57 Dens of axis (odontoid
   peg of second cervical
   vertebra)
58 Body of axis
59 C 2/3 Intervertebral disc
60 Atlanto-axial joint
61 Glossopharyngeal
   nerve (IX)
62 Vagus nerve (X)
63 Spinal accessory nerve (XI)
64 Hypoglossal nerve (XII)
65 Posterior wall of pharynx
66 Thyroid cartilage
67 Sternocleidomastoid
68 Platysma

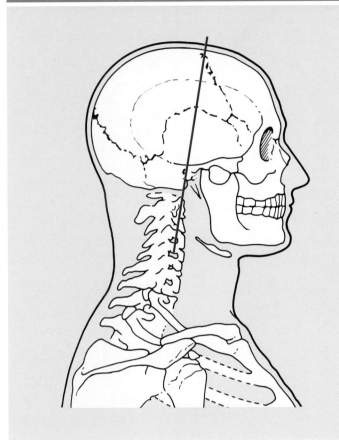

Section level

Orientation guide

SUPERIOR

RIGHT ← → LEFT

INFERIOR

Notes

This section passes through the external auditory meatus (**46**). This is about (37 mm) long, and has a peculiar S-shaped course, being directed first medially upwards and backwards, then medially and backwards and finally medially forwards and downwards. The outer one third of the canal is cartilaginous and somewhat wider than the medial osseous portion. It leads to the tympanic membrane, or ear drum, (**47**) which faces laterally inferiorly and anteriorly.

This section provides a clear view of the dens (**57**) in coronal section and its articulation with the anterior arch of the atlas (**56**).

It also illustrates the importance of the transverse ligament of the atlas keeping the dens of the axis (odontoid peg of second cervical vertebra) (**57**) in intimate contact with the atlas (first cervical vertebra).

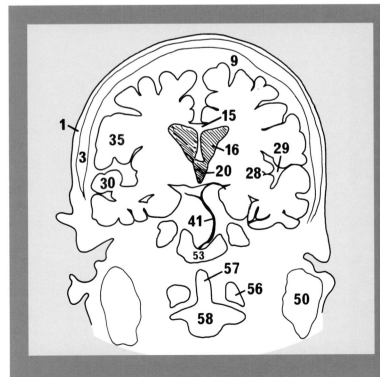

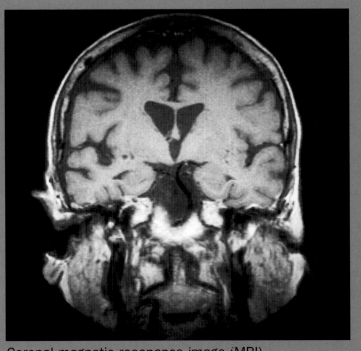

Coronal magnetic resonance image (MRI)

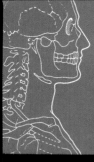

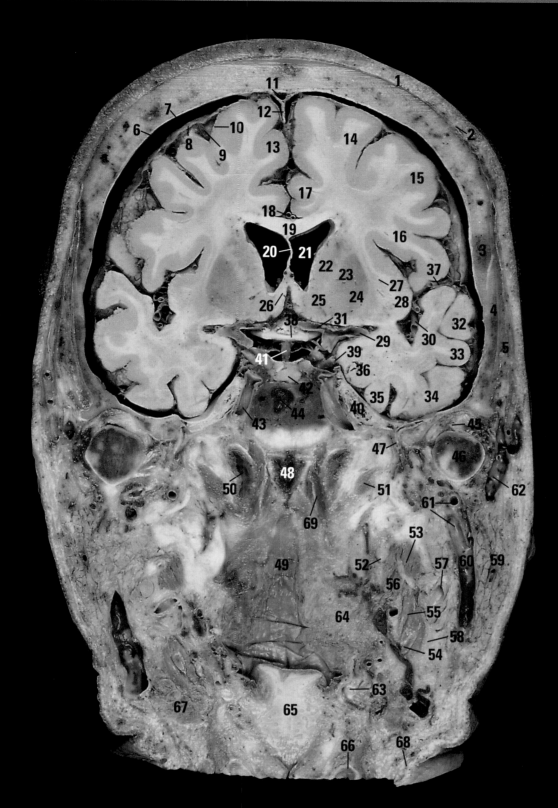

1 Skin and dense subcutaneous tissue	**21** Lateral ventricle	**38** Optic chiasma (II)	**51** Levator veli palatini
2 Epicranial aponeurosis (galea aponeurotica)	**22** Head of caudate nucleus	**39** Oculomotor nerve (III)	**52** Internal carotid artery
	23 Anterior limb of internal capsule	**40** Trigeminal ganglion	**53** Styloglossus
3 Parietal bone	**24** Putamen	**41** Pituitary stalk	**54** Tendon of digastric
4 Squamous part of temporal bone	**25** Nucleus accumbens	**42** Pituitary gland within pituitary fossa (sella turcica)	**55** Stylohyoid
5 Temporalis	**26** Anterior column of fornix		**56** Stylopharyngeus
6 Dura mater	**27** Claustrum		**57** External carotid artery
7 Subdural space	**28** Insula	**43** Internal carotid artery within cavernous sinus	**58** Hypoglossal nerve (XII)
8 Arachnoid mater	**29** Origin of middle cerebral artery (see 30)	**44** Body of sphenoid bone and sphenoidal sinus	**59** Parotid gland
9 Subarachnoid space	**30** Middle cerebral artery branches (see 29)		**60** Retromandibular vein
10 Pia mater		**45** Intra-articular disc of temporomandibular joint	**61** Maxillary artery and vein
11 Superior sagittal sinus	**31** Origin of anterior cerebral artery (see 18)	**46** Head of mandible	**62** Superficial temporal vein
12 Falx cerebri	**32** Superior temporal gyrus	**47** Middle meningeal artery within foramen spinosum of sphenoid bone	**63** Greater horn of hyoid bone
13 Medial frontal gyrus	**33** Middle temporal gyrus		**64** Constrictor muscles of pharynx
14 Superior frontal gyrus	**34** Inferior temporal gyrus		
15 Middle frontal gyrus	**35** Lateral occipitotemporal gyrus	**48** Posterior wall of nasopharynx	**65** Cartilage of epiglottis
16 Inferior frontal gyrus		**49** Posterior wall of oropharynx	**66** Superior margin of lamina of thyroid cartilage
17 Cingulate gyrus	**36** Medial occipitotemporal gyrus	**50** Auditory (Eustachian) tube	**67** Submandibular gland
18 Pericallosal artery	**37** Lateral sulcus		**68** Platysma
19 Body of corpus callosum			**69** Longus capitis
20 Septum pellucidum			

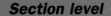

Section level

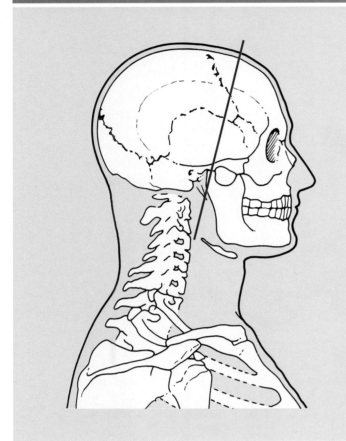

Orientation guide

SUPERIOR

RIGHT ←→ LEFT

INFERIOR

Notes

The plane of this section passes through the head of the mandible (**46**) and the temporomandibular joint. The articular surfaces of the joint are covered with fibrocartilage (not hyaline cartilage as is usual in a synovial joint). The joint contains a prominent fibro-cartilaginous intra-articular disc (**45**), which divides it into an upper and lower compartment. The parotid gland (**59**) and the submandibular salivary gland (**67**) are in contact with each other, separated only by a sheet of fascia, the stylo-mandibular ligament.

The anterior limb of the internal capsule (**23**) relates medially to the head of the caudate nucleus (**22**) and laterally to the putamen (**24**). See also the note on the posterior limb of the internal capsule in Section 6.

The pituitary gland (**42**) can be seen lying within its fossa, in close relationship to the optic chiasma. An enlarging tumour of the pituitary gland classically produces the visual disturbance of bitemporal hemianopia because of pressure on the medial aspect of the chiasma. The modern pernasal trans-sphenoidal fibreoptic approach for pituitary surgery via the sphenoid sinus (**44**) can be appreciated in this section.

On this T1 weighted MR image the sphenoid (**44**) is very bright because there is virtually no sinus aeration; this is very variable; the bright signal reflects a high marrow content of bone.

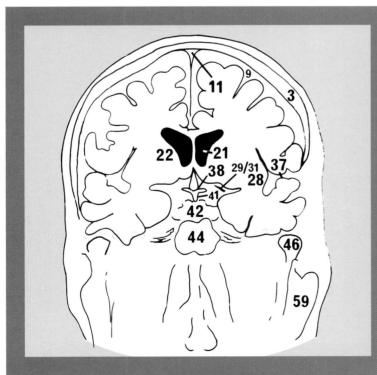

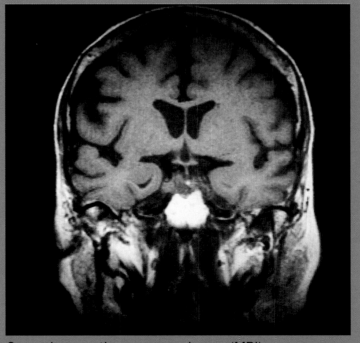

Coronal magnetic resonance image (MRI)

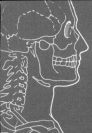

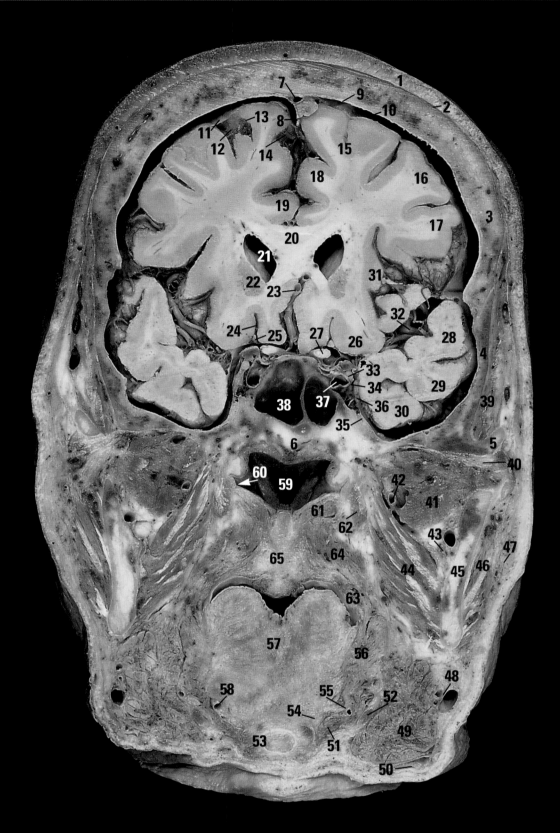

1 Skin and dense subcutaneous tissue	**16** Middle frontal gyrus	**36** Ophthalamic nerve (III) with trochlear nerve (IV)	**53** Body of hyoid bone
2 Epicranial aponeurosis (galea aponeurotica)	**17** Inferior frontal gyrus	**37** Internal carotid artery in cavernous sinus	**54** Lesser horn of hyoid bone
3 Parietal bone	**18** Medial frontal gyrus	**38** Sphenoidal sinus	**55** Stylohyoid ligament
4 Squamous part of temporal bone	**19** Cingulate gyrus	**39** Temporalis	**56** Styloglossus
5 Zygomatic process of temporal bone	**20** Body of corpus callosum	**40** Intra-articular disc of temporomandibular joint	**57** Intrinsic muscle of tongue
6 Body of sphenoid bone	**21** Anterior horn of lateral ventricle	**41** Lateral pterygoid	**58** Lingual artery
7 Superior sagittal sinus	**22** Head of caudate nucleus	**42** Maxillary artery	**59** Nasopharynx
8 Falx cerebri	**23** Anterior cerebral artery	**43** Inferior alveolar nerve and artery	**60** Opening of auditory (Eustachian) tube (arrowed)
9 Dura mater	**24** Olfactory sulcus	**44** Medial pterygoid	**61** Levator veli palatini
10 Subdural space	**25** Olfactory tract (I)	**45** Ramus of mandible	**62** Tensor veli palatini
11 Arachnoid mater	**26** Orbital gyri	**46** Masseter	**63** Palatoglossus
12 Subarachnoid space	**27** Optic nerve (II)	**47** Parotid gland	**64** Superior constrictor of pharynx
13 Pia mater	**28** Superior temporal gyrus	**48** Facial artery and vein	**65** Soft palate
14 Callosomarginal branch of anterior cerebral artery in longitudinal fissure	**29** Middle temporal gyrus	**49** Submandibular gland	
	30 Inferior temporal gyrus	**50** Platysma	**66** Internal carotid artery
	31 Insula	**51** Hyoglossus	**67** Anterior clinoid process of sphenoid bone
15 Superior frontal gyrus	**32** Middle cerebral artery	**52** Tendon of digastric	**68** Temporal lobe
	33 Oculomotor nerve (III)		
	34 Abducent nerve (VI)		
	35 Maxillary nerve (V^{II})		

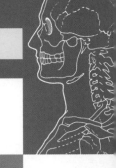

Section level

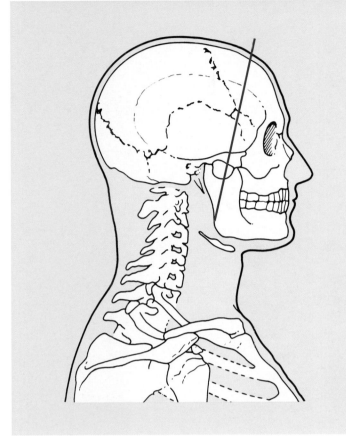

Orientation guide

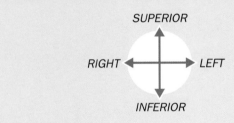

SUPERIOR

RIGHT   LEFT

INFERIOR

Notes

The line of this section passes through the zygomatic process of the temporal bone (**5**), the posterior part of the tongue (**57**) and the body of the hyoid bone (**53**). We peer into the nasopharynx (**59**) with the termination of the auditory, or Eustachian, tube (**60**) just visible.

The oculomotor nerve (III) (**33**) passes through the sharp edge of the tentorium cerebelli to enter the cavernous sinus (**37**). The cerebral hemisphere, compressed by an extradural or subdural clot, presses upon the nerve at the tentorial edge and produces dilatation of the pupil. Hence the neurosurgical aphorism 'explore the side with the dilated pupil'. Damage to the internal carotid artery within the cavernous sinus (**37**) usually as a result of trauma, may produce a carotico-cavernous fistula and results in a pulsating exophthalmos.

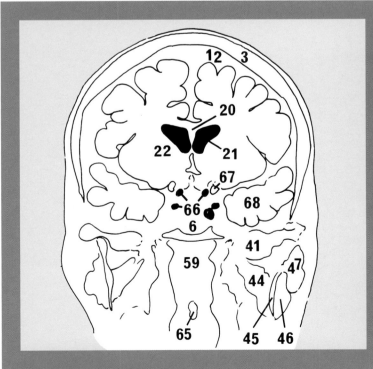

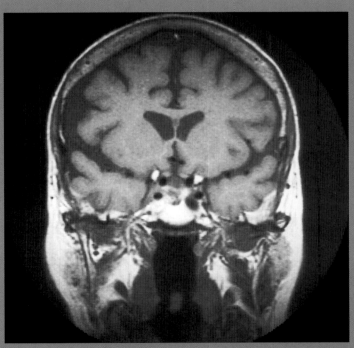

Coronal magnetic resonance image (MRI)

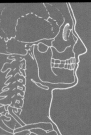

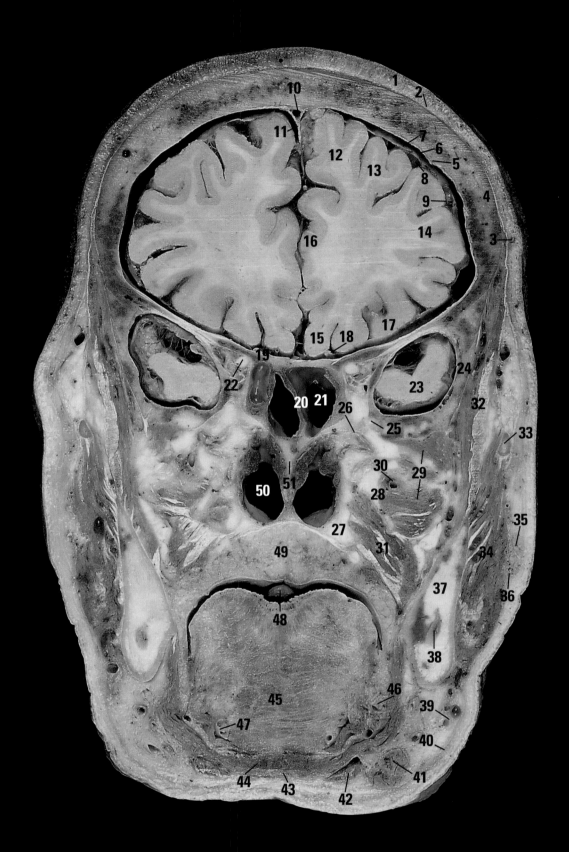

1 Skin and dense subcutaneous tissue	**17** Medial orbital gyrus	**28** Lateral pterygoid plate of sphenoid bone	**44** Geniohyoid
2 Epicranial aponeurosis (galea aponeurotica)	**18** Olfactory tract (I)	**29** Lateral pterygoid	**45** Transverse fibres of intrinsic muscle of tongue
3 Branch of superficial temporal artery	**19** Lesser wing of sphenoid bone	**30** Maxillary artery	**46** Sublingual gland
4 Frontal bone	**20** Septum between sphenoidal sinuses	**31** Medial pterygoid	**47** Lingual artery
5 Dura mater	**21** Sphenoidal sinus	**32** Temporalis	**48** Uvula
6 Subdural space	**22** Optic nerve (II)	**33** Zygomatic arch	**49** Palatine glands of soft palate
7 Arachnoid mater	**23** Temporal lobe of brain within middle cranial fossa	**34** Masseter	**50** Nasal cavity
8 Subarachnoid space	**24** Greater wing of sphenoid bone	**35** Accessory parotid gland	**51** Nasal septum (vomer)
9 Pia mater	**25** Maxillary nerve within foramen rotundum of greater wing of sphenoid bone	**36** Parotid duct	**52** Anterior clinoid process (lesser wing of sphenoid bone)
10 Superior sagittal sinus		**37** Body of mandible	**53** Ramus of mandible
11 Falx cerebri	**26** Pterygopalatine ganglion	**38** Inferior alveolar artery and nerve within mandibular canal	**54** Nasopharynx
12 Superior frontal gyrus	**27** Medial pterygoid plate of sphenoid bone	**39** Facial artery and nerve	
13 Middle frontal gyrus		**40** Platysma	
14 Inferior frontal gyrus		**41** Submandibular gland	
15 Gyrus rectus		**42** Anterior belly of digastric	
16 Cingulate gyrus		**43** Mylohyoid	

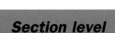

Section level

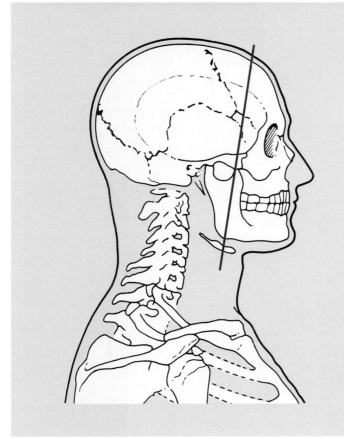

Orientation guide

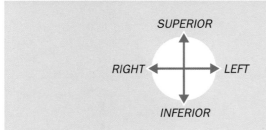

SUPERIOR

RIGHT ◄────► LEFT

INFERIOR

Notes

Do not be deceived! This section passes through the tip of the temporal lobe of the cerebrum (**23**), lying inferior to the lesser wing of the sphenoid (**19**) and **not** the orbit! Note that the plane of this section lies immediately anterior to the anterior horn of the lateral ventricle.

The parotid duct (**36**) can be palpated easily in the living subject by tensing the masseter muscle (**34**) and feeling along the upper part of the anterior border of this muscle just inferior to the zygomatic arch (**33**). The accessory parotid gland (**35**) or pars accessoria, is usually completely detached from the main gland and lies between the parotid duct and the zygomatic arch. It accounts for an occasionally very anteriorly placed parotid tumour.

The paired sphenoidal sinuses (**21**) lie within the body of the sphenoid bone and vary quite considerably in size and shape. They are rarely symmetrical, one often being much larger than the other and extending across the midline behind the other. Occasionally one overlaps the other sinus superiorly. Usually the septum (**20**) between the two sinuses is intact, although occasionally they communicate with each other.

Besides the main salivary glands, many other accessory ones are found, some in the tongue, some between the crypts of the palatine tonsils and some on the inner aspects of the lip and cheeks. Large numbers are found in the posterior hard palate and the soft palate (**49**). They are mainly mucous in type and are occasional sites for the development of a pleomorphic salivary tumour.

The CT image is purposefully displayed at optimal setting for bony structure.

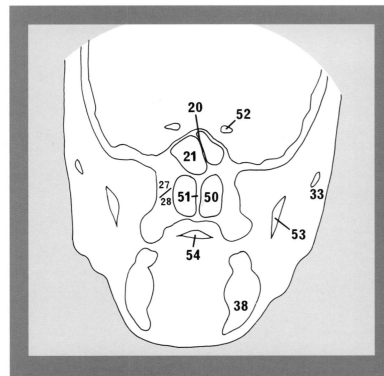

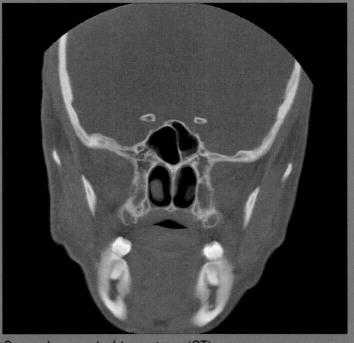

Coronal computed tomogram (CT)

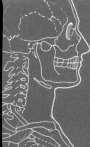

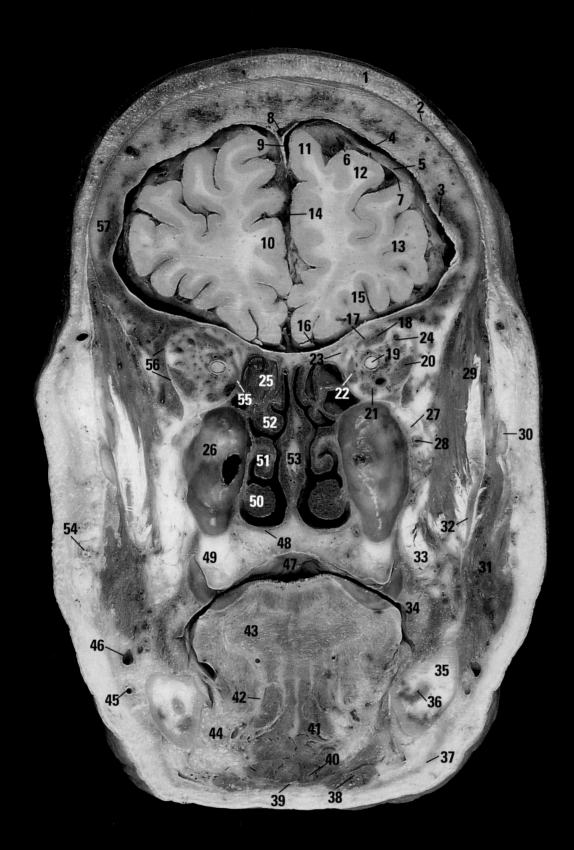

1 Skin and dense subcutaneous tissue	**17** Levator palpebrae superioris	**32** Ramus of mandible
2 Epicranial aponeurosis (galea aponeurotica)	**18** Superior rectus	**33** Buccal pad of fat
3 Dura mater	**19** Optic nerve (II) in dural sheath	**34** Buccinator
4 Subdural space	**20** Lateral rectus	**35** Body of mandible
5 Arachnoid mater	**21** Inferior rectus	**36** Inferior alveolar nerve in mandibular canal
6 Subarachnoid space	**22** Medial rectus	**37** Platysma
7 Pia mater	**23** Superior oblique	**38** Anterior belly of digastric
8 Superior sagittal sinus	**24** Branches of ophthalmic artery and vein	**39** Mylohyoid
9 Falx cerebri	**25** Ethmoidal air cells	**40** Geniohyoid
10 Medial frontal gyrus	**26** Maxillary sinus	**41** Genioglossus
11 Superior frontal gyrus	**27** Maxillary nerve	**42** Lingual artery
12 Middle frontal gyrus	**28** Maxillary artery	**43** Transverse fibres of intrinsic muscle of tongue
13 Inferior frontal gyrus	**29** Temporalis	**44** Sublingual gland
14 Longitudinal fissure	**30** Zygomatic arch	**45** Facial artery
15 Orbital gyri	**31** Masseter	**46** Facial vein
16 Olfactory tract (I)		**47** Soft palate

48 Horizontal plate of palatine bone	
49 Tuberosity of maxilla	
50 Inferior nasal concha	
51 Middle nasal concha	
52 Superior nasal concha	
53 Nasal septum	
54 Parotid duct	
55 Orbital part of ethmoid bone	
56 Greater wing of sphenoid bone – orbital surface	
57 Frontal bone	
58 Zygoma	
59 Dental artefacts (see notes)	

Section level

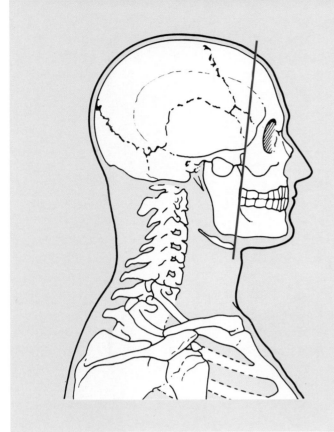

Orientation guide

SUPERIOR

RIGHT ⟷ LEFT

INFERIOR

Notes

This section does indeed pass through the posterior part of the cavity of the orbit and demonstrates the close packing of the extrinsic muscles (**17**, **18**, **20–23**) and blood vessels (**24**) with the orbital fat and optic (II) nerve (**19**). Note that the optic nerve is surrounded by an extension of the dura mater and is therefore bathed in cerebrospinal fluid. Raised intracranial pressure is thus transmitted in the C.S.F. along the sheath and results in the changes of papilloedema.

The ethmoidal air cells, or sinuses (**25**), are small, thin-walled cavities in the ethmoidal labyrinth. They range in number from three large to 18 small cells on either side and are separated from the orbit by the paper-thin orbital plate of the ethmoid. Orbital cellulitis can thus easily result from ethmoid sinusitis (see (**54**) section 13, page 74).

The three nasal conchae, (still often called by ENT surgeons the turbinate bones), project inferiorly like three scrolls from the lateral wall of the nasal cavity. The lowest, the inferior (**50**) is the largest and broadest. It is a separate bone, unlike the middle (**51**) and superior (**52**), which are part of the ethmoid bone (**55**). The middle and superior conchae are joined anteriorly, but diverge away from each other posteriorly so that the superior concha can only be visualised at posterior rhinoscopy and is invisible on viewing through the anterior nares. Beneath each concha is a space, termed the superior, middle and inferior meatus respectively.

Metallic material, used in dental fillings, create substantial problems for coronal CT. Even with careful positioning and gantry angulation they may be unavoidable.

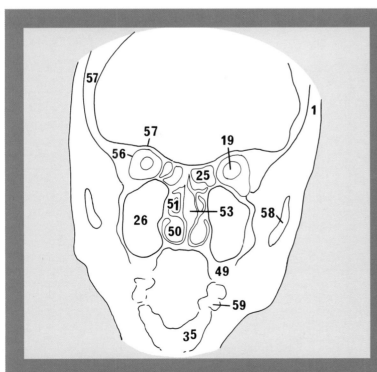

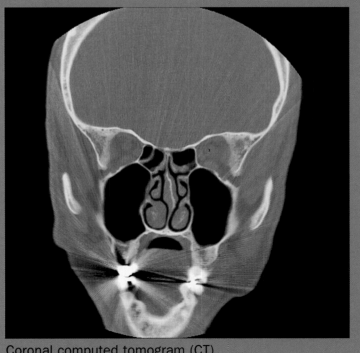

Coronal computed tomogram (CT)

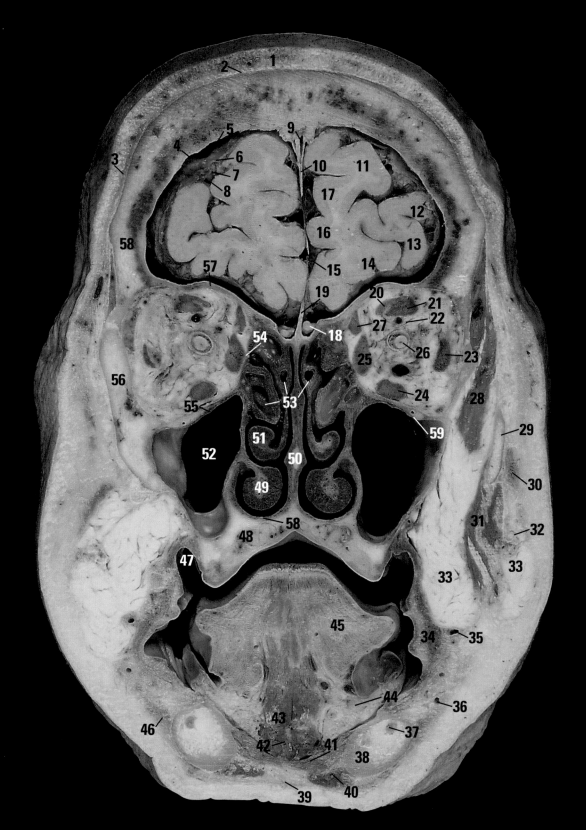

1 Skin and dense subcutaneous tissue	**18** Posterior portion of olfactory bulb (I) lying on cribriform plate of ethmoid bone	**30** Zygomaticus major	**48** Palatine glands of soft palate
2 Epicranial aponeurosis (galea aponeurotica)		**31** Masseter	**49** Inferior nasal concha
3 Frontal belly of occipitofrontalis	**19** Posterior part of crista galli	**32** Parotid duct	**50** Nasal septum
4 Dura mater	**20** Levator palpebrae superioris	**33** Buccal fat	**51** Middle nasal concha
5 Subdural space		**34** Buccinator	**52** Maxillary sinus
6 Arachnoid mater	**21** Superior rectus	**35** Facial vein	**53** Ethmoidal air cells
7 Subarachnoid space	**22** Branches of ophthalmic artery and vein	**36** Facial artery	**54** Orbital part of ethmoid bone
8 Pia mater		**37** Inferior alveolar nerve in mandibular canal	
9 Superior sagittal sinus	**23** Lateral rectus		**55** Orbital surface of maxilla
10 Falx cerebri	**24** Inferior rectus	**38** Body of mandible	**56** Zygomatic bone
11 Superior frontal gyrus	**25** Medial rectus	**39** Platysma	**57** Orbital part of frontal bone
12 Middle frontal gyrus	**26** Optic nerve (II) in dural sheath	**40** Anterior belly of digastric	**58** Palatine process of maxilla
13 Inferior frontal gyrus		**41** Mylohyoid	**59** Infra-orbital artery and nerve within infra-orbital canal of maxilla
14 Orbital gyri	**27** Superior oblique	**42** Geniohyoid	
15 Longitudinal fissure	**28** Temporalis	**43** Genioglossus	
16 Cingulate gyrus	**29** Temporal process cf zygomatic bone	**44** Sublingual gland	**60** Teeth arising from mandible
17 Medial frontal gyrus		**45** Intrinsic muscle of tongue	
		46 Depressor anguli oris	**61** Globe
		47 Buccal vestibule	

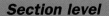

Section level

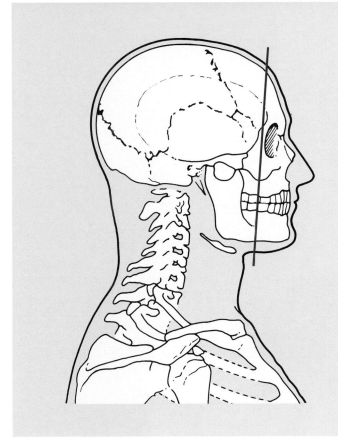

Orientation guide

SUPERIOR

RIGHT ← → LEFT

INFERIOR

Notes

From the roof of the nasal cavity, some 20 olfactory nerve (I) filaments on each side perforate the dura and arachnoid over the cribriform plate and pass superiorly through the subarachnoid space to enter the olfactory bulb (**18**). From here, the olfactory tract passes posteriorly on the inferior surface of the frontal lobe. Fractures crossing the anterior cranial fossa, with tearing of the overlying dura, may result in cerebrospinal rhinnorrhoea; watery fluid draining into the nose. Untreated, this communication between the nasal cavity and the subarachnoid space inevitably results in meningitis.

The maxillary sinus, or antrum (**52**), occupying most of the body of the maxilla, is the largest of the nasal accessory sinuses. In dentulous subjects, conical elevations, which correspond to the roots of the first and second molar teeth project into the floor of the sinus, which they occasionally perforate. Less commonly, the roots of the two pre-molars, the third molar and, rarely, the canine may also project into the sinus. Upper dental infection may thus involve the sinus and dental extraction may result in an oro-maxillary fistula. The sinus opens into the nasal cavity in the lowest part of the hiatus semilunaris below the middle concha (**51**). A second orifice is often present in or just below the hiatus.

CT in the coronal plane is used to demonstrate the anatomy of the maxillary sinus and its drainage into the nasal cavity. Some ENT surgeons now perform FESS (flexible endoscopic sinus surgery) to improve matters. This CT projection is also useful for assessing fractures of the floor of the orbit (blow-out fracture – see notes (**54**), section 13, page 74).

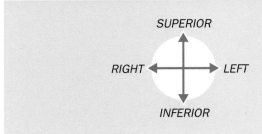

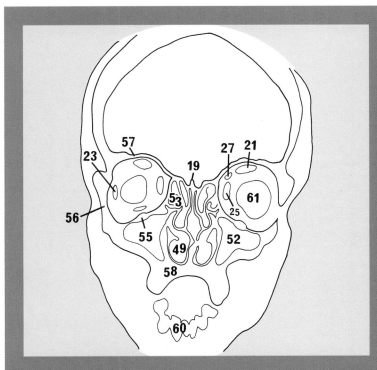

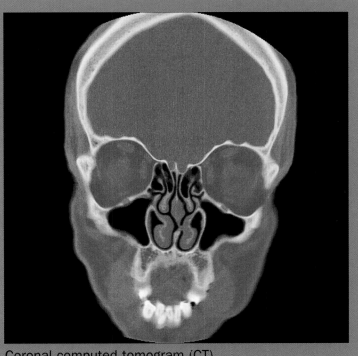

Coronal computed tomogram (CT)

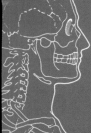

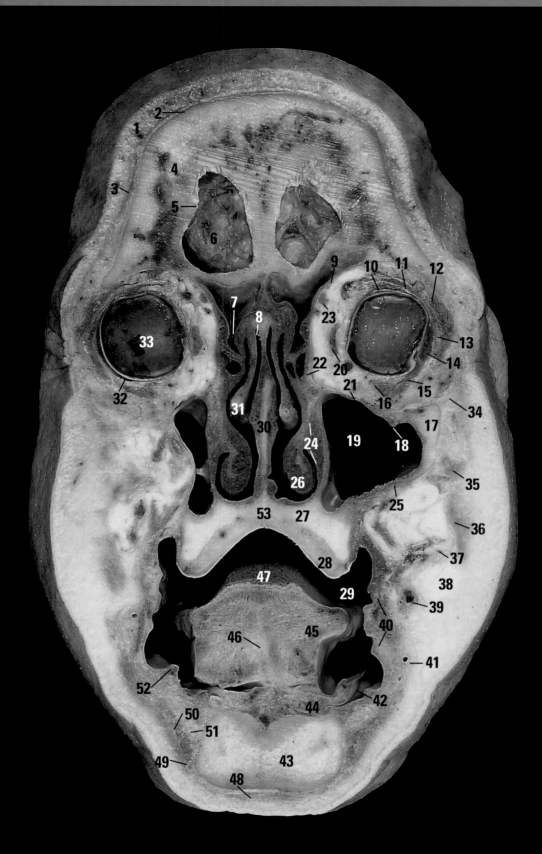

1	Skin and dense subcutaneous tissue
2	Epicranial aponeurosis (galea aponeurotica)
3	Occipital belly of occipitofrontalis
4	Frontal bone
5	Dura mater
6	Frontal lobe of brain covered with arachnoid mater and blood vessels within the anterior cranial fossa
7	Infundibulum draining frontal sinus
8	Roof of nasal cavity
9	Orbital part of frontal bone
10	Superior rectus
11	Levator palpebrae superioris
12	Lacrimal gland (orbital part)
13	Lacrimal gland (palpebral part)
14	Lateral rectus
15	Inferior oblique
16	Inferior rectus
17	Orbital margin of zygomatic bone
18	Infra-orbital artery and nerve within infra-orbital canal of maxilla
19	Maxillary sinus
20	Medial rectus
21	Orbital surface of maxilla
22	Lacrimal bone
23	Tendon of superior oblique
24	Nasolacrimal duct
25	Maxilla
26	Inferior nasal concha
27	Palatine process of maxilla
28	Alveolar process of maxilla
29	Vestibule of mouth
30	Nasal septum
31	Middle nasal concha
32	Scleral layer of orbit
33	Vitreous humour
34	Orbicularis oculi
35	Zygomaticus minor
36	Zygomaticus major
37	Parotid duct
38	Buccal fat pad
39	Facial vein
40	Buccinator
41	Facial artery
42	Mucous membrane of mouth
43	Mandible
44	Sublingual gland
45	Genioglossus
46	Median septum of tongue
47	Dorsum of tongue
48	Platysma
49	Depressor anguli oris
50	Depressor labii inferioris
51	Mental nerve
52	Sublingual papilla
53	Hard palate
54	Orbital margin of ethmoid bone
55	Crista galli of ethmoid bone

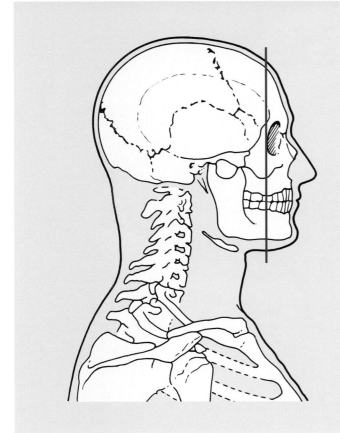

Section level

Orientation guide

SUPERIOR

RIGHT — LEFT

INFERIOR

Notes

The orbital part of the lacrimal gland (**12**) lies in the lacrimal fossa on the lateral part of the roof of the orbit supported by the lateral margin of levator palpebrae superioris (**11**). It projects around the lateral margin of this muscle and turns forward to form the palpebral part of the gland (**13**), which is visible through the superior fornix of the conjunctiva. Its dozen or so ducts drain into the superior fornix.

The nasolacrimal duct (**24**), about 2 cm in length, runs downwards and laterally to open into the inferior meatus below the inferior nasal concha (**26**) about 2 cm behind the nostril. Its mucosa is raised into several folds, which act as valves. These prevent air or nasal mucus being forced up the duct into the lacrimal sac on blowing the nose.

The buccal pad of fat (**38**) protrudes anterior to masseter to lie on buccinator (**40**) immediately inferior to the parotid duct (**37**). It is well developed in babies, where it forms a prominent elevation over the external surface of the face (the sucking pad). This helps to prevent collapse of the cheeks in vigorous sucking. It persists through life and is relatively 'protected' in that it does not decrease much even in emaciated subjects.

Note the paper thin (lamina papyricea) (**54**) orbital margin of the ethmoid bone. This portion and the relatively thin orbital margin of maxilla are liable to be damaged by a 'blow out' injury; the globe being tougher than bone, transmits trauma to the walls of the orbit; the squash ball is a particular culprit; the exstrinsic eye muscles may get trapped between the fracture margins.

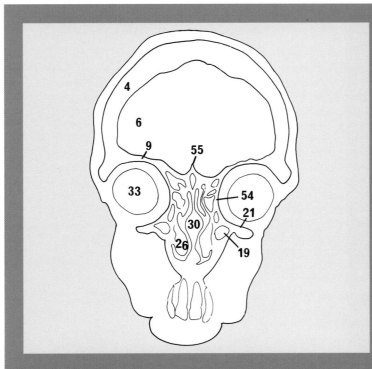

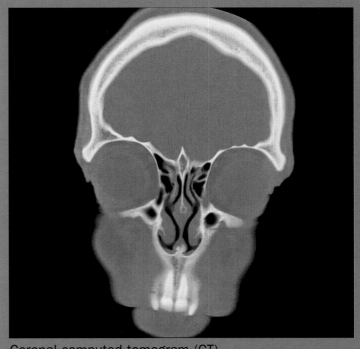

Coronal computed tomogram (CT)

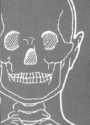

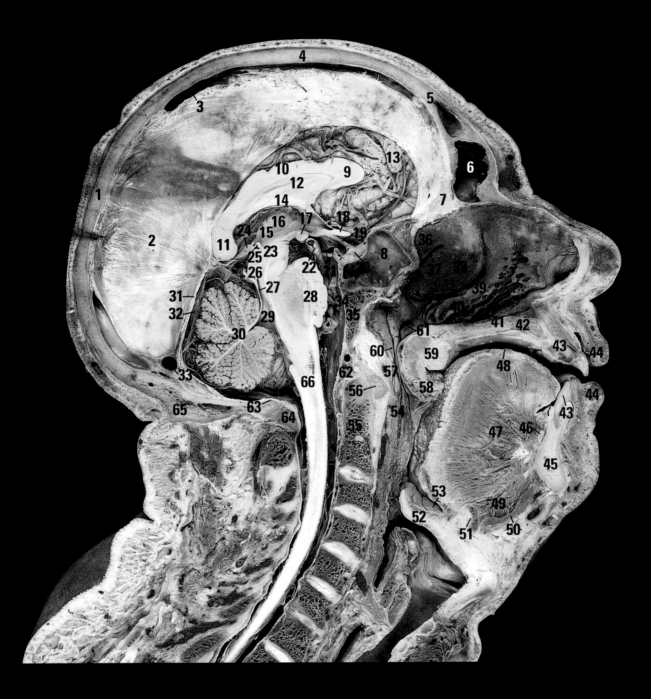

1 Occipital bone	**21** Oculomotor nerve (III)	**39** Middle meatus	**56** Anterior arch of atlas
2 Falx cerebri	**22** Posterior cerebral artery	**40** Inferior nasal concha	(first cervical vertebra)
3 Superior sagittal sinus	**23** Midbrain	**41** Inferior meatus	**57** Nasal part of pharynx
4 Parietal bone	**24** Pineal body	**42** Hard palate	(nasopharynx)
5 Frontal bone	**25** Superior colliculus	**43** Central incisor	**58** Uvula
6 Frontal sinus	**26** Inferior colliculus	(upper and lower)	**59** Soft palate
7 Crista galli of ethmoid bone	**27** Aqueduct (of Sylvius)	**44** Lip (upper and lower)	**60** Pharyngeal recess
8 Sphenoid sinus	connecting third and	**45** Body of mandible	**61** Opening of auditory
9 Genu of corpus callosum	fourth ventricles	**46** Sublingual gland	(Eustachian) tube
10 Body of corpus callosum	**28** Pons	**47** Genioglossus	**62** Anterior margin
11 Splenium of corpus	**29** Fourth ventricle	**48** Dorsum of tongue	of foramen magnum
callosum	**30** Cerebellum	**49** Geniohyoid	**63** Posterior margin
12 Septum pellucidum	**31** Tentorium cerebelli	**50** Mylohyoid	of foramen magnum
13 Anterior lobe gyrus	**32** Straight sinus	**51** Body of hyoid bone	**64** Posterior arch of atlas
14 Body of fornix	**33** Transverse sinus	**52** Epiglottis	**65** External occipital
15 Third ventricle	**34** Basilar artery	**53** Vallecula	protuberance
16 Hypothalamus	**35** Clivus (basioccipital and	**54** Oral part of pharynx	**66** Medulla oblongata
17 Mamillary body	basisphenoid bones)	(oropharynx)	
18 Optic chiasm	**36** Superior nasal concha	**55** Dens of axis (odontoid	**67** Lateral ventricle
19 Pituitary stalk	**37** Superior meatus	peg of second cervical	
20 Pituitary gland	**38** Middle nasal concha	vertebra)	

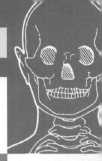

Section level

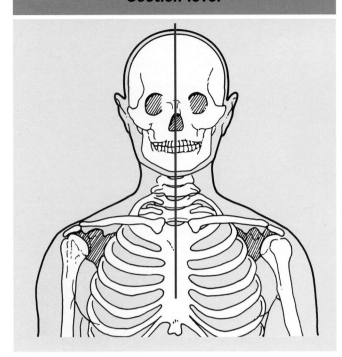

Orientation guide

SUPERIOR

POSTERIOR ←→ ANTERIOR

INFERIOR

Notes

Note that the nasal septum has been removed from this section in order to display the nasal conchae on the lateral wall.

The roof of the hard palate (**42**) lies at the level of the atlas (first cervical vertebra). Note that a clear AP view of the dens of the axis (second cervical vertebra) can be obtained on radiological examination by asking the patient to open the mouth widely.

This section illustrates the approach to the pituitary gland (**20**) via the transnasal trans-sphenoidal sinus (**8**) route at firbreoptic endoscopic surgery.

The frontal sinuses (**6**) vary considerably in size and are rarely symmetrical, the septum between the two usually being deviated to one or the other side. Each may be further divided by incomplete bony septa. One or both may occasionally be absent. (See notes (**21**), Coronal head section 10, page 68.)

These two sagittal T1 weighted MR images (a and b) are very close to the median sagittal plane. Indeed image (a) is so midline that the falx cerebri has been traversed. Image (b) is minimally lateral to the median sagittal plane and thus cerebral gyri and sulci are visible. The anatomy of the cerebral aqueduct and fourth ventricle is well demonstrated. So too is the important close relationship of the pituitary gland to the optic chiasm.

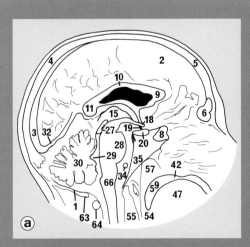

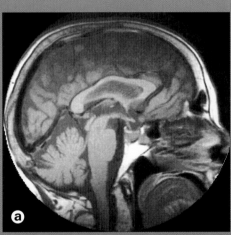

Sagittal magnetic resonance image (MRI)

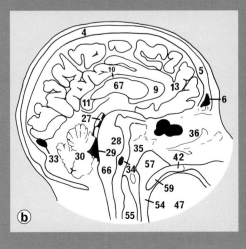

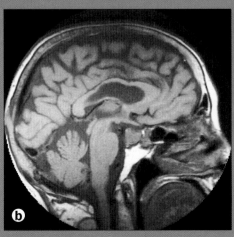

Sagittal magnetic resonance image (MRI)

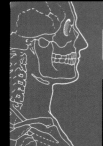

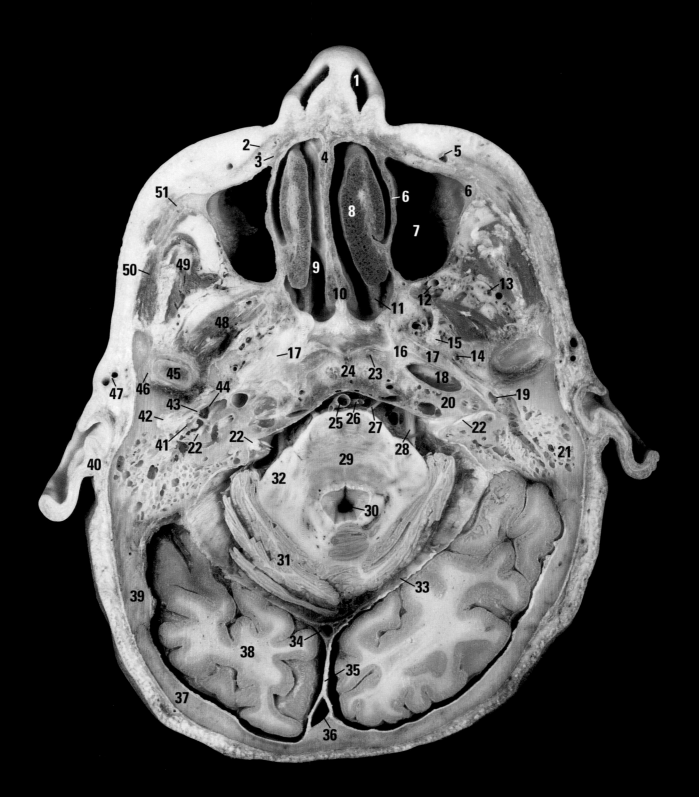

1 Vestibule of nose
2 Levator labii superioris alaeque nasi
3 Levator labii superioris
4 Cartilage of nasal septum
5 Facial vein
6 Maxilla
7 Maxillary sinus (antrum of Highmore)
8 Inferior nasal concha
9 Middle meatus
10 Vomer
11 Middle nasal concha
12 Maxillary artery
13 Pterygoid branch of maxillary artery
14 Middle meningeal artery
15 Mandibular nerve (V^{iii})

16 Greater wing of sphenoid
17 Cartilaginous roof of auditory (Eustachian) tube
18 Internal carotid artery
19 Junction of internal auditory tube and tympanic cavity
20 Petrous temporal bone
21 Mastoid air cells
22 Facial nerve (VII)
23 Longus capitis
24 Body of sphenoid
25 Basilar artery
26 Anterior inferior cerebellar artery
27 Abducent nerve (VI)
28 Trigeminal nerve (V)
29 Pons cerebri

30 Fourth ventricle
31 Cerebellum
32 Middle cerebellar peduncle
33 Tentorium cerebelli
34 Straight sinus
35 Falx cerebri
36 Superior sagittal sinus
37 Occipital bone (squamous part)
38 Occipital lobe of cerebrum
39 Squamous part of temporal bone
40 Pinna of ear
41 Malleus and incus
42 External auditory meatus
43 Tympanic membrane
44 Cavity of middle ear

45 Head of mandible
46 Temporomandibular joint
47 Superficial temporal artery and vein
48 Lateral pterygoid
49 Temporalis and tendon
50 Masseter
51 Zygomatic process of maxilla

52 Internal jugular vein (at origin)
53 Occipital bone (basilar part)
54 Postnasal space
55 Coronoid process of mandible
56 Medulla oblongata

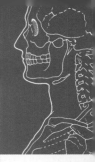

Section level

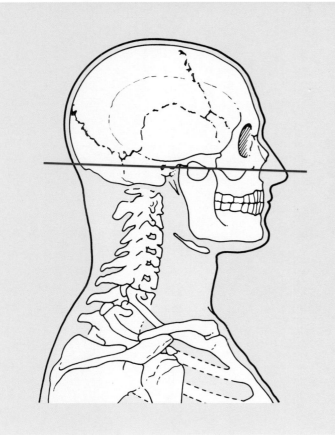

Orientation guide

ANTERIOR

RIGHT ←→ LEFT

POSTERIOR

Notes

This section passes through the vestibule of the nose (**1**), the inferior nasal concha (**8**), the temporo-mandibular joint (**46**), the pons (**29**) and the occipital lobe of the cerebrum (**38**).

The angulation of this MR image does not tally exactly with this section; some of the anatomical features of the neck on this and subsequent sections are therefore better seen on other images.

The maxillary sinus (the antrum of Highmore) within the maxilla (**7**) is well demonstrated. Its orifice lies at a more superior plane and drains into the middle meatus (**9**) inferior to the bulla ethmoidalis. The fact that the opening of this antrum is situated at this high level accounts for the poor drainage and consequent frequency of infection.

Note that the lateral pterygoid muscle (**48**) inserts not only into a depression on the front of the neck of the mandible, but also into the articular capsule of the temporomandibular joint (**46**) and also its articular disc.

The postnasal space (**54**) lies between the nasopharynx and the basi-occiput (**53**) together with the anterior arch of the atlas. As well as containing the prevertebral muscles, this space also contians variable quanities of lymphoid tissue (the pharyngeal tonsil, or adenoids). The size of the space is readily assessed on a lateral radiograph of the region. It is usually very narrow in adults (see section 4, page 83), but can be very prominent in young children, whose adenoids are often very large.

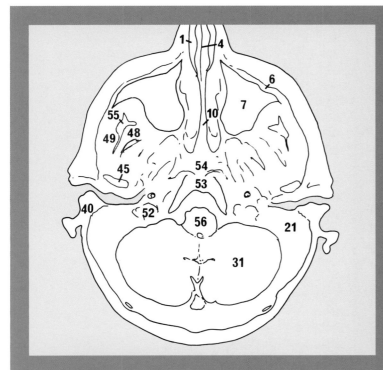

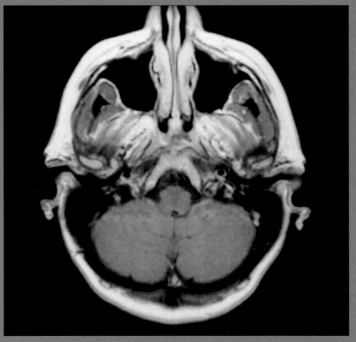

Axial magnetic resonance image (MRI)

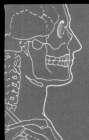

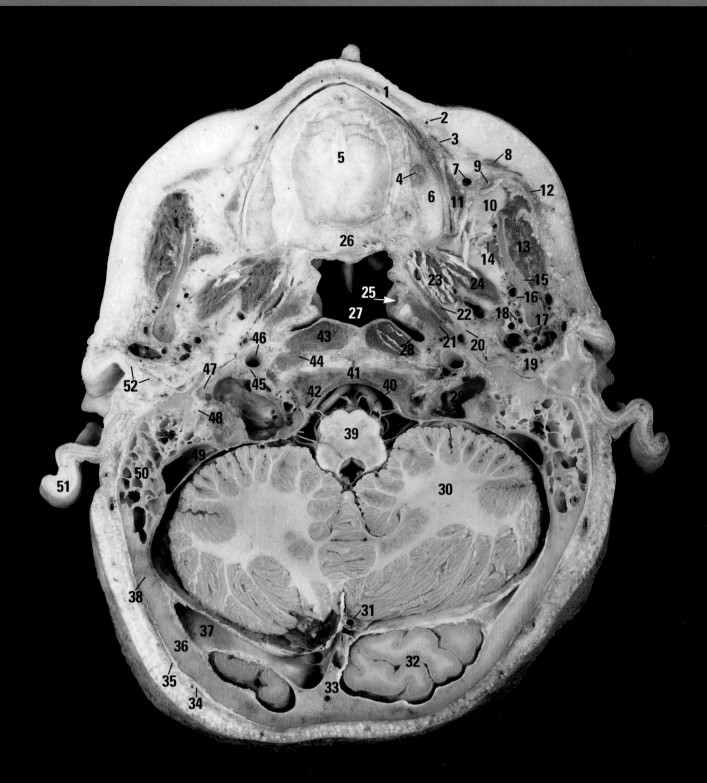

1 Orbicularis oris
2 Facial artery
3 Levator labii superioris
4 Mucosa of maxillary antrum
5 Hard palate
6 Alveolar process of maxilla
7 Facial vein
8 Zygomaticus major
9 Parotid duct
10 Buccal fat pad
11 Buccinator
12 Accessory parotid gland
13 Masseter
14 Temporalis and tendon
15 Ramus of mandible
16 Inferior alveolar artery and vein
17 Superficial temporal artery and vein

18 Maxillary artery and vein
19 Parotid gland
20 Lingual nerve, inferior alveolar nerve and nerve to mylohyoid (V^iii)
21 Levator veli palatini
22 Tensor veli palatini
23 Medial pterygoid
24 Lateral pterygoid
25 Orifice of auditory tube (Eustachian tube) arrowed
26 Soft palate
27 Nasopharynx
28 Pharyngeal recess (fossa of Rosenmuller)
29 Internal jugular vein at origin
30 Cerebellum

31 Straight sinus at junction of tentorium cerebelli, falx cerebri and falx cerebelli
32 Occipital lobe of cerebrum
33 Internal occipital crest
34 Occipital artery and vein
35 Occipitofrontalis
36 Squamous part of occipital bone
37 Transverse sinus
38 Occipitomastoid suture
39 Medulla oblongata
40 Vertebral artery
41 Clivus of the basilar part of the occipital bone
42 Hypoglossal nerve (XII)
43 Longus capitis

44 Rectus capitis anterior
45 Glossopharyngeal nerve (IX), vagus nerve (X) and accessory nerve (XI)
46 Internal carotid artery
47 Styloid process
48 Facial nerve (VII)
49 Sigmoid sinus
50 Mastoid air cells of the temporal bone
51 Pinna of ear
52 Cartilage of external auditory meatus

53 Tonsil of cerebellum
54 Occipital bone (condyle)

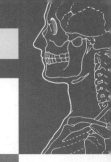

Section level

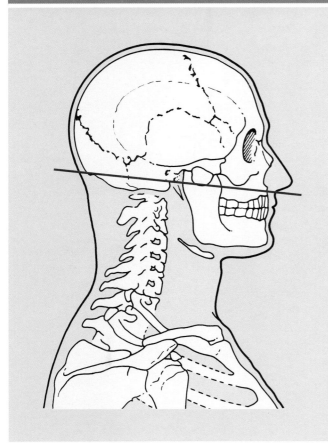

Orientation guide

ANTERIOR

RIGHT ←→ LEFT

POSTERIOR

Notes

This section passes through the alveolar process of the maxilla (**6**) to reveal the hard palate (**5**) in its entirety. It then traverses the upper part of the ramus of the mandible (**15**), the mastoid air cells (**50**), the medulla oblongata (**39**), cerebellum (**30**) and the posterior tip of the occipital lobe (**32**).

The floor of the maxillary sinus is formed by the alveolar process of the maxilla; several conical elevations, corresponding to the roots of the first and second molar teeth, project into the floor. An example of this is demonstrated here (**4**). Indeed, the floor is sometimes perforated by one or more of these molar roots.

This section gives a good view of the parotid duct (**9**) as it arches medially to penetrate buccinator (**11**) and to enter the mouth at the level of the second upper molar tooth. The parotid duct is accompanied by a small, more or less detached, part of the gland which lies above the duct as it crosses masseter; this is named the accessory part of the gland (**12**).

This section passes through the junctional zone between the falx cerebri, separating the occipital lobes of the brain (**32**), the falx cerebelli, separating the lobes of the cerebellum (**30**) and the tentorium cerebelli, which roofs the cerebellum. The straight sinus (**31**) is seen in section as it lies in the line of junction of the falx cerebri and tentorium cerebelli. The transverse sinus (**37**) lies in the attached margin of the tentorium cerebelli.

The facial nerve (within the stylomastoid foramen) is well demonstrated (**48**) in its immediate lateral relationship to the root of the styloid process (**47**).

Note that the orifice of the auditory tube (**25**) lies anterior to a depression – the pharyngeal recess (**28**). This helps to keep the orifice of the tube clear of secretions in the supine position.

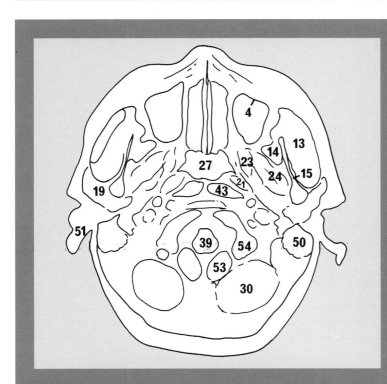

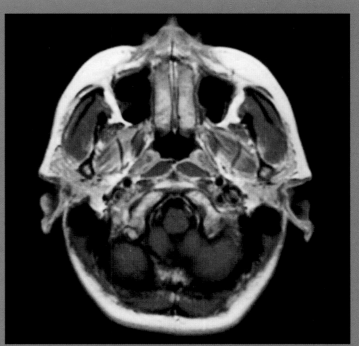

Axial magnetic resonance image (MRI)

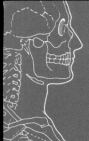

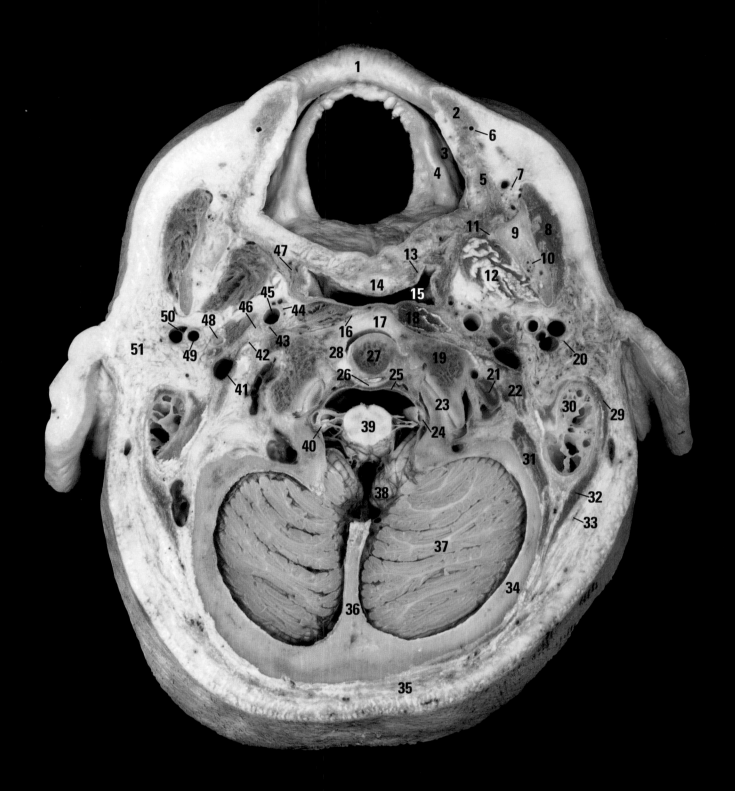

1 Upper lip	**17** Anterior arch of atlas	**28** Atlanto-axial joint	**41** Internal jugular vein
2 Orbicularis oris	(first cervical vertebra)	**29** Sternocleidomastoid	**42** Accessory nerve (XI)
3 Vestibule of mouth	**18** Longus capitis	**30** Mastoid air cells of	and hypoglossal nerve
4 Alveolus	**19** Lateral mass of atlas	temporal bone	(XII)
5 Buccinator	(first cervical vertebra)	**31** Posterior belly of	**43** Vagus nerve (X)
6 Superior labial artery	**20** Facial nerve (VII)	digastric	**44** Sympathetic chain
7 Facial artery and vein	**21** Roof of third part of	**32** Longissimus capitis	**45** Internal carotid artery
8 Masseter	vertebral artery	**33** Splenius capitis	**46** Glossopharyngeal
9 Ramus of mandible	**22** Rectus capitis lateralis	**34** Squamous part of	nerve (IX)
10 Inferior alveolar artery	**23** Atlanto-occipital joint	occipital bone	**47** Superior constrictor
vein and nerve (V^{iii})	**24** Fourth part of vertebral	**35** Trapezius	muscle of pharynx
within mandibular canal	artery	**36** Internal occipital crest	**48** Styloid process
11 Lingual nerve (V^{iii})	**25** Membrana tectoria	of occipital bone	**49** External carotid artery
12 Medial pterygoid	**26** Superior longitudinal	**37** Hemisphere of	**50** Retromandibular vein
13 Tensor veli palatini	band of cruciform	cerebellum	at bifurcation
14 Soft palate	ligament	**38** Tonsil of cerebellum	**51** Parotid gland
15 Nasopharynx	**27** Dens of axis (odontoid	**39** Spinal cord	
16 Anterior atlanto-	process of second	**40** Spinal root of	
occipital membrane	cervical vertebra)	accessory nerve	

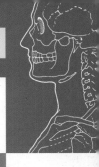

Section level

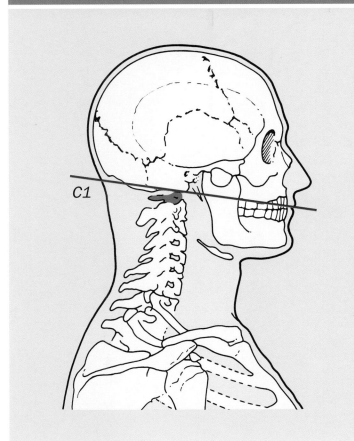

Orientation guide

ANTERIOR

RIGHT ←→ LEFT

POSTERIOR

Notes

This section passes through the mouth at the level of the upper alveolus (**4**), the dens of the axis (**27**) at the articulation (**28**) with the anterior arch of the atlas (**17**) and posteriorly traverses the internal occipital crest of the occipital bone (**36**).

The third part of the vertebral artery (**21**) can be seen as it curves posterior to the lateral mass of the atlas (**19**) as it ascends to enter the vertebral canal by passing below the lower border of the posterior atlanto-occipital membrane. The fourth part (**24**) ascends anterior to the roots of the hypoglossal nerve.

Note how the last four cranial nerves (**42**, **43**, **46**) lie 'line astern' between the internal carotid artery (**45**) and the internal jugular vein (**41**) at the base of the skull.

The retromandibular vein (**50**) sperates the parotid gland (**51**) into a superficial and deep lobe; it also demarcates the plane through which the facial nerve (**20**) and branches run.

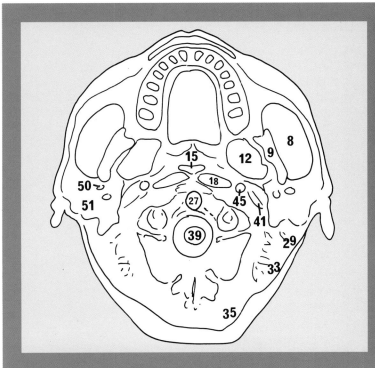

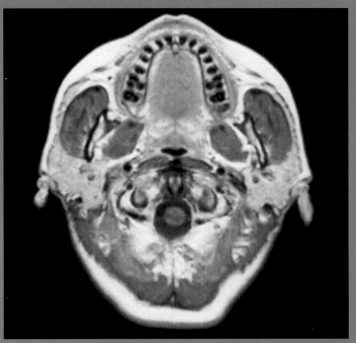

Axial magnetic resonance image (MRI)

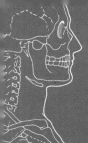

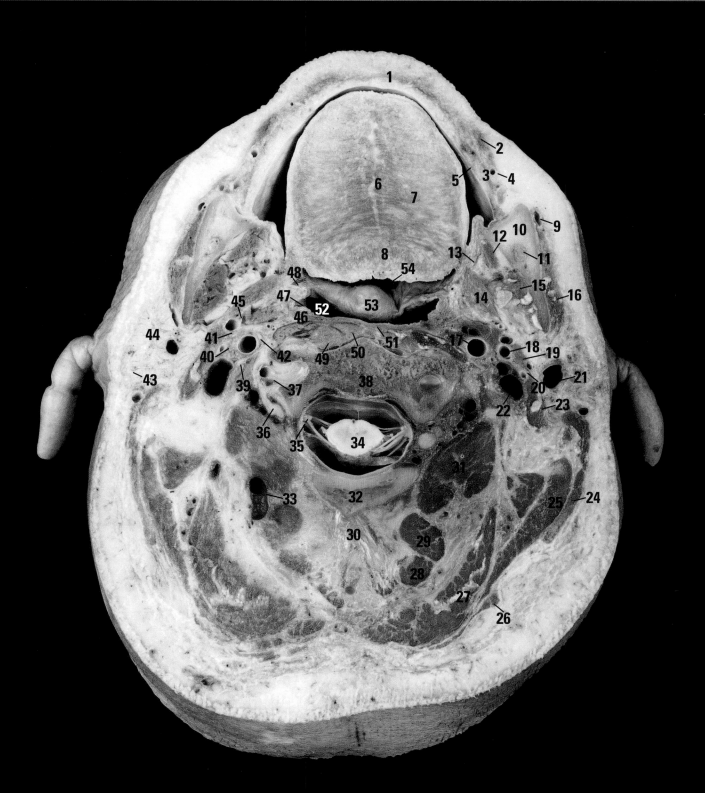

1 Orbicularis oris in lower lip	**14** Styloglossus	**30** Ligamentum nuchae	**41** Hypoglossal nerve (XII)
2 Depressor anguli oris	**15** Medial pterygoid	**31** Obliquus capitis inferior	**42** Vagus nerve (X)
3 Buccinator	**16** Masseter	**32** Posterior arch of atlas (first cervical vertebra)	**43** Facial nerve (VII)
4 Anterior facial artery	**17** Internal carotid artery		**44** Parotid gland
5 Mucosa of lower lip	**18** External carotid artery	**33** Occipital vein	**45** Glossopharyngeal nerve (IX)
6 Median raphe of tongue	**19** Stylohyoid	**34** Spinal cord within dural sheath	**46** Palatopharyngeus
7 Intrinsic transverse muscle of tongue	**20** Posterior auricular artery and vein	**35** Dorsal root ganglion of second cervical nerve	**47** Tonsillar fossa
8 Intrinsic superior longitudinal muscle of tongue	**21** External jugular vein	**36** Anterior primary ramus of second cervical nerve	**48** Palatoglossus
	22 Internal jugular vein		**49** Longus capitis
	23 Posterior belly of digastric		**50** Longus colli
9 Facial vein	**24** Sternocleidomastoid	**37** Vertebral artery and vein within foramen transversarium	**51** Superior constrictor muscle of pharynx
10 Ramus of mandible	**25** Splenius capitis		**52** Nasopharynx
11 Inferior alveolar artery vein and nerve (V^{iii}) within the mandibular canal	**26** Trapezius	**38** Body of axis (second cervical vertebra)	**53** Uvula
	27 Semispinalis capitis		**54** Oropharynx
	28 Rectus capitis posterior minor	**39** Sympathetic chain	
12 Mylohyoid	**29** Rectus capitis posterior major	**40** Accessory nerve (XI)	**55** Retromandibular vein
13 Lingual nerve (V^{iii})			

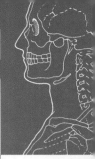

Section level

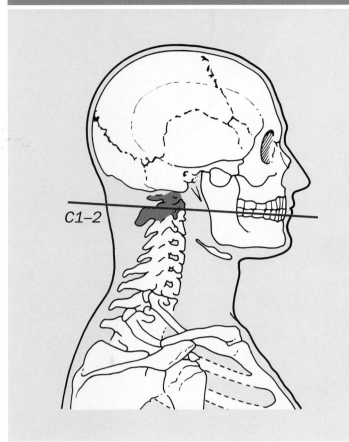

C1–2

Orientation guide

ANTERIOR

RIGHT ←→ LEFT

POSTERIOR

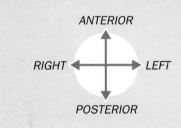

Notes

This section passes through the tongue (**6**) and the body of the axis, the second cervical vertebra (**38**). This section gives a useful appreciation of the inferior alveolar nerve and its accompanying vessels within the mandibular canal (**11**). Note also the vertebral artery in its second part, together with its accompanying vein, within the foramen transversarium (**37**). The further course of this artery, in its third and fourth part, can be seen in section 3.

Note how close the posterior wall of the nasopharynx (**52**) lies to the body of the axis (**38**) – and also to the anterior arch of the atlas in the previous section. The prevertebral space is thus normally very narrow on a lateral radiograph of the adult cervical spine (see section 1, page 77).

This MR image shows the parotid gland (**44**) very well. Note again how the retromandibular vein (**55**) separates the gland into superficial and deep portions.

The medial pterygoids are shown to good effect. The fat lying medially to these muscles in the parapharyngeal space shows up well on both MR and CT imaging. Loss of this fat plane is an important sign when assessing the extent of tumours in this region.

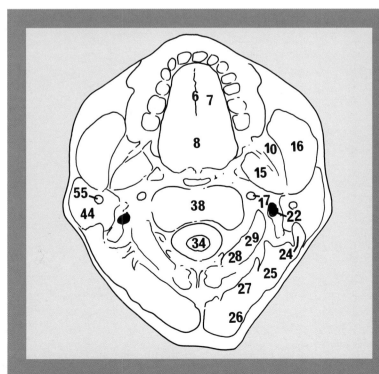

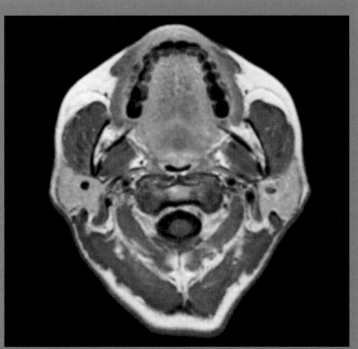

Axial magnetic resonance image (MRI)

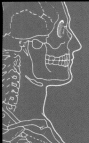

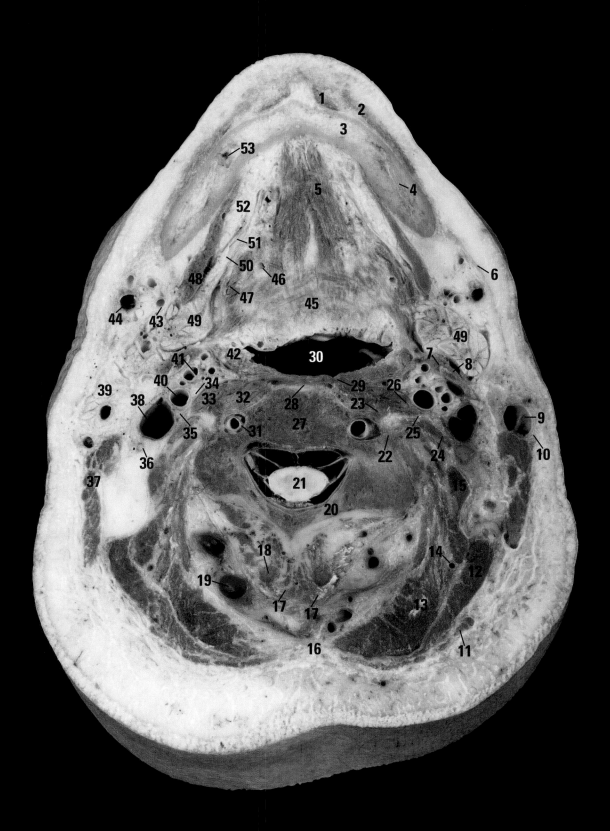

1 Mentalis	**17** Bifid spine of third	**27** Body of third cervical	**40** Internal carotid artery
2 Orbicularis oris	cervical vertebra	vertebra	**41** External carotid artery
3 Mandible	**18** Semispinalis cervicis	**28** Anterior longitudinal	**42** Palatine tonsil
4 Inferior alveolar	**19** Occipital vein	ligament	**43** Facial artery
nerve (V^{iii})	**20** Lamina of third cervical	**29** Superior constrictor	**44** Facial vein
5 Genioglossus	vertebra	muscle of pharynx	**45** Intrinsic transverse
6 Platysma	**21** Spinal cord within	**30** Oropharynx	muscle of tongue
7 Posterior belly of	dural sheath	**31** Vertebral artery and	**46** Lingual artery
digastric	**22** Posterior tubercle of	vein within foramen	**47** Hyoglossus
8 Stylohyoid ligament	transverse process of	transversarium	**48** Mylohyoid
9 External jugular vein	third cervical Vertebra	**32** Longus colli	**49** Submandibular gland
10 Great auricular nerve	**23** Anterior tubercle of	**33** Longus capitis	**50** Lingual nerve (V^{iii})
11 Trapezius	transverse process of	**34** Vagus nerve (X)	**51** Submandibular duct
12 Splenius	third cervical vertebra	**35** Sympathetic chain	**52** Sublingual gland
13 Semispinalis capitis	**24** Scalenus medius	**36** Accessory nerve (XI)	**53** Inferior alveolar artery,
14 Occipital artery	**25** Anterior primary ramus	**37** Sternocleidomastoid	vein and nerve within
15 Levator scapulae	of third cervical nerve	**38** Internal jugular vein	mandibular canal
16 Ligamentum nuchae	**26** Scalenus anterior	**39** Parotid gland	**54** Hyoid

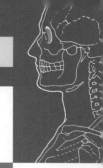

Section level

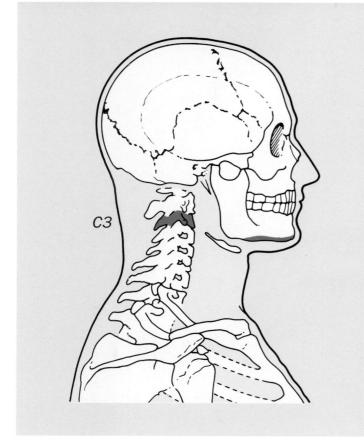

C3

Notes

This section passes through the lower border of the body of the mandible (**3**) the oropharynx (**30**) and the third cervical vertebra (**27**).

It demonstrates how the parotid gland (**39**) projects deeply towards the side wall of the oropharynx (**30**). Indeed, a tumour of the deep portion of the gland may project into the tonsillar fossa and bulge the palatine tonsil (**42**) medially.

Orientation guide

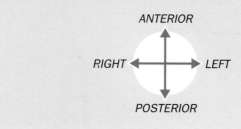

ANTERIOR

RIGHT ←→ LEFT

POSTERIOR

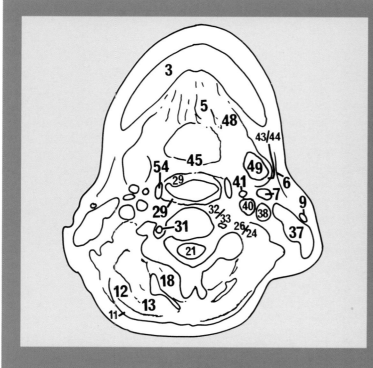

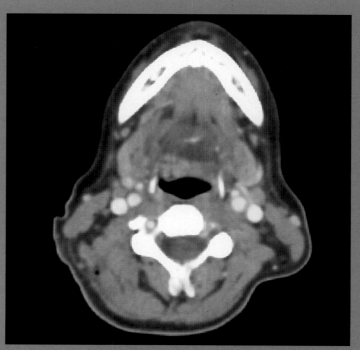

Axial computed tomogram (CT)

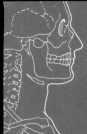

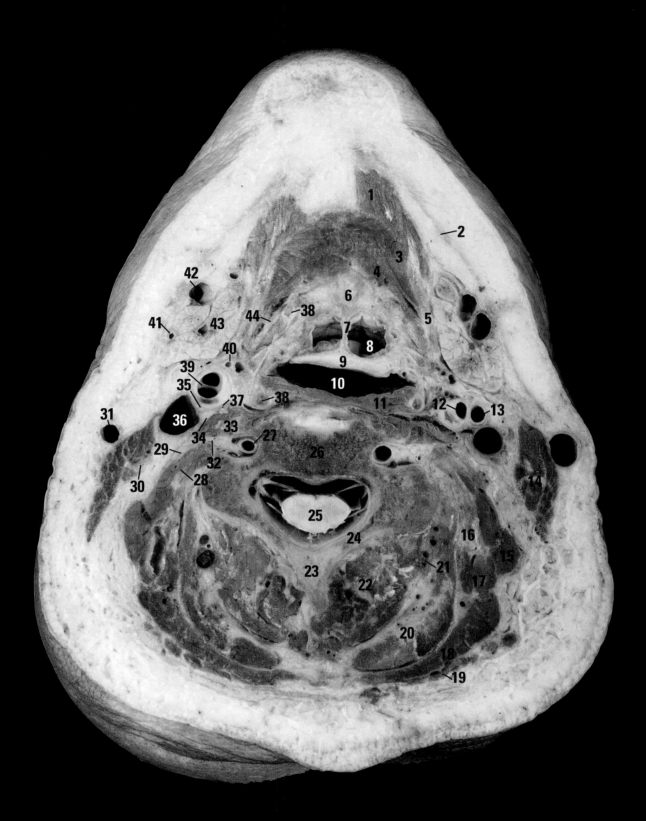

1 Anterior belly of digastric	**14** Sternocleidomastoid	**26** Body of fourth cervical vertebra	**38** Hyoid
2 Platysma	**15** Levator scapulae	**27** Vertebral artery and vein within foramen transversarium	**39** Right common carotid artery at bifurcation
3 Mylohyoid	**16** Longissimus capitis and cervicis		**40** Superior thyroid artery
4 Hyoglossus	**17** Splenius cervicis	**28** Scalenus medius	**41** Facial artery
5 Tendon of digastric	**18** Splenius capitis	**29** Anterior primary ramus of third cervical nerve	**42** Facial vein
6 Base of tongue	**19** Trapezius		**43** Submandibular salivary gland
7 Glosso-epiglottic fold	**20** Semispinalis capitis	**30** Accessory nerve (XI)	
8 Vallecula	**21** Deep cervical artery and vein	**31** External jugular vein	**44** Lingual artery
9 Epiglottis		**32** Anterior primary ramus fourth cervical nerve	
10 Laryngopharynx	**22** Semispinalis cervicis		**45** Mandible
11 Middle constrictor muscle of pharynx	**23** Spine of fourth cervical vertebra	**33** Scalenus anterior	**46** Common carotid artery
		34 Phrenic nerve	**47** Pre-epiglottic space
12 Left internal carotid artery	**24** Lamina of fourth cervical vertebra	**35** Vagus nerve (X)	**48** Superior cornu of thyroid cartilage
	25 Spinal cord within dural sheath	**36** Internal jugular vein	**49** Aryepiglottic fold
13 Left external carotid artery		**37** Sympathetic chain	**50** Piriform fossa

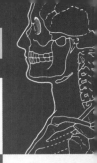

Section level

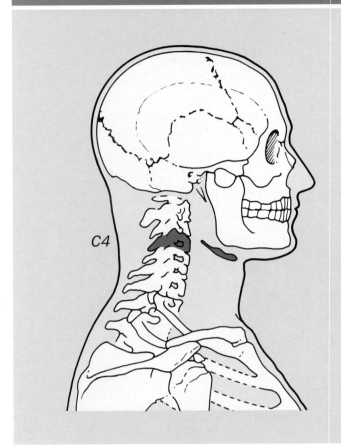

C4

Notes

This section passes through the body of the fourth cervical vertebra (**26**), just shaving the inferior margin of the hyoid bone (**38**).

The fourth cervical vertebra marks the level of bifurcation of the common carotid artery. On the right side, this is just occurring (**39**) and on the left it has already taken place (**12**, **13**). Note the marked atheromatous thickening of the internal carotid artery. On the CT image the plane passes through the common carotid arteries.

The way in which the lingual artery (**44**) passes deep to the hyoglossus muscle (**4**) to supply the tongue is demonstrated. On CT imaging, precise definition of the various intrinsic muscles of the tongue is difficult unless the fat planes are very pronounced.

The precise shape of the laryngopharynx (**10**), and indeed the whole airway system of the head and neck, depends on the phase of respiration, phonation etc. In practice, gentle inspiration is the most appropriate phase for routine CT imaging, but attempts at phonation and the Valsava manoeuvre may be helpful.

Orientation guide

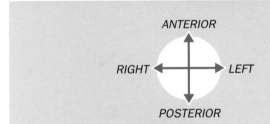

ANTERIOR

RIGHT   LEFT

POSTERIOR

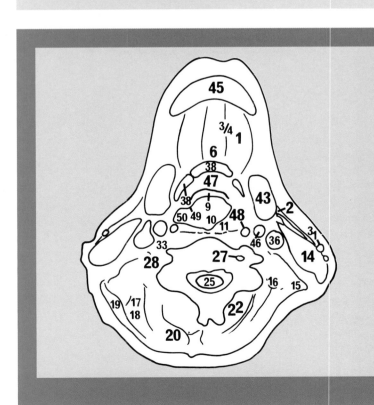

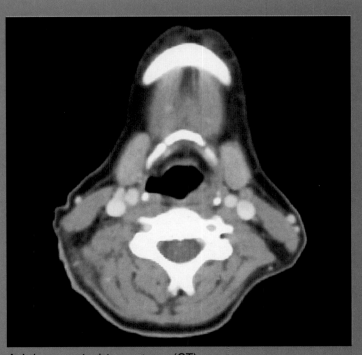

Axial computed tomogram (CT)

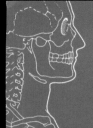

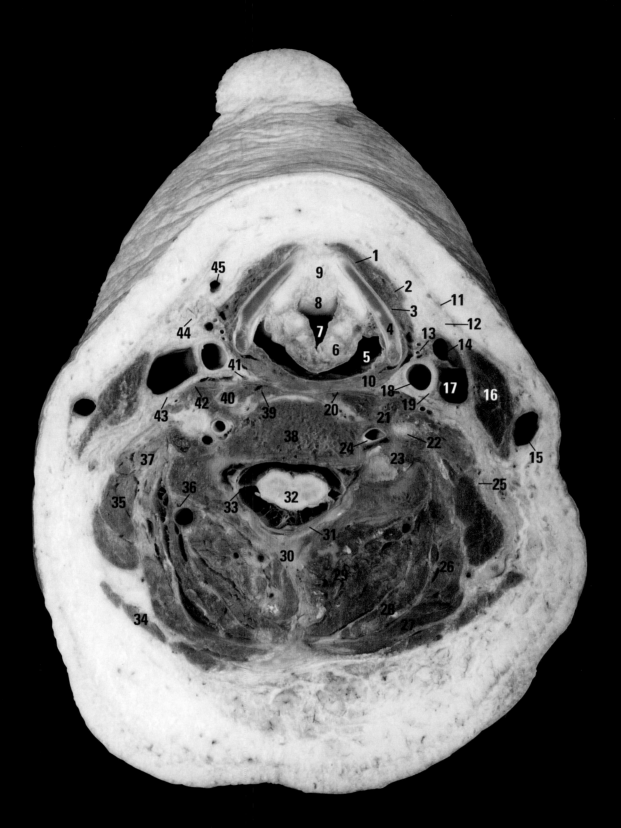

1 Sternohyoid	**15** External jugular vein	**28** Semispinalis capitis	**40** Longus capitis
2 Omohyoid	**16** Sternocleidomastoid	**29** Erector spinae	**41** Sympathetic chain
3 Thyrohyoid	**17** Internal jugular vein	**30** Spine of fifth cervical	**42** Scalenus anterior
4 Lamina of thyroid	**18** Common carotid artery	vertebra	**43** Phrenic nerve
cartilage	**19** Vagus nerve (X)	**31** Lamina of fifth cervical	**44** Submandibular salivary
5 Laryngopharynx	**20** Prevertebral fascia	vertebra	gland
6 Corniculate cartilage	**21** Anterior tubercle of	**32** Spinal cord within	**45** Anterior jugular vein
7 Vestibule of larynx	fifth cervical vertebra	dural sheath	
8 Epiglottis	**22** Ventral ramus of fifth	**33** Ligamentum	
8 Pre-epiglottic space	cervical nerve	denticulatum	**46** Inferior horn of thyroid
(fat filled)	**23** Posterior tubercle of	**34** Trapezius	cartilage
10 Inferior constrictor	fifth cervical vertebra	**35** Levator scapulae	**47** Arytenoid cartilage
muscle of pharynx	**24** Vertebral artery and	**36** Deep cervical artery	**48** Cricoid cartilage
11 Platysma	vein within foramen	and vein	**49** Vocal fold
12 Investing fascia of neck	transversarium	**37** Scalenus medius	**50** Anterior border of
13 Superior thyroid artery	**25** Accessory nerve (XI)	**38** Body of fifth cervical	thyroid cartilage
and vein	**26** Splenius cervicis	vertebra	
14 Common facial vein	**27** Splenius capitis	**39** Longus colli	

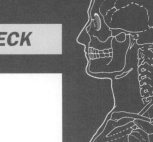

Section level

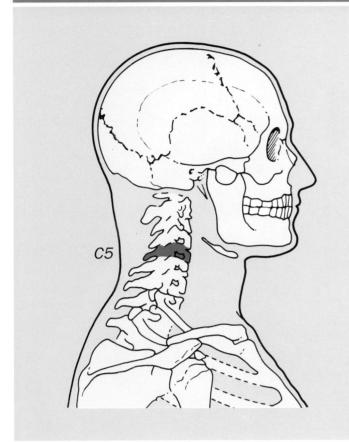

C5

Orientation guide

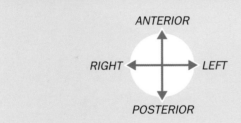

ANTERIOR

RIGHT ←→ LEFT

POSTERIOR

Notes

This section passes through the body of the fifth cervical vertebra (**38**) and the lamina of the thyroid cartilage (**4**).

The attachment of the stem of the cartilage of the epiglottis (**8**) to the angle formed by the two laminae of the thyroid cartilage (**4**) is demonstrated at this level.

This section gives an excellent demonstration of the ligamentum denticulatum (**33**). This is a narrow fibrous sheet situated on each side of the spinal cord. Its medial border is continuous with the pia mater at the side of the spinal cord while its lateral border presents a series of triangular tooth-like processes whose points are fixed at intervals to the dura mater. There are 21 such processes on each side, the last lies between the exits of the twelfth thoracic and first lumbar nerves.

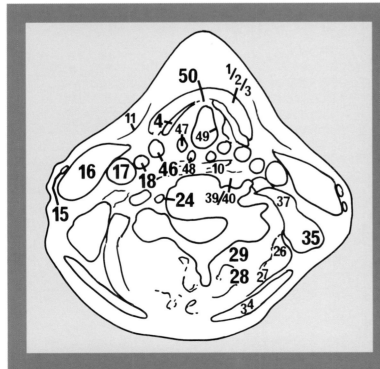

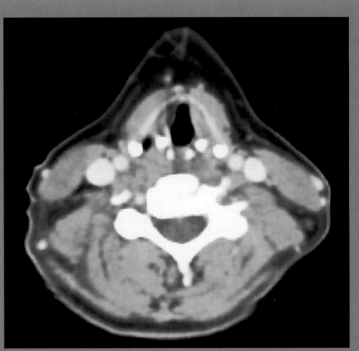

Axial computed tomogram (CT)

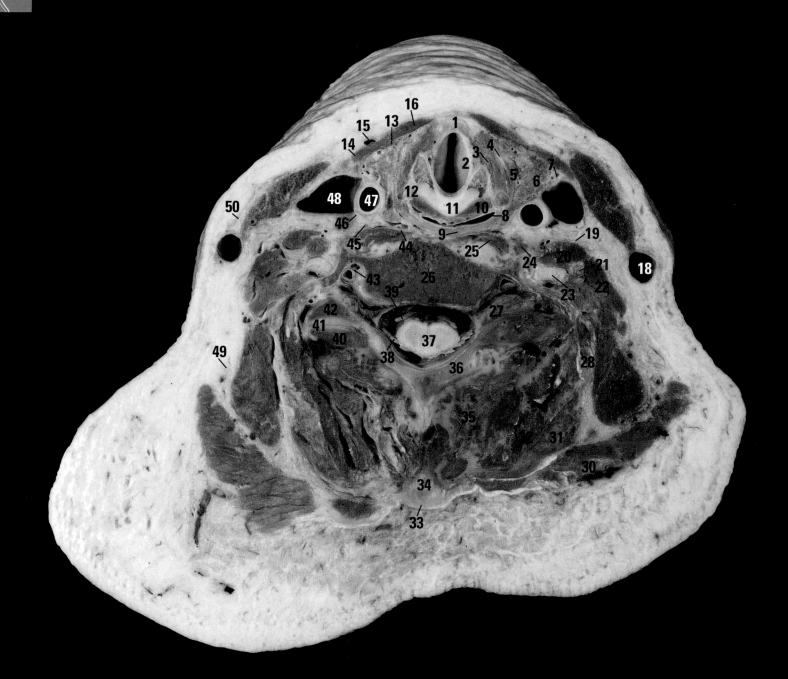

			seventh cervical
1 Anterior border of	**14** Omohyoid	**30** Trapezius	vertebrae
thyroid cartilage	**15** Anterior jugular vein	**31** Splenius capitis	**42** Superior articular facet
2 Vocal fold	**16** Sternohyoid	**32** Semispinalis	of seventh cervical
3 Lateral cricoarytenoid	**17** Sternocleidomastoid	**33** Ligamentum nuchae	vertebra
4 Lamina of thyroid	**18** External jugular vein	**34** Tip of spinous process	**43** Vertebral artery and
cartilage	**19** Phrenic nerve	of seventh cervical	vein within foramen
5 Cricothyroid	**20** Scalenus anterior	vertebra	transversarium
6 Lateral lobe of thyroid	**21** Ventral ramus of fifth	**35** Erector spinae	**44** Prevertebral fascia
gland	cervical nerve	**36** Lamina of sixth cervical	**45** Sympathetic trunk
7 Superior thyroid artery	**22** Scalenus medius	vertebra	**46** Vagus nerve (X)
and vein	**23** Ventral ramus of sixth	**37** Spinal cord within	**47** Common carotid artery
8 Laryngopharynx	cervical nerve	dural sheath	**48** Internal jugular vein
9 Inferior constrictor	**24** Longus capitis	**38** Dorsal nerve root of	**49** Accessory nerve (XI)
muscle of pharynx	**25** Longus colli	seventh cervical nerve	**50** Platysma
10 Posterior	**26** Body of sixth cervical	**39** Ventral nerve root of	
crico-arytenoid	vertebra	seventh cervical nerve	
11 Cricoid cartilage	**27** Dorsal root ganglion of	**40** Inferior articular facet of	**51** Outline of subglottic
12 Inferior cornu of	seventh cervical nerve	sixth cervical vertebra	space
thyroid cartilage	**28** Splenius cervicis	**41** Interarticular facet joint	
13 Sternothyroid	**29** Levator scapulae	between sixth and	

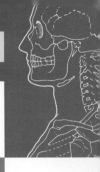

Section level

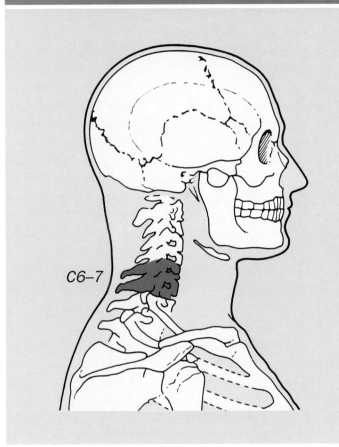

C6–7

Orientation guide

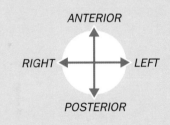

ANTERIOR

RIGHT ← → LEFT

POSTERIOR

Notes

This section passes through the body of the sixth cervical vertebra (**26**) and traverses the cricoid cartilage (**11**). The cricoid is the only complete ring of cartilage throughout the respiratory system, but the plane of this section is above the narrow arch of the cricoid and only passes through its posterior lamina.

This section, together with the following one, provides a good appreciation of the relationships of the lateral lobe of the thyroid gland (**6**). Here, it is seen to be overlapped superficially by the strap muscles – the sternohyoid (**16**), omohyoid (**14**) and, on a deeper plane, the sternothyroid (**13**). Medially, it lies against the larynx and laryngopharynx (**8**) and posteriorly it lies against the common carotid artery (**47**) and internal jugular vein (**48**). (See CT image section 9, page 94.)

Note the demonstration of the relationship of the phrenic nerve (**19**) to the anterior aspect of scalenus anterior (**20**). The nerve is bound down to the underlying muscle by the overlying prevertebral fascia (**44**).

The ventral rami (**21** and **23**) of C5 and 6 together with C7, C8 and T1, form the brachial plexus; those of C1–4 form the cervical plexus.

The inferior surfaces of the vocal folds (**2**) can be seen within the larynx (see CT image section 7, page 90). The vestibular folds (false cords), which lie cranial to the vestibule of the larynx, are situated more cranially to this section.

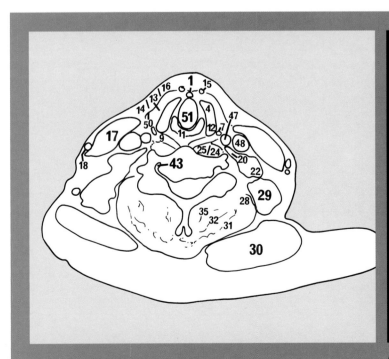

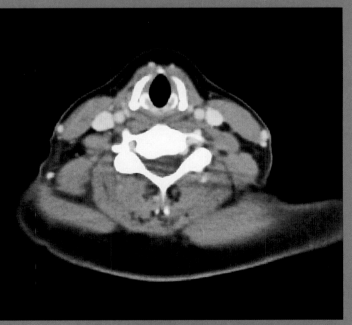

Axial computed tomogram (CT)

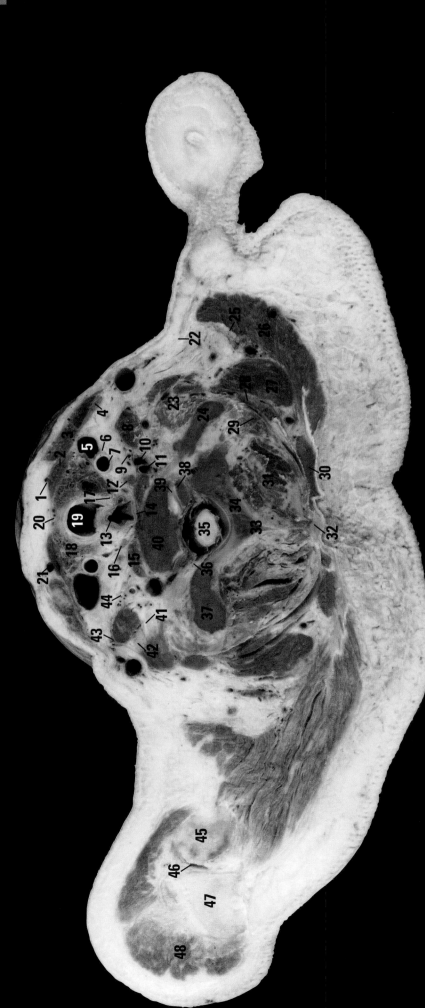

1 Sternohyoid
2 Sternothyroid
3 Sternocleidomastoid
4 Omohyoid
5 Internal jugular vein
6 Vagus nerve (X)
7 Common carotid artery
8 Scalenus anterior
9 Inferior thyroid artery
10 Vertebral vein
11 Vertebral artery
12 Deep cervical lymph node
13 Oesophagus
14 Prevertebral fascia
15 Longus colli
16 Parathyroid gland

17 Recurrent laryngeal nerve
18 Lateral lobe of thyroid gland
19 Trachea
20 Isthmus of thyroid gland
21 Anterior jugular vein
22 Investing (deep) fascia of the neck
23 Scalenus medius and posterior
24 Left first rib
25 Accessory nerve (XI)
26 Trapezius
27 Levator scapulae
28 Splenius
29 Semispinalis
30 Rhomboideus minor
31 Erector spinae

32 Ligamentum nuchae
33 Spinous process of first thoracic vertebra
34 Lamina of first thoracic vertebra
35 Spinal cord within dural sheath
36 Dorsal root ganglion of eighth cervical nerve
37 Transverse process of first thoracic vertebra
38 Part of body of first thoracic vertebra
39 Uncovertebral synovial joint between lip of T1 body and inferior aspect of C7
40 Body of seventh cervical vertebra

41 Ventral ramus of seventh cervical nerve
42 Ventral ramus of sixth cervical nerve
43 Phrenic nerve
44 Cervical sympathetic chain
45 Clavicle
46 Acromioclavicular joint
47 Acromion
48 Deltoid

49 External jugular vein

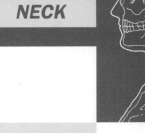

C7–T1

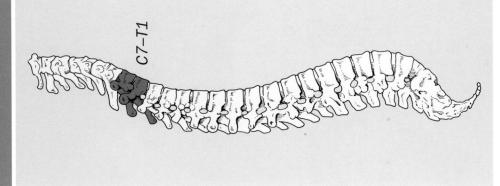

ANTERIOR

LEFT

RIGHT

POSTERIOR

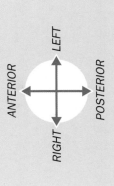

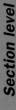

Axial computed tomogram (CT)

Notes

This section passes through the body of the seventh cervical vertebra (**40**) and through the tip of the shoulder, so that a sliver of the clavicle (**45**) and adjacent acromioclavicular joint (**46**) are shown.

Taken in conjunction with the previous section, the relationships of the lateral lobe of the thyroid gland (**18**) are demonstrated. In this section, it is overlapped by the strap muscles (**1**, **2**, **4**) and by sternocleidomastoid (**3**). Medially it lies against the trachea (**19**) and oesophagus (**13**), while posteriorly it rests against the common carotid artery (**7**) and internal jugular vein (**5**). The inferior thyroid artery (**9**) passes transversely behind the common carotid artery

to reach the thyroid gland. Note also the important posterior relationship of the lobe of the thyroid gland to the recurrent laryngeal nerve (**17**), lying in the tracheo-oesophageal groove.

The parathyroid glands (**16**) are usually four in number but vary from two to six. The superior glands are fairly constant in position, at the middle of the posterior border of the thyroid lobe above the level at which the inferior thyroid artery crosses the recurrent laryngeal nerve. The inferior glands are most usually situated near the lower pole of the thyroid gland below the inferior thyroid artery, but aberrant glands may be found in front of the trachea, behind the oesophagus,

buried in the thyroid gland or descended into the superior mediastinum in company with thymic tissue.

On the CT image, the vertebral artery (**11**) is seen as it passes towards the gap between the foramina transversarium of the sixth and seventh cervical vertebrae.

The bodies of the cervical vertebrae and the superior aspect of T1 have raised lips (uncinate processes) on each lateral margin of their superior surfaces. These processes enclose the intervertebral disc and articulate (**39**) with the inferior aspect of the adjacent vertebral body; they are prone to degenerative disease which can lead to neurological problems.

94

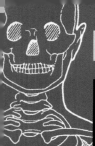

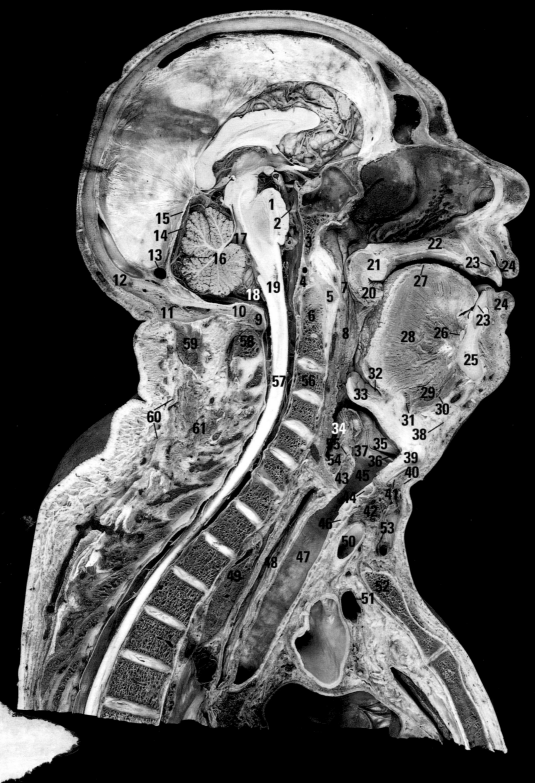

1 Pons	**11** External occipital protuberance	**29** Geniohyoid
2 Basilar artery	**12** Occipital bone	**30** Mylohyoid
3 Clivus (basioccipital and basisphenoid bones)	**13** Transverse sinus	**31** Body of hyoid bone
	14 Straight sinus	**32** Vallecula
4 Anterior margin of foramen magnum	**15** Tentorium cerebelli	**33** Epiglottis
5 Anterior arch of atlas (first cervical vertebra)	**16** Cerebellum	**34** Laryngeal part of pharynx
	17 Fourth ventricle	**35** Vestibular fold
6 Dens of axis (odontoid peg of second cervical vertebra)	**18** Cisterna magna	**36** Ventricle of larynx
	19 Medulla oblongata	**37** Vocal fold (vocal cord)
	20 Uvula	**38** Platysma
7 Nasal part of pharynx (nasopharynx)	**21** Soft palate	**39** Lamina of thyroid cartilage
	22 Hard palate	
8 Oral part of pharynx (oropharynx)	**23** Central incisor (upper and lower)	**40** Sternohyoid
		41 Sternothyroid
9 Posterior arch of atlas (first cervical vertebra)	**24** Lip (Upper and lower)	**42** Isthmus of thyroid gland
	25 Body of mandible	**43** Lamina of cricoid cartilage
	26 Sublingual gland	
10 Posterior margin of foramen magnum	**27** Dorsum of tongue	**44** Arch of cricoid cartilage
	28 Genioglossus	**45** Lower part of larynx

46 Second tracheal ring	
47 Trachea	
48 Oesophagus	
49 Superior lobe of left lung	
50 Brachiocephalic trunk	
51 Brachiocephalic vein	
52 Manubrium of sternum	
53 Anterior jugular vein	
54 Posterior crico-arytenoid	
55 Arytenoid cartilage	
56 Body of third cervical vertebra	
57 Spinal cord	
58 Spinous process of second vertebra	
59 Semispinalis capitis	
60 Trapezius	
61 Semispinalis cervicis	
62 Occipital lobe of brain	

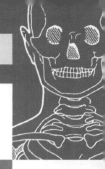

Section level

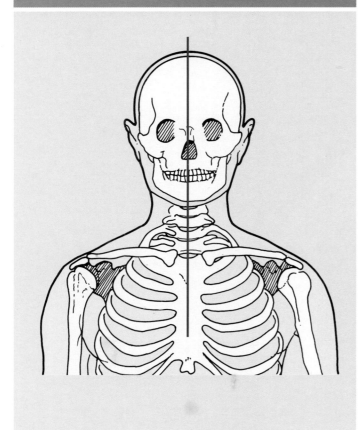

Orientation guide

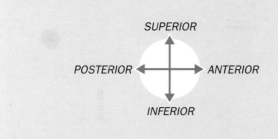

SUPERIOR

POSTERIOR ← → ANTERIOR

INFERIOR

Notes

The nasal septum has been removed from this section in order to display the nasal conchae on the lateral wall.

Cricothyroid puncture is performed between the thyroid cartilage (**39**) and the isthmus of the cricoid cartilage (**44**). Note that a tube inserted at this site will lie below the vocal folds (**37**),which are therefore free of danger. Note that the junction of the larynx and trachea (**46**) lies at the level of the sixth cervical vertebra. This level also marks the junction of the pharynx (**34**) and the oesophagus (**48**).

These midline sagittal MR images (a – T1 and b – T2 weighted) clearly demonstrate the normal relationship of the pons, medulla and cervical spinal cord to the base of the skull, foramen magnum, dens of the axis (odontoid peg) and cervical canal. The anterior and posterior margins of the foramen magnum, the tip of the basioccipital part of the clivus and the anterior margin of the occipital bone, can be well appreciated. Note the size of the cervical cord in relation to the spinal canal compared with the ratio more caudally; of course the cervical cord carries many more white matter fibres than the lumbar cord. On T2 weighting (image b) there is only a relatively small amount of cerebrospinal fluid surrounding the cord. Hence the diameter of the spinal canal in this region is of key importance. If the canal is too narrow, the inevitable 'degenerative' changes of middle/old age occuring in the vertebral column can affect nerve roots supplying the arms (brachalgia) or even affect the cord to cause upper motor neurone signs.

The relationship of the anterior arch of the atlas (first cervical vertebra) to the dens (odontoid peg) of the axis (the body of the first cervical vertebra assimilated onto the body of the second cervical vertebra – the axis) is well shown.This pivot synovial joint allows rotation of the head and C1 on C2.

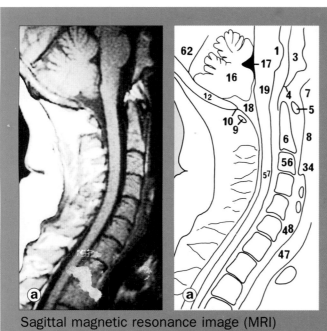

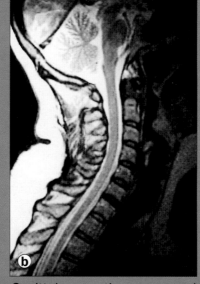

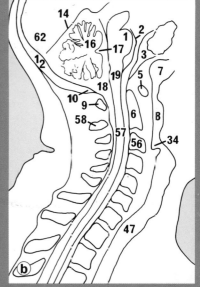

Sagittal magnetic resonance image (MRI)   Sagittal magnetic resonance image (MRI)

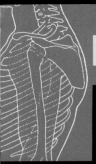

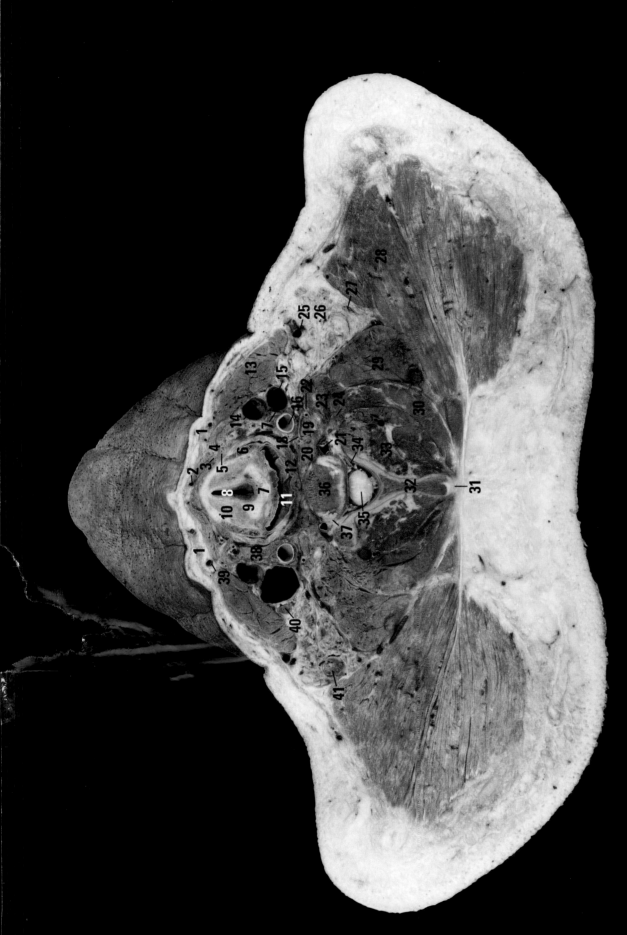

1 Platysma
2 Anterior jugular vein
3 Sternohyoid
4 Omohyoid
5 Sternothyroid
6 Thyroid cartilage
7 Cricoid cartilage
8 Rima glottidis
9 Arytenoid cartilage
10 Thyro-arytenoid
11 Pharynx (laryngeal part)
12 Inferior constrictor
   muscle of pharynx

13 Sternocleidomastoid
14 Common facial vein
15 Internal jugular vein
16 Common carotid artery
17 Vagus nerve (X)
18 Sympathetic chain
19 Longus capitis
20 Longus colli
21 Vertebral artery and vein within
   foramen transversarium
22 Phrenic nerve
23 Scalenus anterior
24 Scalenus medius and posterior

25 External jugular vein
26 Fat of posterior triangle
27 Accessory nerve (XI)
28 Trapezius
29 Levator scapulae
30 Splenius
31 Ligamentum nuchae
32 Spine of fifth cervical
   vertebra
33 Erector spinae
34 Root of sixth cervical nerve
35 Spinal cord within dural sheath
36 Body of fifth cervical vertebra

37 Neurocentral or uncovertebral
   synovial joint (of Lushka)
38 Lateral lobe of thyroid gland
39 Accessory anterior jugular vein
40 Lymph node of internal
   jugular chain
41 Cervical lymph node

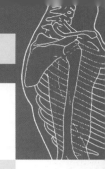

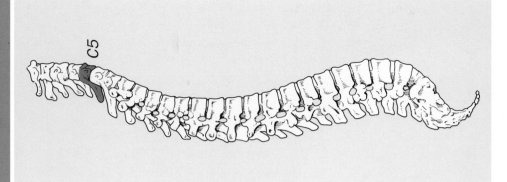

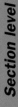

C5

Orientation guide

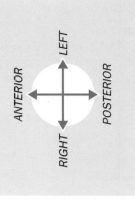

ANTERIOR

LEFT

POSTERIOR

RIGHT

Axial computed tomogram (CT)

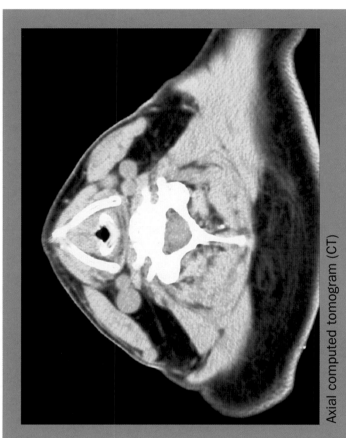

Notes

This section passes through the body of the 5th cervical vertebra (**36**), immediately above the level of the shoulder joint. Here the fibres of the trapezius muscle (**28**) arch over the posterior extremity of the posterior triangle. Just below this level, at C6, lies the junction between the pharynx (**11**) and oesophagus, and the larynx (**6,7,9**) and the trachea. In both the section and CT image the laryngeal part of the pharynx (**11**) has a narrow antero-posterior diameter; it distends consider-ably during deglutition. On the CT image, the vocal cords of the rima glottidis (**8**) are adducted.

Not unusually, as in this subject, the external jugular vein (**39**) is double.

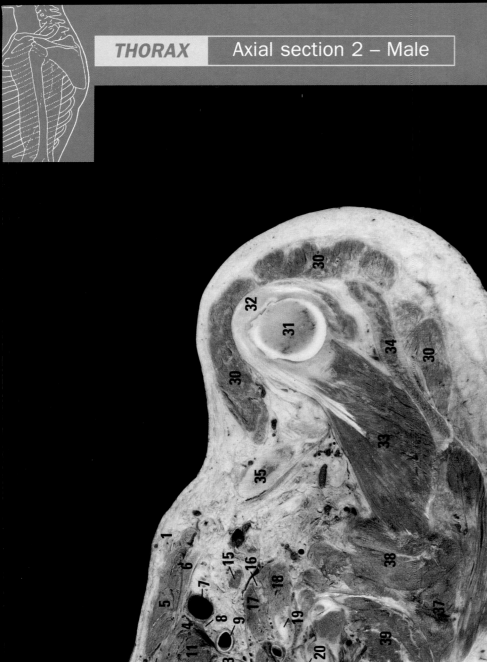
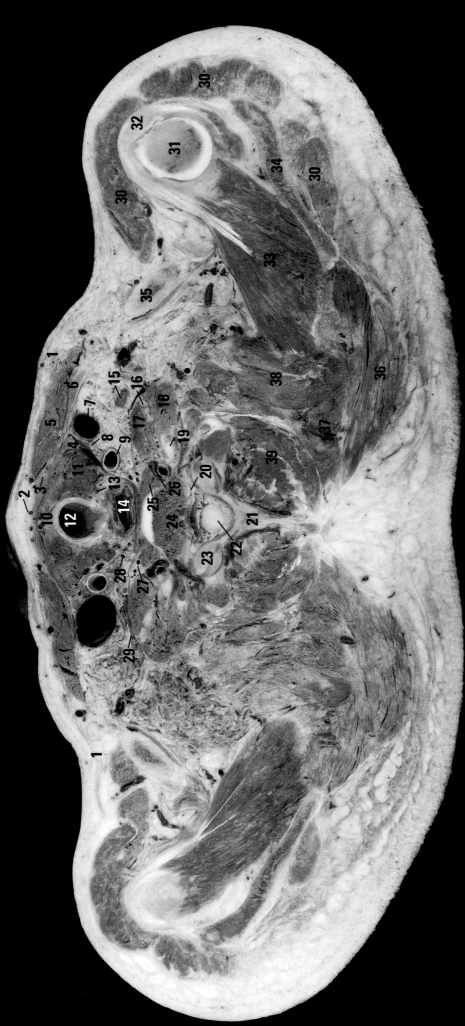

1 Platysma
2 Anterior jugular vein
3 Sternohyoid
4 Sternothyroid
5 Sternocleidomastoid
6 Omohyoid
7 Internal jugular vein
8 Vagus nerve (X)
9 Common carotid artery
10 Isthmus of thyroid gland
11 Lateral lobe of thyroid gland
12 Trachea
13 Recurrent laryngeal nerve

14 Oesophagus
15 Lymph node
16 Ventral ramus of sixth cervical nerve
17 Scalenus anterior
18 Scalenus medius
19 Ventral ramus of seventh cervical nerve
20 Dorsal root ganglion of eighth cervical nerve
21 Spine of seventh cervical vertebra – vertebra prominens
22 Spinal cord within dural sheath

23 Inferior articular facet of seventh cervical vertebra
24 Body of seventh cervical vertebra
25 Longus colli
26 Vertebral artery and vein
27 Ascending cervical artery and vein
28 Inferior thyroid artery
29 Phrenic nerve
30 Deltoid
31 Head of humerus
32 Capsule of shoulder joint

33 Supraspinatus
34 Spine of scapula
35 Coracoid process of scapula
36 Trapezius
37 Rhomboideus minor
38 Levator scapulae
39 Erector spinae

40 External jugular vein

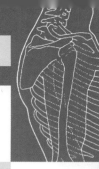

Section level

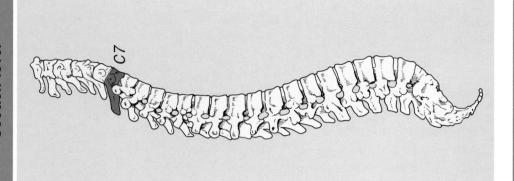

C7

Orientation guide

ANTERIOR

LEFT

RIGHT

POSTERIOR

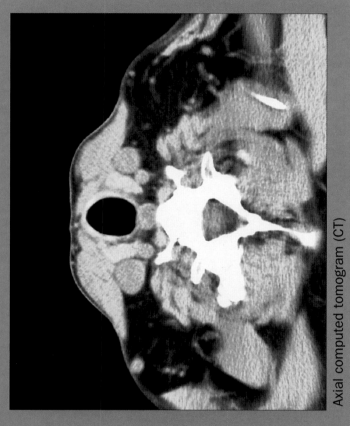

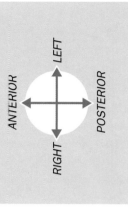

Axial computed tomogram (CT)

Notes

This section traverses the body of the seventh cervical vertebra which bears the longest spine of the cervical series, the vertebra prominens (**21**). However, this is shorter than the spine of T1 as can easily be ascertained by feeling the back of your own neck.

Two important relationships are well demonstrated. The recurrent laryngeal nerve (**13**) lies in the groove between trachea (**12**) and oesophagus (**14**). The phrenic nerve (**29**) hugs the anterior aspect of scalenus anterior (**17**) beneath the prevertebral fascia.

100

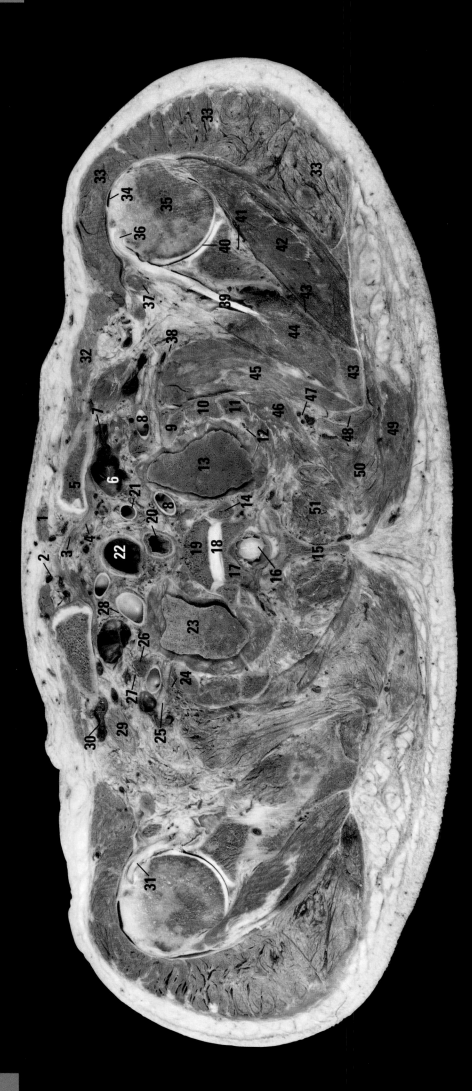

1 Sternocleidomastoid sternal head
2 Anterior jugular vein
3 Sternohyoid
4 Sternothyroid
5 Clavicle
6 Internal jugular vein – junction with left subclavian vein
7 Left subclavian vein
8 Subclavian artery
9 First rib
10 Intercostal muscles
11 Second rib
12 Intercostal neurovascular bundle
13 Apex of left lung

14 Head of second rib
15 Spine of first thoracic vertebra
16 Spinal cord within dural sheath
17 Part of body of second thoracic vertebra
18 Part of intervertebral disc between first and second thoracic vertebra
19 Part of body of first thoracic vertebra
20 Oesophagus
21 Common carotid artery
22 Trachea
23 Right lung apex
24 Scalenus medius
25 Root of first thoracic nerve

26 Scalenus anterior
27 Phrenic nerve
28 Vagus nerve (X)
29 Subclavius
30 Right subclavian vein
31 Tendon of right biceps long head
32 Pectoralis major
33 Deltoid
34 Subdeltoid bursa
35 Head of humerus
36 Tendon of biceps long head
37 Coracoid process of scapula
38 Nerve to serratus anterior
39 Tendon of subscapularis
40 Glenoid fossa of scapula

41 Suprascapular artery and vein
42 Infraspinatus
43 Scapula
44 Subscapularis
45 Serratus anterior
46 Serratus posterior superior
47 Superficial (transverse) cervical artery and vein
48 Rhomboideus minor
49 Trapezius
50 Rhomboideus major
51 Erector spinae

52 Supraspinatus
53 Pectoralis minor

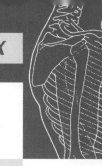

Section level

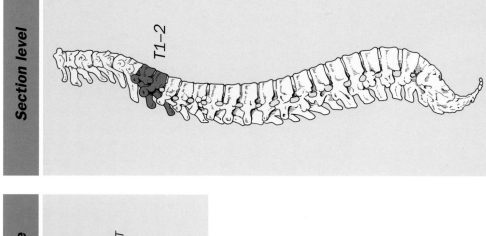

T1–2

Orientation guide

ANTERIOR

LEFT

RIGHT

POSTERIOR

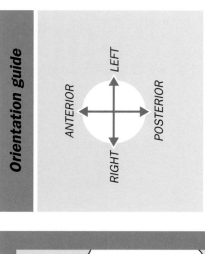

Axial computed tomogram (CT)

Axial computed tomogram (CT)

Notes

This section, through the intervertebral disc between the 1st and 2nd thoracic vertebra (**18**), enters the apex of the thorax and traverses the extra pleural space around the upper lobes of the lungs (**13, 23**). There are considerable differences between the section and CT images at this level because the CT is performed with the arms elevated alongside the head in order to reduce artefacts from the humeri.

(**6**) joins with the subclavian vein (**7**) to form the brachiocephalic vein (see section 4, page 103).

The intercostal neurovascular bundle (**12**) is well seen. Note that it comprises the intercostal vein, artery and nerve from above downwards; the nerve corresponds to the number of its overlying rib, and lies protected within the subcostal groove.

Only in transverse section is the extreme thinness of the blade of the scapula (**43**) fully appreciated.

Here, posterior to the medial end of the clavicle (**5**), the internal jugular vein

One CT (a) is displayed at soft tissue settings (window level and width of grey scale), the other CT (b) at lung windows.

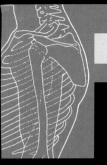

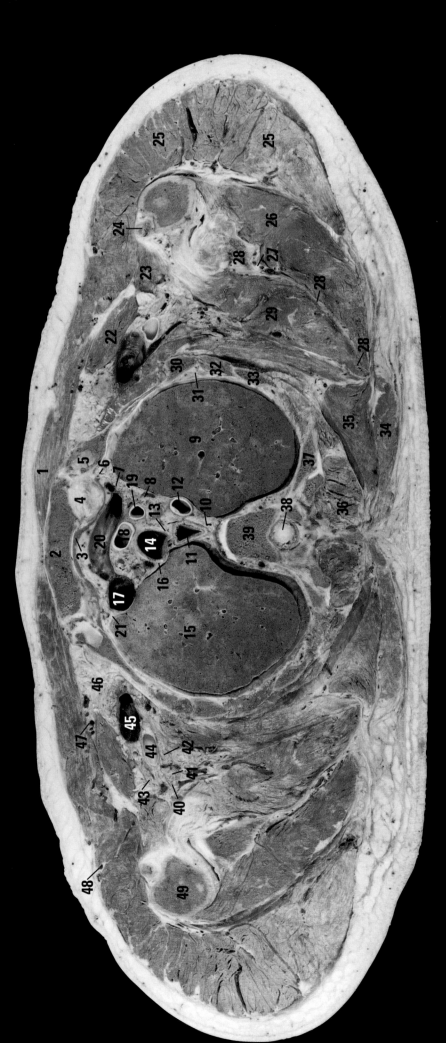

1 Pectoralis major
2 Manubrium of sternum
3 Sternothyroid
4 Sternoclavicular joint
5 First rib
6 Internal thoracic artery
7 Left phrenic nerve
8 Left vagus nerve (X)
9 Upper lobe of left lung
10 Thoracic duct
11 Oesophagus
12 Left subclavian artery
13 Left recurrent laryngeal nerve
14 Trachea

15 Upper lobe of right lung
16 Right vagus nerve (X)
17 Right brachiocephalic vein
18 Brachiocephalic artery
19 Left common carotid artery
20 Left brachiocephalic vein
21 Right phrenic nerve
22 Pectoralis minor
23 Coracobrachialis and biceps
   (short head)
24 Long head of biceps tendon
25 Deltoid
26 Infraspinatus
27 Suprascapular artery and vein

28 Scapula
29 Subscapularis
30 Second rib
31 Intercostal artery and
   vein and nerve
32 External and internal
   intercostal muscles
33 Third rib
34 Trapezius
35 Rhomboideus major
36 Erector spinae
37 Fourth rib with articulation of its
   head with body of third thoracic
   vertebra transverse process

38 Spinal cord within dural sheath
39 Body of third thoracic vertebra
40 Axillary nerve
41 Radial nerve
42 Ulnar nerve
43 Median nerve
44 Right axillary artery
45 Right axillary vein
46 Axillary fat
47 Pectoral branch of the
   acromiothoracic artery and vein
48 Cephalic vein
49 Shaft of humerus

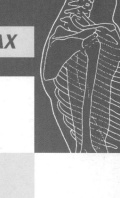

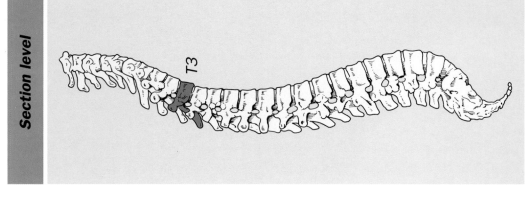

Section level

T3

Orientation guide

ANTERIOR

LEFT

RIGHT

POSTERIOR

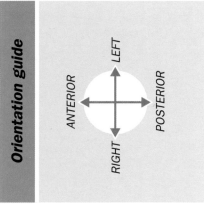

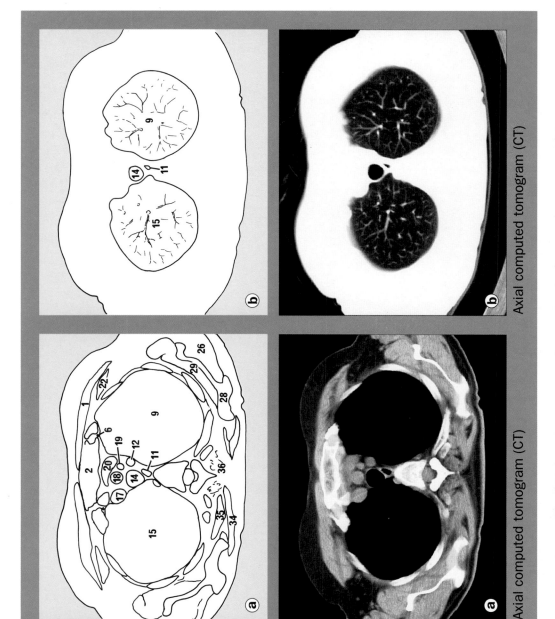

Axial computed tomogram (CT)

Axial computed tomogram (CT)

Notes

The contents of the upper mediastinum – including oesophagus, trachea and great vessels – are demonstrated in this section, which traverses the manubrium and the third thoracic vertebra; these are also shown in section, 5 page 105. This section also shows the walls and contents of the axilla.

Note that the cephalic vein (**48**) runs in the deltopectoral groove between the medial edge of deltoid and the lateral edge of pectoralis major.

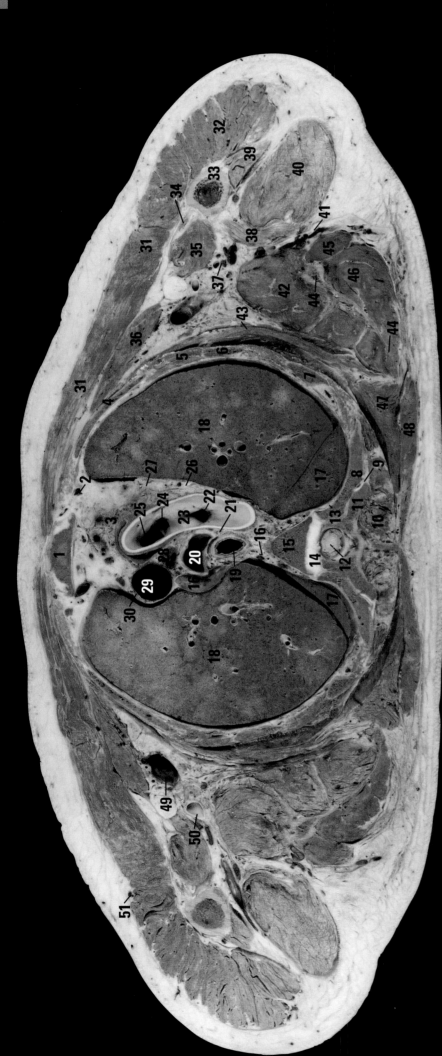

1 Manubriosternal joint (angle of Louis)
2 Internal thoracic artery and vein
3 Thymic residue within anterior mediastinal fat
4 Second rib
5 Intercostal
6 Third rib
7 Fourth rib
8 Fifth rib
9 Fifth costotransverse joint
10 Erector spinae
11 Transverse process of fifth thoracic vertebra
12 Spinal cord within dural sheath
13 Sympathetic chain
14 Part of intervertebral disc between fourth and fifth thoracic vertebra
15 Part of body of fourth thoracic vertebra
16 Azygos vein
17 Apical segment lower lobe lung separated by oblique fissure from (18)
18 Upper lobe of lung
19 Oesophagus
20 Trachea at bifurcation
21 Recurrent laryngeal nerve
22 Left subclavian artery orifice
23 Aortic arch
24 Left common carotid artery orifice

25 Brachiocephalic artery orifice
26 Left vagus nerve (X)
27 Left phrenic nerve
28 Pretracheal lymph node
29 Superior vena cava
30 Right phrenic nerve
31 Pectoralis major
32 Deltoid
33 Shaft of humerus
34 Biceps – long head
35 Biceps – short head and coracobrachialis
36 Pectoralis minor
37 Subscapular artery vein and nerve
38 Latissimus dorsi

39 Triceps – lateral head
40 Triceps – long head
41 Circumflex scapular artery and vein
42 Subscapularis
43 Serratus anterior
44 Body of scapula
45 Teres minor
46 Infraspinatus
47 Rhomboideus
48 Trapezius
49 Axillary vein
50 Axillary artery
51 Cephalic vein
52 Oblique fissure

Section level

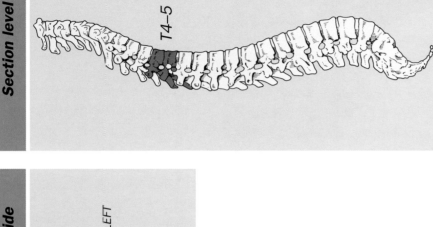

T4–5

Orientation guide

ANTERIOR

LEFT

RIGHT

POSTERIOR

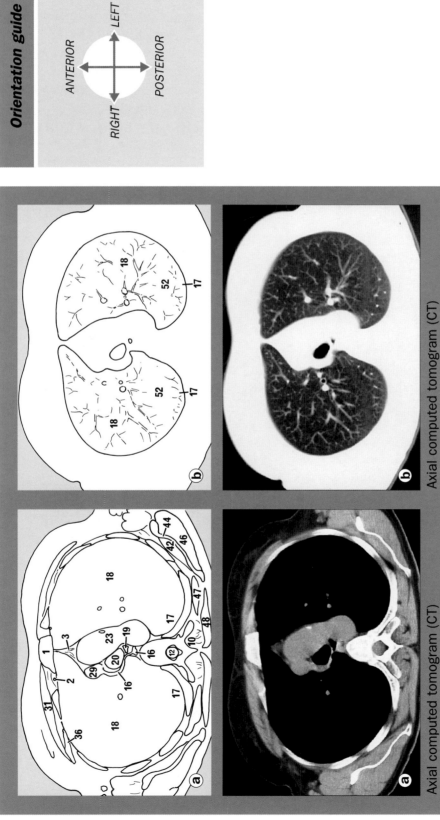

Axial computed tomogram (CT)

Axial computed tomogram (CT)

Notes

This section passes through the important anatomical level of the manubriosternal joint, the angle of Louis (**1**). At this joint articulate the second costal cartilage and rib (**4**) and it is from here that the ribs can be conveniently counted in clinical practice. Posteriorly this plane passes through the T4/5 intervertebral disc (**14**).

This plane demarcates the junction between the superior mediastinum and the lower, which is subdivided into the anterior mediastinum, in front of the pericardium, the middle mediastinum, occupied by the pericardium and its contents, and the posterior mediastinum, behind the pericardium.

The trachea bifurcates at this level (**20**). However, in the living upright subject, the bifurcation may be as low as the level of T6, particularly in deep inspiration.

The cranial portions of the oblique fissures of the lungs (**17, 52**) are traversed on this section. The normal oblique fissures are often not seen on conventional CT images of the lung parenchyma. However, the position can be inferred (see above CT image b) by the paucity of blood vessels; only small terminal vessels are present in the lung parenchyma adjacent to a fissure.

Pretracheal nodes (**28**) may become enlarged due to a wide variety of disease processes. They are accessible for biopsy via mediastinoscopy.

Subscapularis (**42**) arises not only from the periosteum of the medial two/thirds of the subscapular fossa of the scapula, but also from tendinous laminae in the muscle itself which are attached to prominent transverse ridges on the subscapular fossa. This is clearly shown in this section.

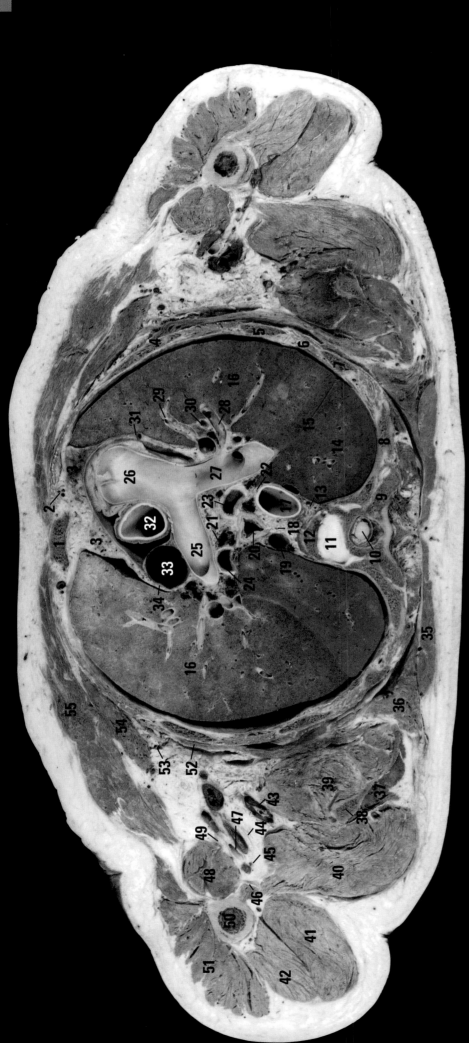

1 Body of sternum
2 Internal thoracic artery and vein
3 Thymic residue within anterior mediastinal fat
4 Third rib
5 Fouth rib
6 Intercostal muscles
7 Fifth rib
8 Sixth rib
9 Transverse process of sixth thoracic vertebra
10 Spinal cord within dural sheath
11 Part of intervertebral disc between fifth and sixth thoracic vertebra
12 Part of body of fifth thoracic vertebra

13 Intercostal artery and vein
14 Lower lobe of lung
15 Oblique fissure
16 Upper lobe of lung
17 Descending aorta
18 Thoracic duct
19 Azygos vein
20 Oesophagus
21 Lymph node
22 Left vagus nerve (X)
23 Left main bronchus
24 Right intermediate bronchus
25 Right pulmonary artery
26 Pulmonary trunk
27 Left pulmonary artery
28 Pulmonary artery branch

29 Pulmonary vein tributary
30 Segmental bronchus
31 Left phrenic nerve with pericardiacophrenic artery
32 Ascending aorta
33 Superior vena cava
34 Right phrenic nerve
35 Trapezius
36 Rhomboideus major
37 Infraspinatus
38 Scapula
39 Subscapularis
40 Teres major
41 Triceps – long head
42 Triceps – lateral head
43 Subscapular artery and vein

44 Ulnar nerve
45 Radial nerve
46 Latissimus dorsi tendon
47 Axillary artery and vein
48 Biceps and coracobrachialis
49 Median nerve
50 Shaft of humerus
51 Deltoid
52 Serratus anterior
53 Lateral thoracic artery and vein
54 Pectoralis minor
55 Pectoralis major
56 Superior pulmonary vein
57 Left basal pulmonary artery
58 Breast

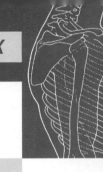

Section level

T5–6

Orientation guide

ANTERIOR

LEFT

POSTERIOR

RIGHT

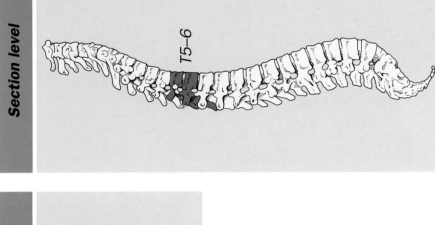

Axial computed tomogram (CT)

Axial computed tomogram (CT)

Notes

This section, traversing the upper body of the sternum (**1**) and the lower part of the body of the fifth thoracic vertebra (**12**) passes through the great arterial trunks as these emerge from the heart, the pulmonary trunk (**26**) and the ascending aorta (**32**).

On the CT images the left main bronchus gives off its common upper lobe/lingular branch at this level. On the right, the upper lobe bronchus has alrady originated more cranially (on both CT images and section). Hence the term 'intermediate bronchus' (**24**) is applied to that portion of the right bronchus between its upper lobe and middle lobe branches.

At the left hilum the superior pulmonary vein (**56**) lies anterior to the bronchus (**23**) which lies, in turn, anterior to the left basal pulmonary artery (**57**). On the right side, the vein (**56**) lies anterior to the right pulmonary artery which lies anterior to the right intermediate bronchus (**24**).

In this subject, the right and left pulmonary arteries (**25**, **27**) lie in the same axial plane. In most subjects, the left pulmonary artery is at a more cranial level than the right, hence the discrepancy between the section and CT image appearances. The branches of the pulmonary artery (**28**) which accomp-

any the segmental and subsegmental bronchi (**30**) usually lie dorsolaterally to these structures; each pulmonary segment receives an independent arterial supply. The bronchi usually separate the dorsolateral pulmonary artery branch from the ventromedially situated pulmonary vein tributary (**29**). Peripherally, many pulmonary venous tributaries run between, and drain adjacent, pulmonary segments. Thus an individual bronchopulmonary segment will have its own bronchus and artery but not an individual pulmonary venous drainage.

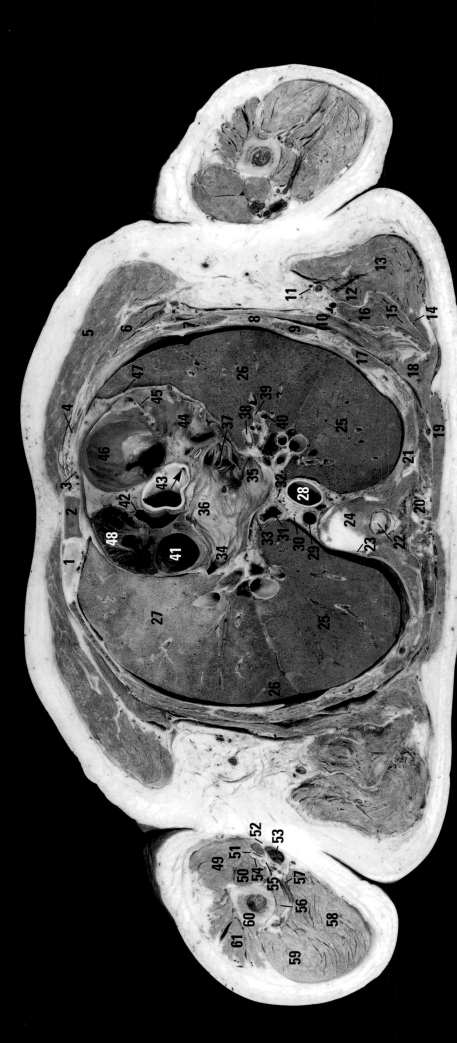

1 Third costal cartilage with adjacent sternocostal joint – (see note)
2 Body of sternum
3 Internal thoracic artery and vein
4 Partially calcified third costal cartilage
5 Pectoralis major
6 Pectoralis minor
7 Third rib
8 Intercostal muscles
9 Fourth rib
10 Serratus anterior
11 Subscapular artery vein and nerve
12 Teres major
13 Latissimus dorsi
14 Infraspinatus
15 Scapula
16 Subscapularis
17 Fifth rib
18 Rhomboideus major
19 Trapezius

20 Erector spinae
21 Sixth rib with adjacent costotransverse joint to transverse process of sixth thoracic vertebra
22 Spinal cord within dural sheath
23 Thoracic sympathetic chain
24 Body of sixth thoracic vertebra with part of intervertebral disc between the sixth and seventh thoracic vertebra
25 Lower lobe lung
26 Upper lobe lung
27 Middle lobe right lung
28 Descending aorta
29 Azygos vein
30 Thoracic duct
31 Oesophagus
32 Left vagal plexus
33 Right vagal plexus
34 Right superior pulmonary vein
35 Left superior pulmonary vein

36 Left atrium
37 Left auricle (atrial appendage)
38 Left pulmonary vein tributary to lingula
39 Left bronchus segmental branch to lingula
40 Left pulmonary artery branch to lingula
41 Superior vena cava
42 Artifactual gap within the pericardial space
43 Ascending aorta with orifice of left coronary artery (arrowed)
44 Left ventricle wall
45 Coronary artery (left anterior interventricular branch)
46 Infundibulum of right ventricle with pulmonary valves
47 Fibrous pericardium
48 Right auricle (atrial appendage)

49 Biceps
50 Coracobrachialis
51 Axillary artery and vein
52 Medial cutaneous nerves of arm and forearm
53 Basilic vein
54 Median nerve
55 Ulnar nerve
56 Triceps – medial head
57 Radial nerve with profunda brachii artery and vein
58 Triceps – long head
59 Triceps – lateral head
60 Shaft of humerus
61 Deltoid

62 Hemiazygos vein
63 Right coronary artery
64 Oblique fissure

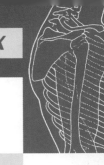

Section level

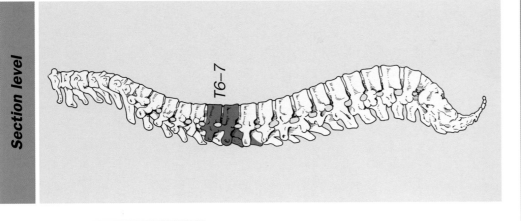

T6–7

Orientation guide

LEFT

ANTERIOR — POSTERIOR

RIGHT

Axial computed tomogram (CT)

(b)

Axial computed tomogram (CT)

(b)

(a)

Axial computed tomogram (CT)

(a)

Notes

The plane of this section traverses the lower part of the body of the sixth thoracic vertebra (**24**). Anteriorly, it passes through the body of the sternum (**2**) at the level of the third costal cartilage (**1**). Note the adjacent sternocostal joint. These vary; the first lacks a synovial cavity, its costal cartilage being attached by fibrocartilage to the manubrium. The 2nd to 7th joints are usually synovial, (as in this subject), with the fibrocartilaginous articular surfaces on both the chondral and the sternal components of the joint. However, in some or all of these joints, a similar arrangement may be found to that of the 1st joint.

The presence of a pericardial effusion in this subject has produced an artefactual gap in the superior reflection of the pericardial space (**42**). The aorta at its origin (**43**) shows the orifice of the left coronary artery. The descending aorta (**28**) is normally more circular in outline than in this subject. Note that

this section passes through the infundibulum of the right ventricle and demonstrates the pulmonary valves (**46**).

On the above CT images, both the ascending aorta (**43**) and the region of the pulmonary valves (**46**) have indistinct outlines due to pulsation (compliance) of their walls during the one second data acquisition time. (See also the ascending aorta; image (a), section 6, page 108).

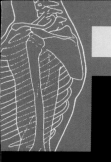

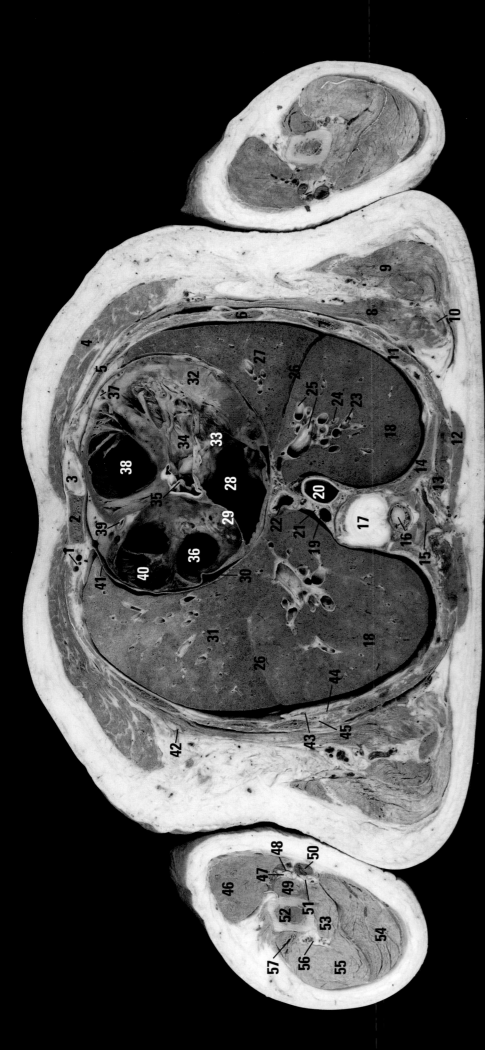

1 Internal thoracic artery and vein
2 Body of sternum
3 Fourth costal cartilage
4 Pectoralis major
5 Fourth rib
6 Fifth rib
7 Sixth rib
8 Serratus anterior
9 Latissimus dorsi
10 Scapula inferior angle
11 Seventh rib
12 Trapezius
13 Erector spinae
14 Eighth rib
15 Lamina of seventh thoracic
   vertebra
16 Spinal cord within dural sheath

17 Intervertebral disc between seventh
   and eighth thoracic vertebrae
18 Lower lobe of lung
19 Azygos vein
20 Descending aorta
21 Thoracic duct
22 Oesophagus
23 Pulmonary artery branch
24 Branches of left lower lobe bronchus
25 Pulmonary vein tributaries
26 Oblique fissure
27 Upper lobe of left lung
28 Left atrium
29 Interatrial septum
30 Phrenic nerve with pericardiacophrenic artery and vein
31 Middle lobe of right lung

32 Wall of left ventricle
33 Mitral valve
34 Vestibule of left ventricle (outflow
   tract) leading to root of aorta
35 Divided cusp of aortic valve
36 Right atrium
37 Anterior interventricular (descending) branch left coronary artery
38 Right ventricle cavity
39 Right coronary artery
40 Right auricle (atrial appendage)
41 Fibrous pericardium
42 Nerve to serratus anterior
43 Intercostal neurovascular bundle
44 Innermost intercostal
45 External and internal intercostal
   muscles

46 Biceps
47 Median nerve with musculocuta-
   neous nerve (lateral to it)
48 Brachial artery with two venae
   comitantes
49 Coracobrachialis
50 Basilic vein
51 Ulnar nerve
52 Shaft of humerus
53 Triceps – short head
54 Triceps – long head
55 Triceps – lateral head
56 Radial nerve with profunda
   brachii artery and vein
57 Deltoid

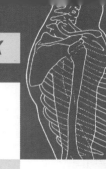

Section level

T7-8

Orientation guide

ANTERIOR

LEFT

RIGHT

POSTERIOR

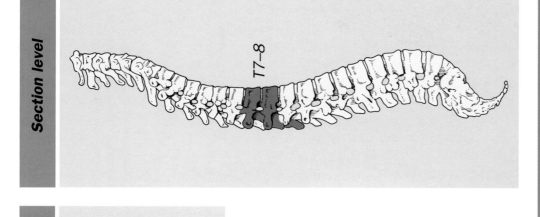

Axial computed tomogram (CT)

Axial computed tomogram (CT)

Notes

This section lies at the level of the intervertebral disc between the seventh and eighth thoracic vertebra (**17**) and passes through the body of the sternum (**2**) at the level of the fourth costal cartilage (**3**). All four cardiac chambers can be seen, and their relationships to each other appreciated. Note that the right atrium (**36**) forms the right border of the heart. The left atrium (**28**) is the major contribution to the posterior aspect of the heart and lies immediately anterior to the oesophagus (**22**) and is separated by the pericardium. The left ventricle (**32**) forms the bulk of the left border of the heart and the right ventricle (**38**) constitutes the major component of the anterior cardiac surface.

In this subject, the left ventricular wall (**32**) becomes thinner in the region of the apex of the left ventricle, due to a previous myocardial infarction.

The interatrial septum (**29**) has a rather curious convexity. This has been caused by extensive post- mortem thrombus in the right atrium (**36**). The septum is normally straighter.

The lower four or five digitations of serratus anterior (**8**) converge to insert on the costal aspect of the inferior angle of the scapula. This component of the muscle, together with the trapezius, powerfully pulls the inferior angle of the scapula forwards and upwards in raising the arm above the head.

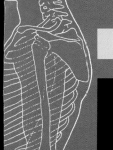

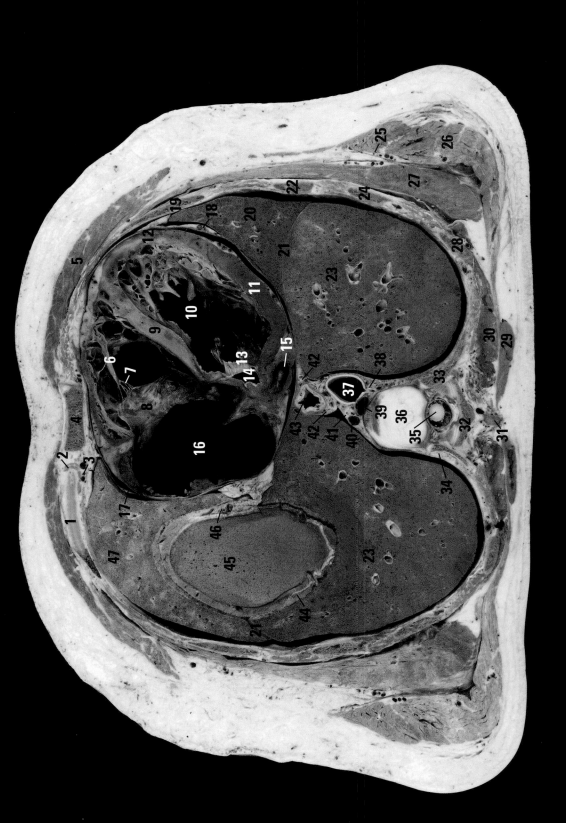

1 Fifth costal cartilage
2 Sternocostal joint
3 Internal thoracic artery and vein
4 Body of sternum
5 Pectoralis major
6 Papillary muscle
7 Chordae tendinae within right ventricular cavity
8 Triscupid valve
9 Interventricular septum
10 Left ventricular cavity
11 Normal left ventricular wall
12 Thinned left ventricular wall
13 Mitral valve

14 Left atrium
15 Coronary sinus
16 Right atrium
17 Fibrous pericardium
18 Left phrenic nerve with pericardiacophrenic artery and vein
19 Fifth rib
20 Upper lobe of left lung (lingula)
21 Oblique fissure
22 Sixth rib
23 Lower lobe of lung
24 Seventh rib
25 Lateral thoracic artery and vein
26 Latissimus dorsi

27 Serratus anterior
28 Eighth rib
29 Trapezius
30 Erector spinae
31 Spine of eighth thoracic vertebra
32 Lamina of eighth thoracic vertebra
33 Ninth rib
34 Right sympathetic chain
35 Spinal cord within dural sheath
36 Intervertebral disc between eighth and ninth thoracic vertebra
37 Aorta
38 Origin of eighth intercostal artery
39 Hemiazygos vein

40 Azygos vein
41 Thoracic duct
42 Oesophageal vagal plexus
43 Oesophagus
44 Dome of right hemidiaphragm
45 Apex of right lobe liver
46 Right phrenic nerve with pericardiacophrenic artery and vein
47 Middle lobe of right lung

48 Inferior vena cava
49 Right ventricular cavity

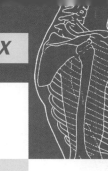

Section level

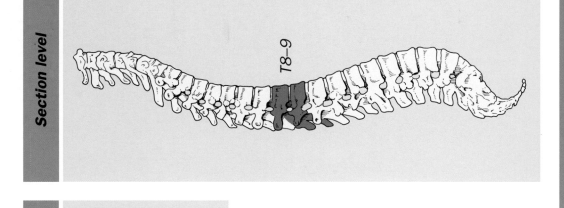

T8–9

Orientation guide

ANTERIOR
RIGHT — LEFT
POSTERIOR

Axial computed tomogram (CT) — (b)

Axial computed tomogram (CT) — (a)

Notes

This section traverses the intervertebral disc between the eighth and ninth thoracic vertebrae (**36**) and slices through the dome of the right hemidiaphragm (**44**) and a sliver of the underlying right lobe of the liver (**45**).

In this section, there is considerable thinning and discoloration of the left ventricular wall at the apex (**12**), consistent with infarction associated with left anterior descending (interventricular) coronary arterial disease.

Note how only a tiny portion of the left atrium (**14**) is present on this section. This demonstrates that the left atrium is situated more cranially than the other three cardiac chambers.

The terminal fibres of the right phrenic nerve (**46**) usually pass through the vena caval opening in the diaphragm but may traverse the muscle itself.

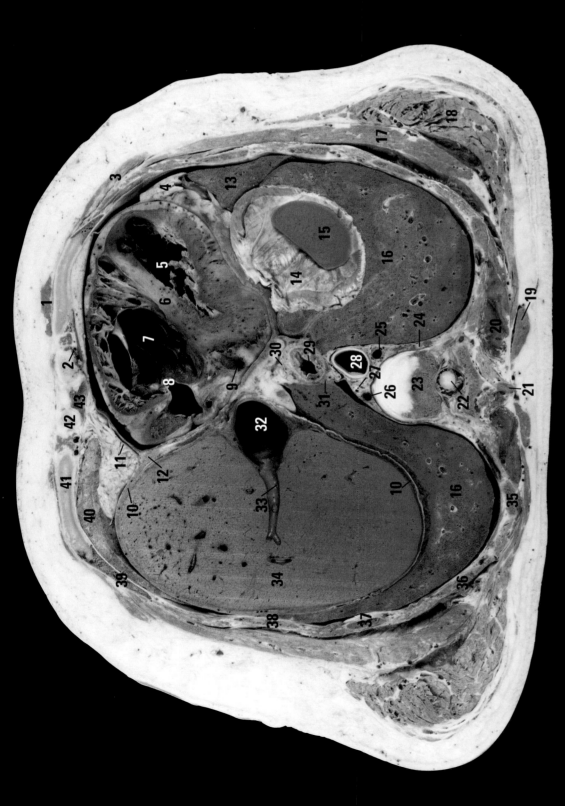

1 Pectoralis major
2 Internal thoracic artery and vein
3 External oblique
4 Extrapericardial pad of fat
5 Left ventricle
6 Interventricular septum
7 Right ventricle
8 Tricuspid valve
9 Coronary sinus
10 Diaphragm
11 Fibrous pericardium
12 Line of fusion of diaphragm
    and pericardium

13 Upper lobe left lung (lingula)
14 Left dome of diaphragm
15 Spleen
16 Lower lobe of lung
17 Serratus anterior
18 Latissimus dorsi
19 Trapezius
20 Erector spinae
21 Tip of spine of eighth thoracic
    vertebra
22 Spinal cord within dural sheath
23 Body of ninth thoracic vertebra
    with part of intervertebral disc

    between ninth and tenth
    thoracic vertebra
24 Left sympathetic chain
25 Hemiazygos vein
26 Azygos vein
27 Thoracic duct
28 Aorta
29 Oesophagus
30 Left vagus nerve (X)
31 Right vagus nerve (X)
32 Inferior vena cava
33 Right hepatic vein
34 Right lobe of liver

35 Tenth rib
36 Ninth rib
37 Eighth rib
38 Seventh rib
39 Sixth rib
40 Middle lobe of right lung
41 Sixth costal cartilage
42 Fifth costal cartilage
43 Sternum

44 Oblique fissure

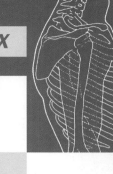

Section level

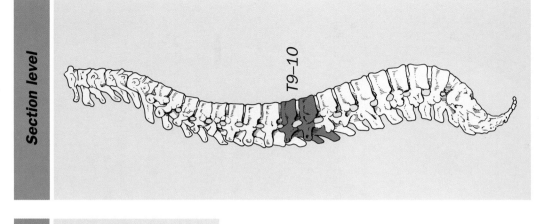

T9–10

Orientation guide

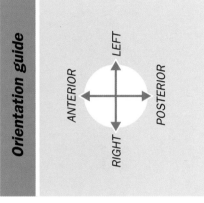

ANTERIOR

LEFT

RIGHT

POSTERIOR

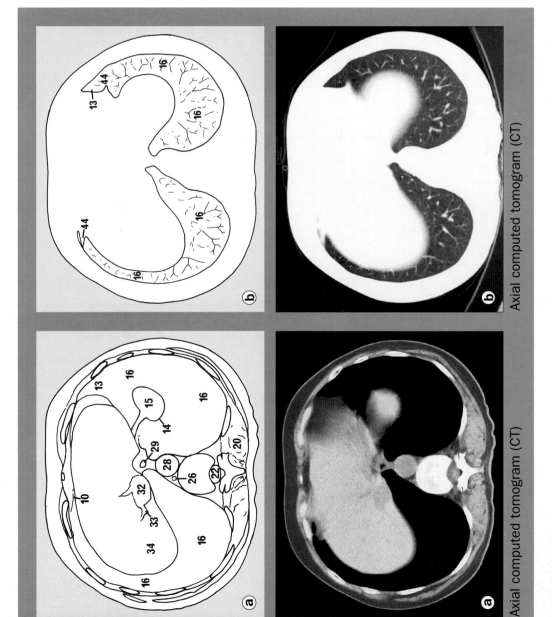

Axial computed tomogram (CT)

Axial computed tomogram (CT)

Notes

This section is at the level of the body of the ninth thoracic vertebra (**23**) and traverses the dome of the left diaphragm (**14**). The cranial portion of the spleen (**15**) is therefore revealed.

The fusion of the diaphragm (**10**) with the base of the fibrous pericardium (**11**) is clearly shown at this point.

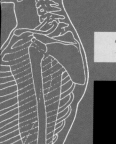

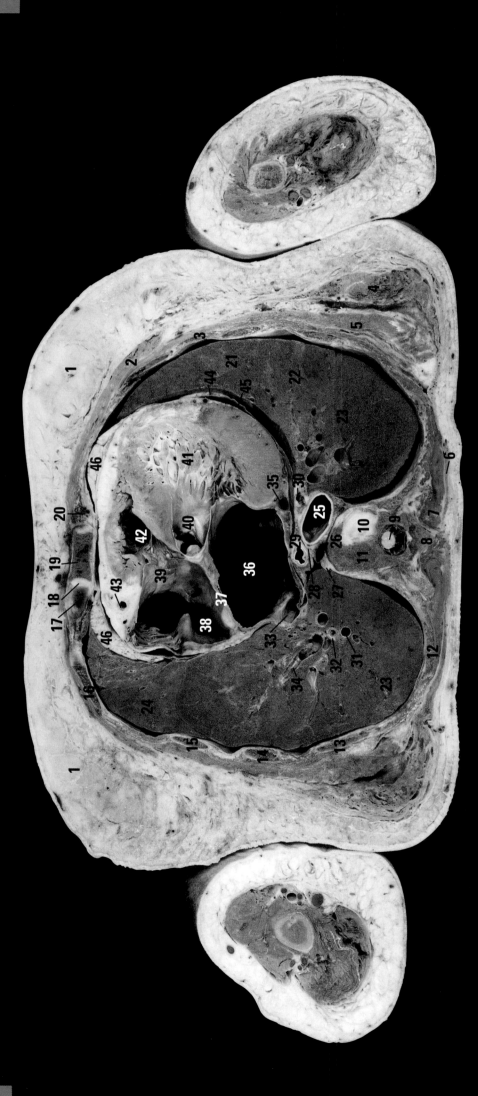

1   Breast
2   Pectoralis major
3   Intercostal muscles
4   Latissimus dorsi
5   Serratus anterior
6   Trapezius
7   Erector spinae
8   Spine of seventh thoracic vertebra
9   Spinal cord within dural sheath
10 Part of intervertebral disc between
    the seventh and eighth thoracic
    vertebrae
11 Body of seventh thoracic vertebra
12 Seventh rib
13 Sixth rib

14 Fifth rib
15 Fourth rib
16 Third rib
17 Third costal cartilage
18 Third sternocostal joint
19 Sternum
20 Internal thoracic artery and vein
21 Upper lobe of left lung (lingula)
22 Left oblique fissure
23 Lower lobe of lung
24 Middle lobe of right lung
25 Aorta
26 Azygos vein
27 Right sympathetic chain
28 Thoracic duct

29 Oesophagus
30 Mediastinal lymph node
31 Pulmonary arterial branch
    in lower lobe
32 Bronchus – segmental
    branch in lower lobe
33 Orifice of right inferior
    pulmonary vein
34 Right inferior pulmonary vein
35 Coronary sinus
36 Left atrium
37 Interatrial septum
38 Right atrium
39 Tricuspid valve
40 Aortic valve

41 Left ventricle
42 Right ventricle
43 Right coronary artery
44 Left phrenic nerve
45 Fibrous pericardium
46 Extrapericardial fat pad

47 Ascending aorta
48 Descending aorta
49 Pulmonary trunk
50 Right pulmonary artery
51 Superior vena cava
52 Left basal pulmonary artery
53 Upper lobe of right lung
54 Carcinoma right breast

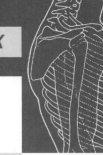

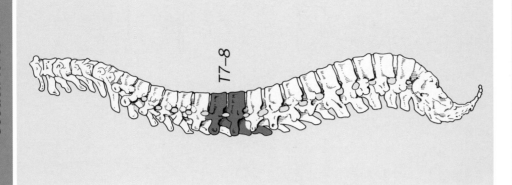

T7–8

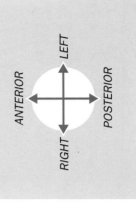

ANTERIOR

LEFT

POSTERIOR

RIGHT

Axial computed tomogram (CT)

Notes

This section of a female subject passes through the body of the seventh thoracic vertebra (**11**) and through the third sternocostal joint (**18**). This elderly subjects kyphosis accounts for the apparent discrepancy between cardiac structures and thoracic landmarks. Note the general smaller configuration of the female thorax and the smaller, less bulky muscles.

The breast (**1**) contains the mammary gland. This extends vertically from the second to the sixth rib and transversely from the side of the sternum to near the mid-axillary line. The gland is situated within the superficial fascia and is separated from the fascia covering pectoralis major, serratus anterior and the external oblique muscle by loose areolar tissue. In old age, as in this subject, the glandular tissue becomes atrophied.

Note that in this section the margin of the mass of left ventricular muscle (**41**) has been cut across.

This CT image shows a patient with a large carcinoma of the right breast, which has ulcerated and has extended into, and infiltrated, a wide area of adjacent skin. The anatomical level is considerably more cranial than the cadaveric section; it corresponds closely to that shown in section 6 Male Thorax, page 107.

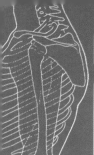

Axial computed tomogram (CT)

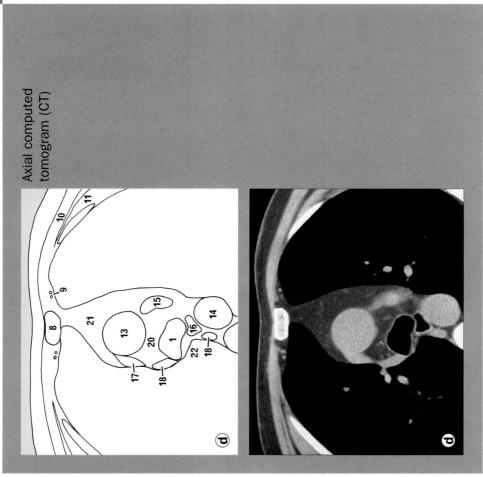

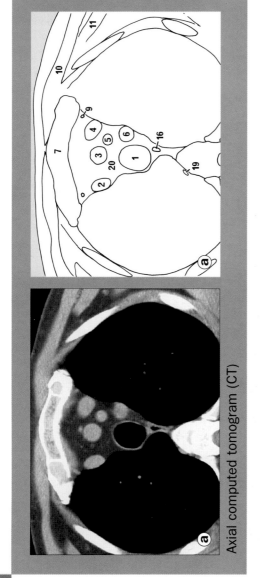

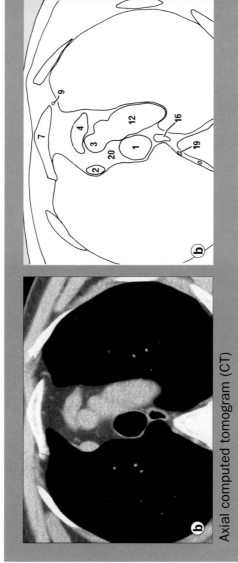

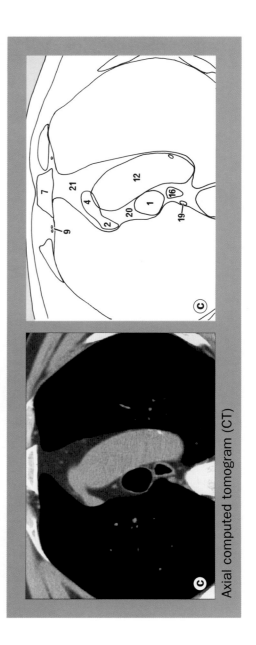

Axial computed tomogram (CT)

Axial computed tomogram (CT)

Axial computed tomogram (CT)

Section level

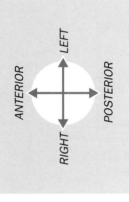

A
B
C
D

Orientation guide

ANTERIOR

LEFT

RIGHT

POSTERIOR

Images A–B

1 Trachea
2 Right brachio-
   cephalic vein
3 Brachiocephalic
   artery
4 Left brachio-
   cephalic vein
5 Left common
   carotid artery
6 Left subclavian
   artery
7 Manubrium of
   sternum
9 Internal thoracic
   artery and vein
10 Pectoralis major
11 Pectoralis minor
16 Oesophagus
19 Right superior
   intercostal vein
20 Fat in pretracheal
   space

Images C–D

1 Trachea
2 Right brachio-
   cephalic vein
4 Left brachio-
   cephalic vein
7 Manubrium of
   sternum
8 Body of sternum
9 Internal thoracic
   artery and vein
10 Pectoralis major
11 Pectoralis minor
12 Aortic arch (with
   fleck of calcifica-
   tion in wall on
   image c)
13 Ascending aorta
14 Descending aorta
15 Left pulmonary
   artery
16 Oesophagus
17 Superior vena cava
18 Azygos vein
19 Right superior
   intercostal vein
20 Fat in pretracheal
   space
21 Fat in anterior
   mediastinal space
   (with thymic
   remnant)
22 Azygo-oesophageal
   recess

Notes

This patient has copious mediastinal fat, which makes the normal structures very conspicuous. Enlarged lymph nodes would show up well in such a patient (see section 6, page 107). If such nodes lie in the pre-tracheal space (**20**), biopsy material can be obtained via mediastinoscopy.

The trachea (**1**) is bifurcating on image (d); this point is known as the carina. The left pulmonary artery (**15**) lies at a more cranial level than the right; it is just entering part of the section shown on image (d). It appears indistinct because only part of the thickness of the slice is occupied by the structure ('partial volume' effect). The space immediatly caudal to the aortic arch and cranial to the bifurcation of the pulmonary artery is know as the subaortic fossa or aortopulmonary window. The ligamentum arteriosum (the obliterated ductus arteriosus passing from the left pulmonary artery to the aorta) runs through this space. This fossa may also contain enlarged lymph nodes.

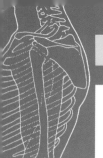

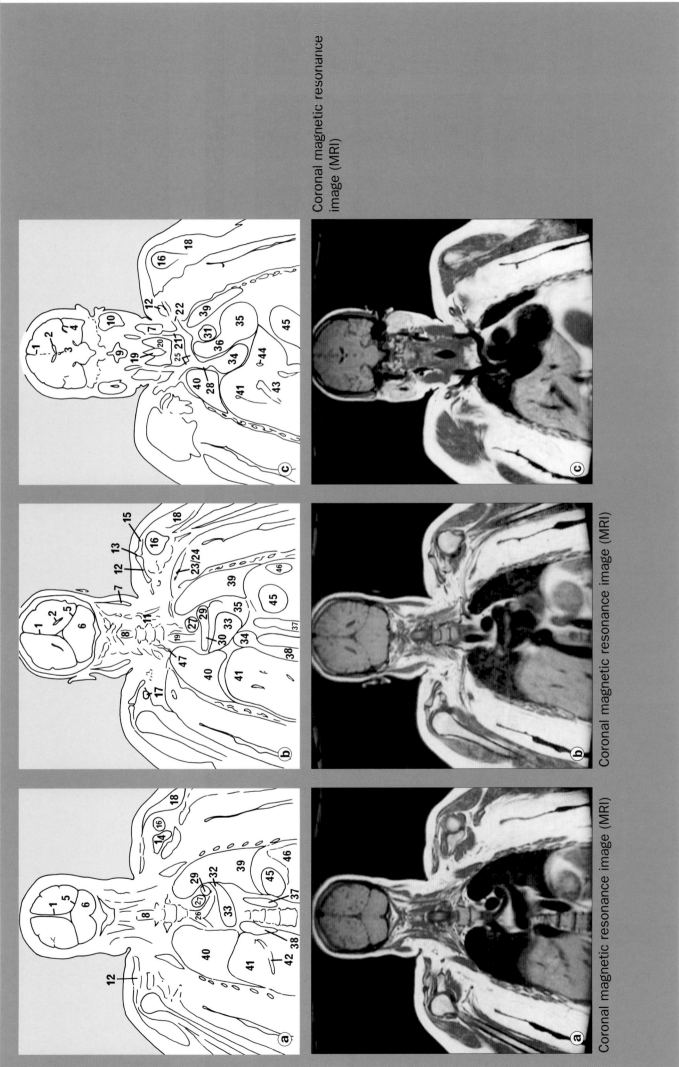

Coronal magnetic resonance image (MRI)

Coronal magnetic resonance image (MRI)

Coronal magnetic resonance image (MRI)

Section level

ABC

Orientation guide

SUPERIOR

LEFT

RIGHT

INFERIOR

1 Falx cerebri
2 Lateral ventricle
3 Third ventricle
4 Lateral sulcus (Sylvian fissure)
5 Tentorium cerebelli
6 Cerebellum
7 Sternocleidomastoid
8 Spinal cord
9 Second cervical vertebra (axis)
10 Parotid gland
11 Scalene muscles
12 Clavicle
13 Acromio-clavicular joint
14 Glenoid fossa of scapula
15 Acromion process of scapula
16 Humeral head
17 Coracoid process of scapula
18 Deltoid
19 Trachea
20 Thyroid gland
21 Internal jugular vein
22 Subclavian vein
23 Axillary vessels
24 Brachial plexus and resulting nerves
25 Brachiocephalic vein
26 Carina (bifurcation of trachea into two main bronchi)
27 Aortic arch
28 Superior vena cava
29 Left pulmonary artery
30 Right pulmonary artery
31 Main pulmonary artery
32 Left superior pulmonary vein
33 Left atrium
34 Right atrium
35 Left ventricle
36 Ascending aorta
37 Descending aorta
38 Inferior vena cava
39 Left lung
40 Right lung
41 Liver
42 Right hepatic vein
43 Middle hepatic vein
44 Left hepatic vein
45 Stomach
46 Spleen
47 Vertebral artery

Notes

These three T1 weighted coronal MR images (a–c: posterior to anterior) are included to show the overall relations of the head, neck, thorax and upper abdomen. Only rarely would such a large field of view be used in clinical practice as the anatomical spatial resolution is inevitably compromised. Of course the exact relations on the coronal plane must depend on the degree of thoracic spine kyphosis, body habitus and degree of inspiration. However the relations in this relatively obese subject are fairly representative.

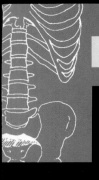

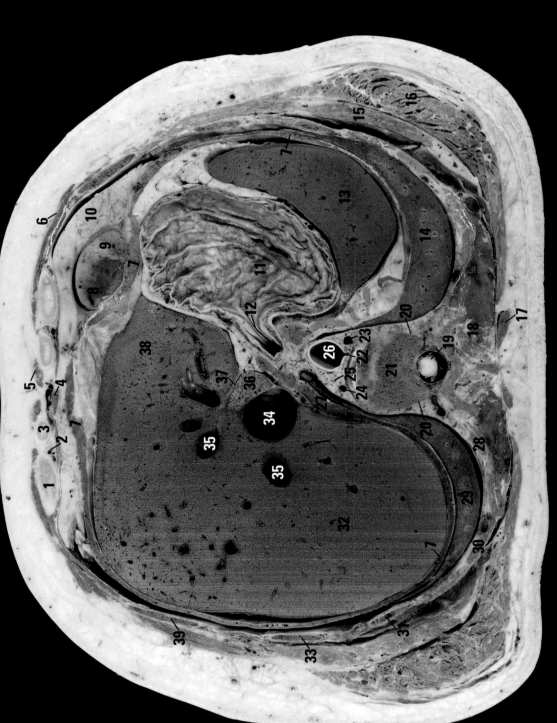

1 Sixth costal cartilage
2 Superior epigastric artery and vein
3 Seventh costal cartilage
4 Xiphoid
5 Rectus abdominis
6 External oblique
7 Diaphragm
8 Right ventricle
9 Left ventricle
10 Extrapericardial fat
11 Fundus of stomach

12 Oesophagogastric junction
13 Spleen
14 Lower lobe of left lung
15 Serratus anterior
16 Latissmus dorsi
17 Trapezius
18 Erector spinae
19 Spinal cord within dural sheath
20 Sympathetic chain
21 Body of tenth thoracic vertebra
22 Origin of intercostal artery

23 Hemiazygos vein
24 Azygos vein
25 Thoracic duct
26 Aorta
27 Right crus of diaphragm
28 Tenth rib
29 Lower lobe of right lung
30 Ninth rib
31 Eighth rib
32 Right lobe of liver
33 Seventh rib

34 Inferior vena cava
35 Hepatic vein
36 Caudate lobe of liver
37 Fissure for ligamentum
      venosum – lesser omentum
38 Left lobe of liver
39 Sixth rib

40 Oesophagus

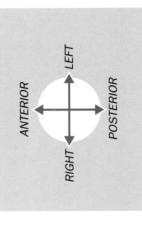

Section level

T10

Orientation guide

ANTERIOR

LEFT

RIGHT

POSTERIOR

Axial computed
tomogram (CT)

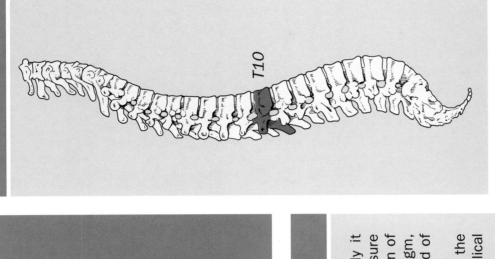

Notes

This section passes through the body of the tenth thoracic vertebra (**21**) and anteriorly transects the xiphoid (**4**).

The oesophagogastric junction (**12**) is seen in longitudinal section. This acts as a physiological sphincter in the prevention of reflux. The fundus of the stomach (**11**) contains air in the erect position but in the supine position is normally full of fluid. It is opaque in the CT image because of the ingested radio-opaque iodinated material.

The lesser omentum is the fold of peritoneum which extends to the liver from the lesser curvature of the stomach and the commencement of the duodenum. Superiorly it attaches to the porta hepatis and to the bottom of the fissure for the ligamentum venosum (**37**). At the cranial margin of this fissure, the lesser omentum reaches the diaphragm, where its two layers separate to surround the lower end of the oesophagus.

The ligamentum venosum is the thrombosed cord of the ductus venosus which, in fetal life, connects the left umbilical vein to the anterior aspect of the inferior vena cava.

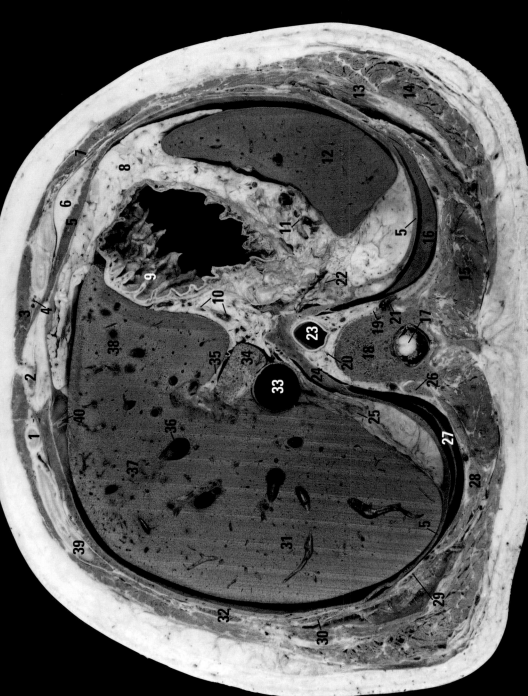

Seventh costal cartilage
Xiphoid
Rectus abdominis
Superior epigastric artery and vein
Diaphragm
Pericardial fat
External oblique
Greater omentum
Body of stomach
Left gastric artery branches
Splenic pedicle
Spleen

13 External oblique
14 Latissimus dorsi
15 Erector spinae
16 Lower lobe of left lung
17 Spinal cord within dural sheath
18 Body of eleventh thoracic vertebra
19 Intercostal artery
20 Thoracic duct
21 Intercostal vein
22 Left suprarenal gland
23 Aorta
24 Right crus of diaphragm

25 Right suprarenal gland
26 Head of eleventh rib
27 Lower lobe of right lung
28 Tenth rib
29 Ninth rib
30 Eighth rib
31 Right lobe of liver
32 Seventh rib
33 Inferior vena cava
34 Caudate lobe of liver
35 Lesser omentum in fissure
   for ligamentum venosum

36 Hepatic vein
37 Left lobe of liver medial segment
38 Left lobe of liver lateral segment
39 Sixth costal cartilage and rib
40 Falciform ligament
41 Portal vein
42 Pancreas
43 Left colic (splenic) flexure
44 Splenic vein
45 Left crus of diaphragm
46 Median arcuate ligament

Section level

T11

Orientation guide

ANTERIOR

LEFT

RIGHT

POSTERIOR

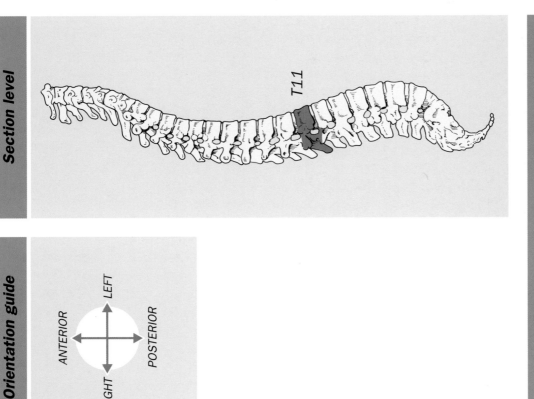

Axial computed tomograms (CTs)

Notes

This section passes through the body of the eleventh thoracic vertebra (**18**) and the xiphoid (**2**).

This is the most caudal section which transects intrathoracic viscera – note the pericardial fat anteriorly (**6**) and the lower lobe of the left lung (**16**).

The suprarenal (adrenal) glands (**22, 25**) have a constant relationship to the diaphragmatic crura (**24, 45**). Note on the CT images that the separate limbs of the suprarenal glands are demarcated.

The right crus of the diaphragm (**24**) on the CT image is often bulky. The crura change shape during respiration; normally they are bulkier on inspiration.

On the CT images the pancreas (**42**) is just visible as it enters the plane of this section. It is better seen in more caudal sections. As the pancreas occupies only part of the section, its outlines are not sharply demarcated. This is another example of the 'partial volume' effect.

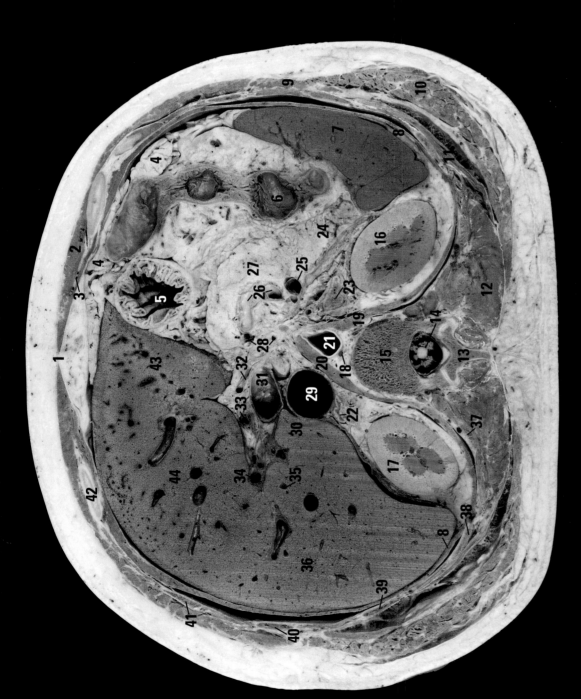

1 Linea alba
2 Rectus abdominis
3 Superior epigastric artery and vein
4 Greater omentum
5 Body of stomach
6 Left colic (splenic) flexure
7 Spleen
8 Diaphragm
9 External oblique
10 Latissimus dorsi
11 Serratus posterior inferior
12 Erector spinae

13 Spine of eleventh thoracic vertebra
14 Conus medullaris surrounded by cauda equina within dural sheath
15 Body of twelfth thoracic vertebra
16 Left kidney
17 Right kidney
18 Thoracic duct
19 Left crus of diaphragm
20 Right crus of diaphragm
21 Aorta
22 Right suprarenal gland

23 Left suprarenal gland
24 Tail of pancreas
25 Splenic vein
26 Splenic artery
27 Body of pancreas
28 Left gastric artery and vein
29 Inferior vena cava
30 Caudate lobe of liver
31 Portal vein
32 Hepatic artery
33 Common bile duct
34 Radicle of portal vein
35 Hepatic artery branch

36 Right lobe of liver
37 Twelfth rib
38 Eleventh rib
39 Tenth rib
40 Ninth rib
41 Eighth rib
42 Seventh costal cartilage
43 Left lobe of liver (lateral segment)
44 Left lobe of liver (medial segment)

45 Gall bladder
46 Ligamentum teres
47 Jejunum

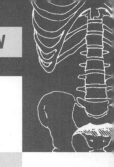

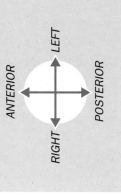

Section level

T12

Orientation guide

ANTERIOR

LEFT

POSTERIOR

RIGHT

Axial computed tomogram (CT)

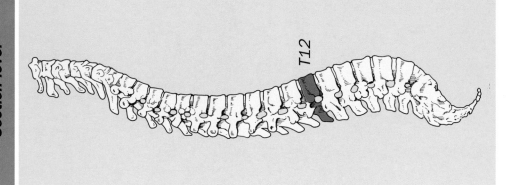

Notes

This section passes through the body of the twelfth thoracic vertebra (**15**). It demonstrates well the relationships of the structures at the porta hepatis – the common bile duct (**33**) anterior and to the right, the hepatic artery (**32**) anterior and to the left and the portal vein (**31**) posterior to these structures. The inferior vena cava (**29**) lies immediately behind the portal vein: between the two is the epiploic foramen, or the aditus to the lesser sac (the foramen of Winslow). The division between the cortex (peripheral) and medulla (central) of the kidneys (**16**, **17**) is well shown: in the plane of this division run the small arcuate vessels which can just be identified in this section. Post mortem changes account for the discrepancy in the differentiation between cortex and medulla in the left kidney.

A Note on the Lobes of the Liver

The gross *anatomical division* of the liver is into a right and left lobe, demarcated by the attachment of the falciform ligament on the anterior surface and by the fissures for the ligamentum teres and ligamentum venosum on its visceral surface. This is simply a gross anatomical descriptive term with no morphological significance. Two subsidiary additional lobes are marked out on the visceral aspect of the liver – the quadrate lobe anteriorly, between the gall bladder fossa and the fissure for the ligamentum teres, and the caudate lobe posteriorly between the groove for the inferior vena cava and the fissure for the ligamentum venosum. The transverse fissure for the porta hepatis separates the quadrate and caudate lobes. The distribution of the right and left branches of the hepatic artery and of the hepatic duct show that the *morphological division* of the liver is into a right and left lobe demarcated by a plane which passes through the fossa of the gall bladder and the fossa of the inferior vena cava (the median plane of the liver). Morphologically, the quadrate lobe and left half of the caudate lobe are part of the morphological left lobe of the liver. Further subdivision into hepatic segments is made by the Couinaud system (segments I–VIII).

128

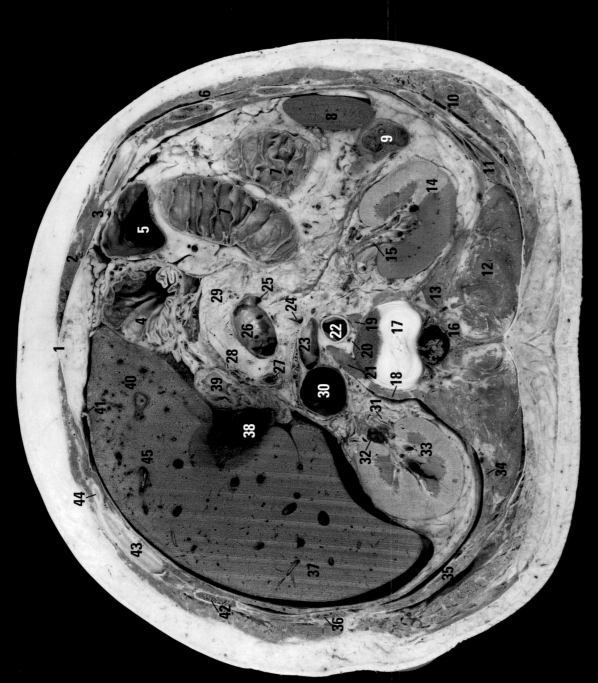

1 Linea alba
2 Rectus abdominis
3 Transversus abdominis
4 Stomach, body/antrum
5 Transverse colon
6 External oblique
7 Jejunum
8 Lower pole of spleen
9 Descending colon
10 Latissimus dorsi
11 Serratus posterior inferior
12 Erector spinae
13 Quadratus lumborum

14 Left kidney
15 Left renal vein (intrarenal portion)
   – *see also* 23
16 Conus medullaris surrounded by
   cauda equina within dural sheath
17 Part of intervertebral disc
   between the twelfth thoracic and
   first lumbar vertebrae with part of
   body of twelfth thoracic vertebra
18 Psoas major
19 Left crus of diaphragm
20 Thoracic duct
21 Right crus of diaphragm

22 Aorta
23 Left renal vein
24 Superior mesenteric artery
25 Splenic vein
26 Portal vein (commencement)
27 Common bile duct
28 Head of pancreas
29 Neck of pancreas
30 Inferior vena cava
31 Right renal artery
32 Right renal vein
33 Right kidney
34 Twelfth rib

35 Eleventh rib
36 Tenth rib
37 Right lobe of liver
38 Gall bladder
39 First part of duodenum (cap)
40 Left lobe of liver (lateral segment)
41 Falciform ligament
42 Ninth rib
43 Eighth costal cartilage
44 Ninth costal cartilage
45 Left lobe of liver (medial
   segment)

46 Right colic (hepatic) flexure

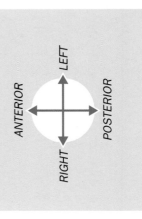

T12–L1

ANTERIOR

LEFT

RIGHT

POSTERIOR

Axial computed tomogram (CT)

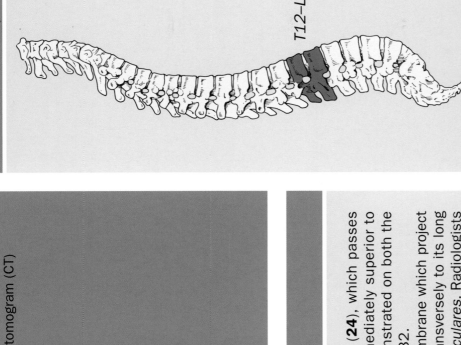

Notes

This section transects the intervertebral disc between the twelfth thoracic and the first lumbar vertebra (**17**). The spinal cord tapers into the conus medullaris (**16**) which terminates, in this subject, at the level of the body of the first lumbar vertebra. The site of termination is variable, the range being from the disc between the twelfth thoracic and first lumbar vertebra to the lower border of the second lumbar vertebra.

The plane of this section passes through the left renal vein (**23**) and demonstrates well the close relationship of this

vein to the superior mesenteric artery (**24**), which passes forward from its aortic origin (**22**) immediately superior to the vein. These features are well demonstrated on both the CT and MRI images, section 5, page 132.

Note the circular folds of mucous membrane which project into the lumen of the small intestine transversely to its long axis (**7**). These are termed the *plicae circulares*. Radiologists and clinicians refer to these as *valvulae conniventes*.

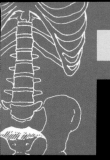

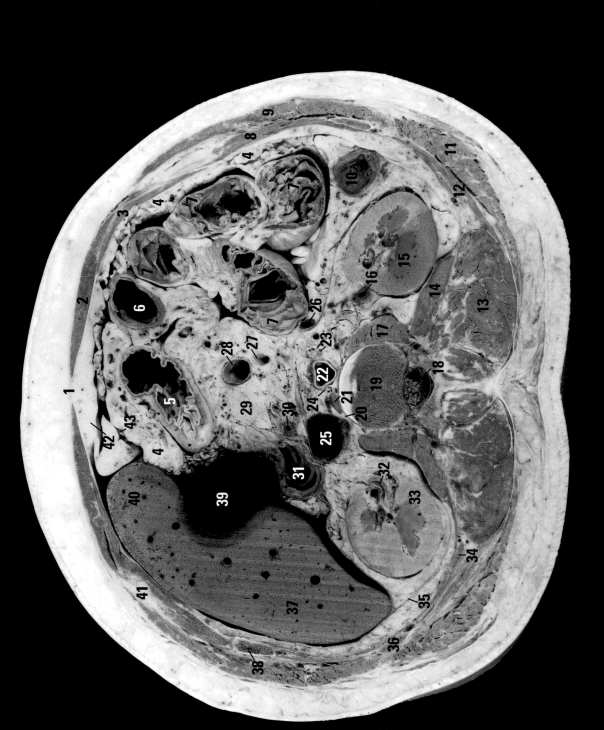

1 Linea alba
2 Rectus abdominis
3 Transversus abdominis
4 Greater omentum
5 Antrum of stomach
6 Transverse colon
7 Jejunum
8 Internal oblique
9 External oblique
10 Descending colon
11 Latissimus dorsi
12 Serratus posterior inferior
13 Erector spinae

14 Quadratus lumborum
15 Left kidney
16 Left ureter
17 Psoas major
18 Cauda equina within dural sheath
19 Body of first lumbar vertebra
   with portion of intervertebral disc
   between the first and second
   lumbar vertebrae
20 Right sympathetic chain
21 Right crus of diaphragm
22 Aorta
23 Para-aortic lymph node

24 Cisterna chyli
25 Inferior vena cava
26 Inferior mesenteric vein
27 Superior mesenteric artery
28 Superior mesenteric vein
29 Head of pancreas
30 Common bile duct
31 Duodenum
32 Commencement of right ureter
33 Right kidney
34 Twelfth rib
35 Renal fascia
36 Eleventh rib

37 Right lobe of liver
38 Tenth rib
39 Gall bladder
40 Left lobe of liver (medial
   segment)
41 Ninth costal cartilage
42 Falciform ligament
43 Left lobe of liver (lateral
   segment)

44 Left renal vein
45 Renal cyst
46 Uncinate process pancreas

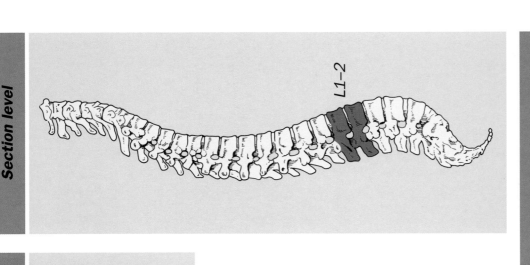

Section level

L1–2

Orientation guide

ANTERIOR

LEFT

RIGHT

POSTERIOR

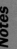

Axial computed tomogram (CT)

Axial magnetic resonance image (MRI)

Notes

This section passes through the body of the first lumbar vertebra (**19**) with a small portion of the intervertebral disc between the first and second lumbar vertebrae.

The kidneys (**15**, **33**) are embedded in a mass of fatty connective tissue termed the perirenal (perinephric) fat, which is thickest at their medial and lateral borders. The fibro-areolar tissue surrounding the kidney and perirenal fat condenses to form a sheath termed the renal fascia (**35**). At the lateral border of the kidney, the two layers of the renal fascia are fused. The anterior layer is carried medially anterior to the kidney and its vessels and merges with the connective tissue anterior to the aorta and inferior vena cava. The posterior layer extends medially in front of the fascia covering quadratus lumborum (**14**)

and psoas major (**17**) and to the vertebrae and intervertebral discs. The perirenal fat and renal fascia (**35**) are surrounded by further retroperitoneal (pararenal) fatty connective tissue. The amount will vary with the relative obesity of the subject.

In this section, a tiny portion of the lateral segment of the left lobe of the liver can be seen (**43**).

132

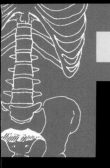

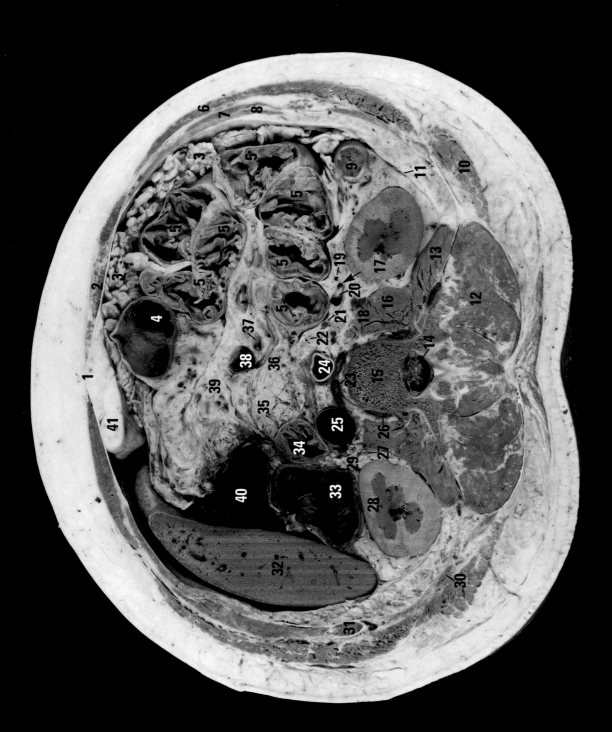

1   Linea alba
2   Rectus abdominis
3   Greater omentum
4   Transverse colon
5   Jejunum
6   External oblique
7   Internal oblique
8   Transversus abdominis
9   Descending colon
10 Latissimus dorsi
11 Renal fascia
12 Erector spinae

13 Quadratus lumborum
14 Cauda equina within dural sheath
15 Body of second lumbar vertebra
16 Psoas major
17 Left kidney
18 Left ureter
19 Left colic artery – ascending branch
20 Inferior mesenteric vein with termi-
    nation of left colic vein (arrowed)
21 Left testicular vein
22 Para-aortic lymph node
23 Left lumbar vein

24 Aorta
25 Inferior vena cava
26 Right lumbar vein
27 Right ureter
28 Right kidney
29 Right testicular vein
30 Twelfth rib
31 Eleventh rib
32 Right lobe of liver
33 Right colic (hepatic) flexure
34 Duodenum second part (with
    ampulla marked with a white bristle)

35 Head of pancreas
36 Uncinate process of pancreas
37 Superior mesenteric artery
38 Superior mesenteric vein
39 Mesentery with mesenteric vessels
40 Gall bladder
41 Falciform ligament

42 Ascending colon
43 Right crus of diaphragm
44 Left renal vein
45 Left renal artery

L2

LEFT

ANTERIOR

POSTERIOR

RIGHT

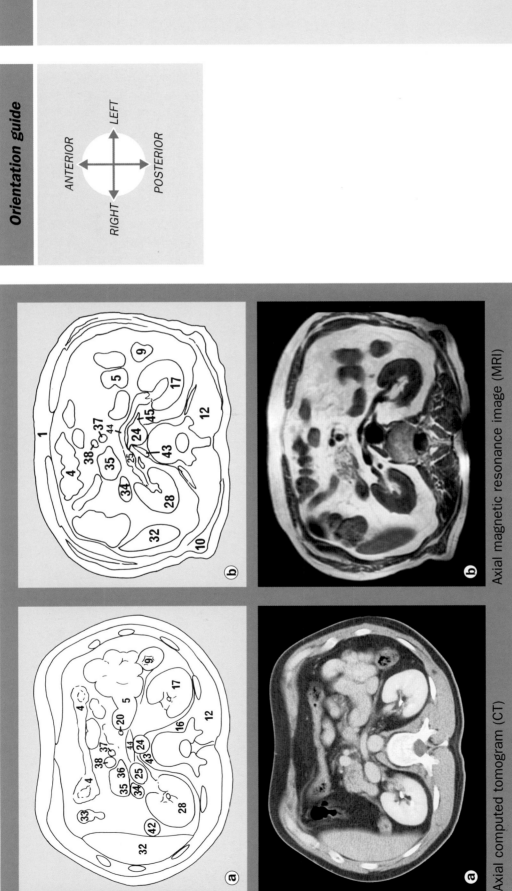

Axial computed tomogram (CT)

Axial magnetic resonance image (MRI)

Notes

This section passes through the body of the second lumbar vertebra (**15**).

The plane of section passes through a prominent left lumbar vein (**23**) as it passes posterior to the aorta (**24**) to drain into the inferior vena cava (**25**). Occasionally it may constitute the principal venous return from the left kidney, when it is termed a retroaortic renal vein.

The right testicular vein (**29**) drains directly into the inferior vena cava, whereas the left testicular vein (**21**) (together with the left suprarenal vein) drains into the left renal vein.

This section passes through the second part of the duodenum (**34**). The orifice of the ampulla of Vater on its papilla is marked with a white bristle.

On both the section and CT image the uncinate process of the pancreas (**36**) is clearly seen. This lies posterior to the superior mesenteric artery and vein (**37**, **38**) and is closely related to the entry point of the left renal vein (**44**) into the inferior vena cava (**25**).

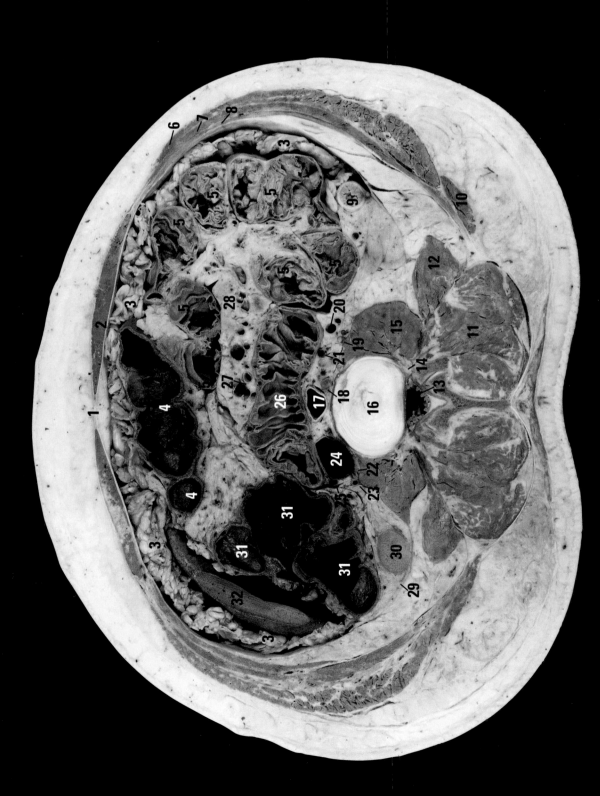

1 Linea alba
2 Rectus abdominis
3 Greater omentum
4 Transverse colon
5 Jejunum
6 External oblique
7 Internal oblique
8 Transversus abdominis
9 Descending colon
10 Latissimus dorsi
11 Erector spinae

12 Quadratus lumborum
13 Cauda equina within dural sheath
14 Root of second lumbar nerve
15 Psoas major
16 Intervertebral disc between the second and third lumbar vertebrae
17 Aorta
18 Para-aortic lymph node
19 Left ureter

20 Inferior mesenteric vein
21 Left testicular artery and vein
22 Right sympathetic chain
23 Right ureter
24 Inferior vena cava
25 Right testicular vein
26 Duodenum third part
27 Superior mesenteric artery and vein
28 Mesentery with mesenteric vessels

29 Renal fascia
30 Right kidney lower pole
31 Ascending colon and right colic (hepatic) flexure
32 Right lobe liver
33 Ascending colon
34 Left kidney
35 Ileum

Section level

L2–3

Orientation guide

ANTERIOR
RIGHT — LEFT
POSTERIOR

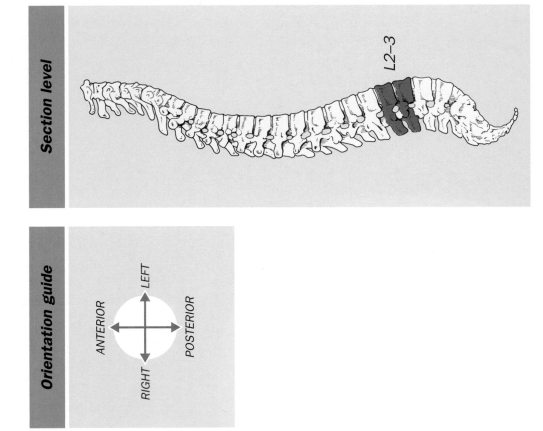

Axial computed tomograms (CTs)

Notes

This section passes through the intervertebral disc between the second and third lumbar vertebrae (**16**). It transects the most caudal part of the right lobe of the liver (**32**). The caudal extent of this lobe is variable and may project downwards in some subjects for a considerable distance as a broad tongue-like process (Riedel's lobe).

Note the third part of the duodenum (**26**) lying in the inverted V between the aorta (**17**) and the superior mesenteric vessels (**27**). Occasionally this produces obstruction of the third part of the duodenum (duodenal ileus).

Clearly seen in this section are the three layers of muscles which constitute the lateral part of the anterior abdominal wall; the external oblique (**6**), internal

oblique (**7**) and transversus abdominis (**8**). Medially, their aponeuroses form the sheath which surrounds the rectus abdominis (**2**). The anterior sheath comprises the aponeurosis of the external oblique together with the split anterior portion of the internal oblique; the posterior sheath is made up of the aponeurosis of the transversus abdominis reinforced by the posterior portion of the internal oblique. Below a line roughly half-way between the umbilicus and the pubis, the posterior sheath is deficient and all three aponeuroses pass in front of rectus to form the anterior sheath. These muscles are well demonstrated on the CT image, section 8, page 138.

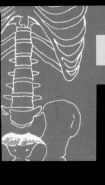

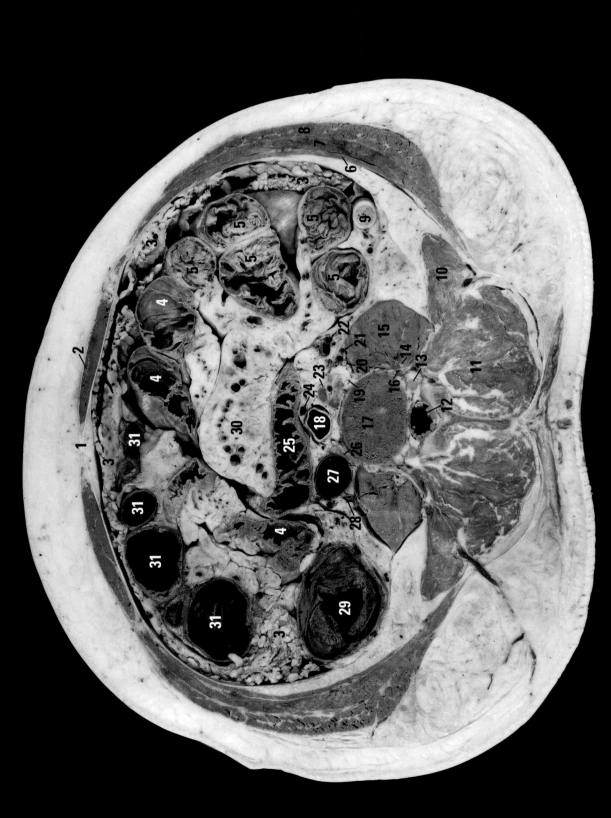

Linea alba
Rectus abdominis
Greater omentum
Ileum
Jejunum
Transversus abdominis
Internal oblique
External oblique
Descending colon

10 Quadratus lumborum
11 Erector spinae
12 Cauda equina within dural
   sheath
13 Dorsal root ganglion of third
   lumbar nerve
14 Ventral ramus of second
   lumbar nerve
15 Psoas major

16 Third lumbar artery
17 Body of third lumbar vertebra
18 Aorta
19 Left sympathetic chain
20 Left ureter
21 Left testicular artery and vein
22 Left colic artery and inferior
   mesenteric vein
23 Para-aortic lymph node

24 Inferior mesenteric artery
25 Duodenum third part
26 Right sympathetic chain
27 Inferior vena cava
28 Right ureter
29 Ascending colon
30 Mesentery with mesenteric
   vessels
31 Transverse colon

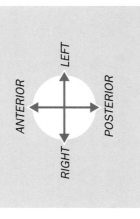

Section level

L3

Orientation guide

ANTERIOR

LEFT

RIGHT

POSTERIOR

Axial computed
tomogram (CT)

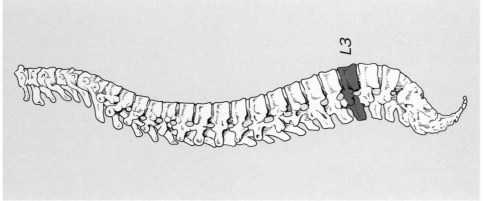

Notes

This section passes through the body of the third lumbar verte-bra (**17**). This is just distal to the origin of the inferior mesen-teric artery (**24**) from the anterior aspect of the aorta (**18**) posterior to the third part of the duodenum (**25**). This section is now caudal to the liver and the kidneys.

The ventral ramus of the second lumbar nerve (**14**) is seen in this section as it passes downwards and laterally into the psoas major (**15**). The first three lumbar nerves and the greater part of the fourth form the lumbar plexus within the posterior part of the psoas major in front of the transverse processes of the lumbar vertebra.

Note the marked disparity between the patulous ascending colon (**29**) and the thick walled narrow descending colon (**9**).

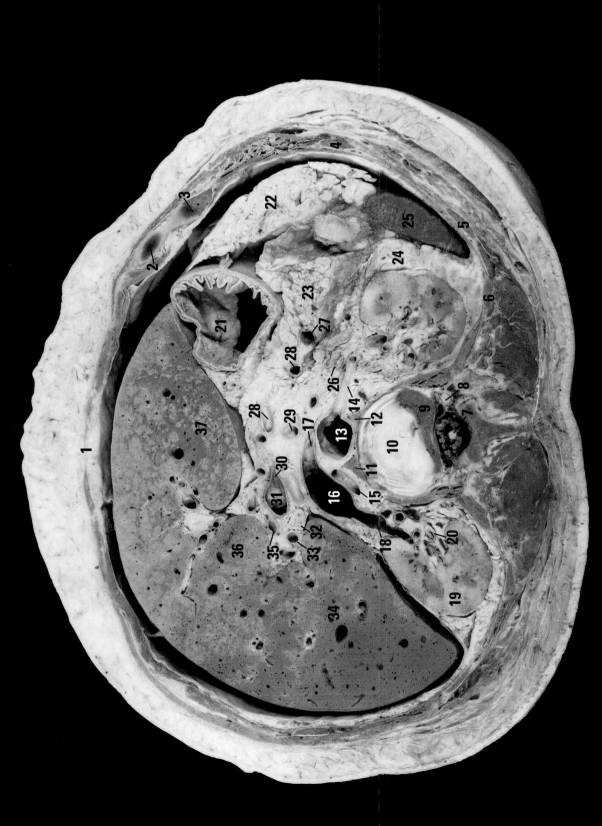

1 Linea alba
2 Eighth costal cartilage
3 Ninth rib/costal cartilage junction
4 Tenth rib
5 Eleventh rib
6 Twelfth rib
7 Cauda equina and termination of spinal cord within dural sheath
8 Dorsal root ganglion of first lumbar nerve
9 Part of body of first lumbar vertebra
10 Part of intervertebral disc between the first and second lumbar vertebrae
11 Right crus of diaphragm
12 Left crus of diaphragm
13 Aorta
14 Left renal artery
15 Right renal artery
16 Inferior vena cava
17 Left renal vein
18 Right renal vein
19 Kidney
20 Right ureter
21 Body of stomach
22 Greater omentum
23 Tail of pancreas
24 Perirenal fat within renal fascia
25 Spleen
26 Left suprarenal gland
27 Splenic vein
28 Splenic artery
29 Superior mesenteric artery
30 Termination of splenic vein
31 Commencement of portal vein
32 Lymph node in porta hepatis
33 Hepatic artery
34 Right lobe of liver
35 Common bile duct
36 Quadrate lobe of medial segment of left lobe of liver
37 Left lobe of liver, lateral segment

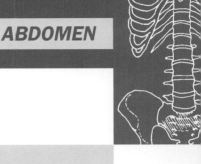

Section level

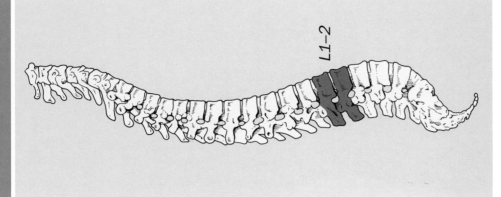

L1–2

Orientation guide

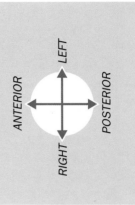

ANTERIOR

LEFT

RIGHT

POSTERIOR

Axial computed
tomogram (CT)

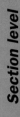

21

13

11

37

36

25

34

Notes

The two sections through the female abdomen (pages 139 & 141), should be compared with the male abdominal sections. There are, of course, wide individual variations in both the sexes, but a comparison of the male and female 'typical' abdomen reveals a greater accumulation of subcutaneous fat in the female in contrast to a higher proportion of intraperitoneal fat in the male subject.

This section passes through the intervertebral disc between the first and second lumbar vertebra.

This section shows well the quadrate lobe of the liver (**36**). Although the common bile duct (**35**) is usually the most anterolateral structure in the free (right) edge of the lesser omentum, variations are common. In this elderly female, the hepatic artery (**33**) is tortuous and thus is unusually lateral. Anomalies of the hepatic artery are common. In around 20% of cases the right hepatic artery derives from the superior mesenteric artery. The left hepatic artery, or an accessory hepatic artery may originate from the left gastric, splenic or superior mesenteric artery. Occasionally, one or other of these vessels derives directly from the aorta.

Note the caudal tip of the left suprarenal gland (**26**), which may extend down to the left renal vein.

140

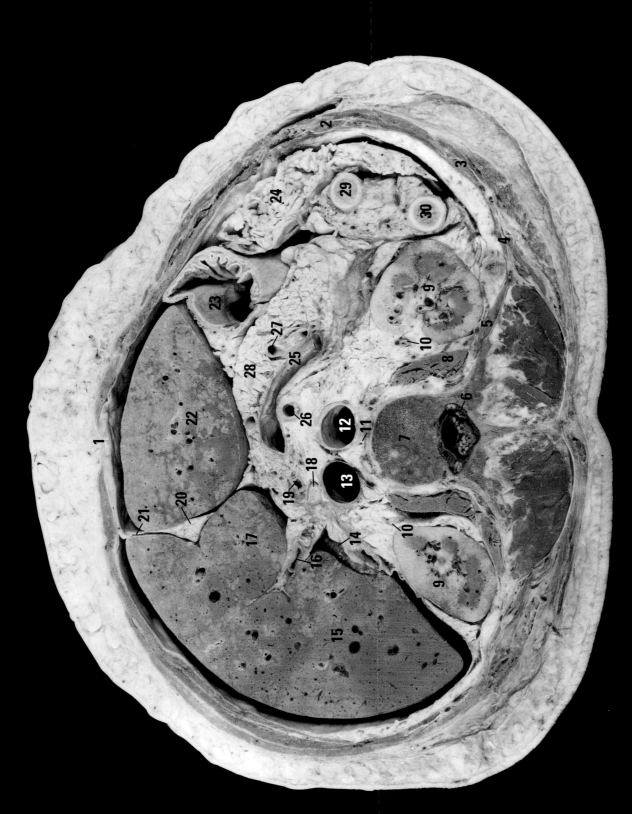

1 Linea alba
2 Tenth rib
3 Eleventh rib
4 Twelfth rib
5 Quadratus lumborum
6 Cauda equina within dural sheath
7 Body of second lumbar vertebra
8 Psoas major
9 Kidney

10 Ureter
11 Cisterna chyli
12 Aorta
13 Inferior vena cava
14 Caudate lobe of liver
15 Right lobe of liver
16 Neck of gall bladder
17 Left lobe of liver (medial segment)

18 Lymph node in porta hepatis
19 Common bile duct
20 Ligamentum teres
21 Falciform ligament
22 Left lobe of liver (lateral segment)
23 Body of stomach
24 Greater omentum
25 Splenic vein

26 Superior mesenteric artery
27 Splenic artery
28 Body of pancreas
29 Transverse colon
30 Descending colon

31 Spleen
32 Right suprarenal gland

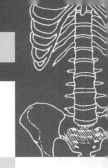

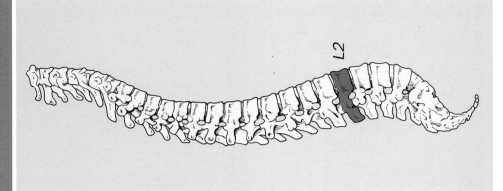

L2

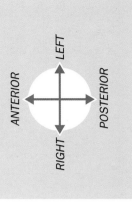

ANTERIOR

LEFT

POSTERIOR

RIGHT

Axial computed
tomogram (CT)

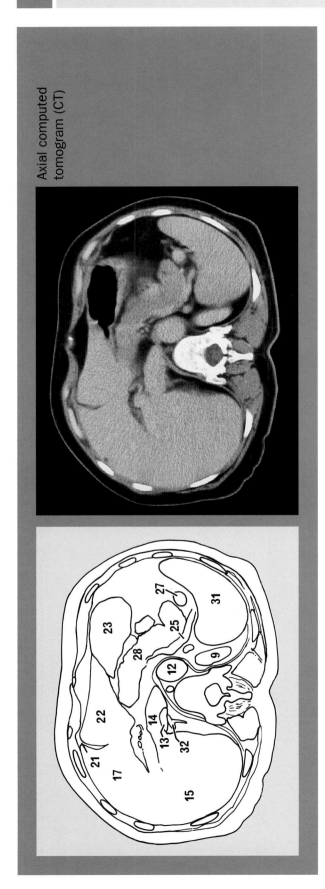

Notes

This section lies just caudal to the left colic (splenic) flexure which joins the transverse colon (**29**) to the descending colon (**30**).

The tip of the papillary process of the caudate lobe of the liver (**14**) can be seen as a separate structure in the gap medial to the right lobe of the liver. The ligamentum teres (**20**) is the fibrotic remnant of the obliterated left umbilical vein.

The falciform ligament divides the morphological left lobe of the liver into a lateral segment (**22**) and medial segment (**17**). The visceral aspect of the medial segment of the left lobe (Couinaud segment IV), between the falciform ligament and the gall bladder bed (**16**) forms the anatomical quadrate lobe.

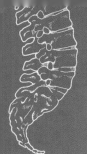

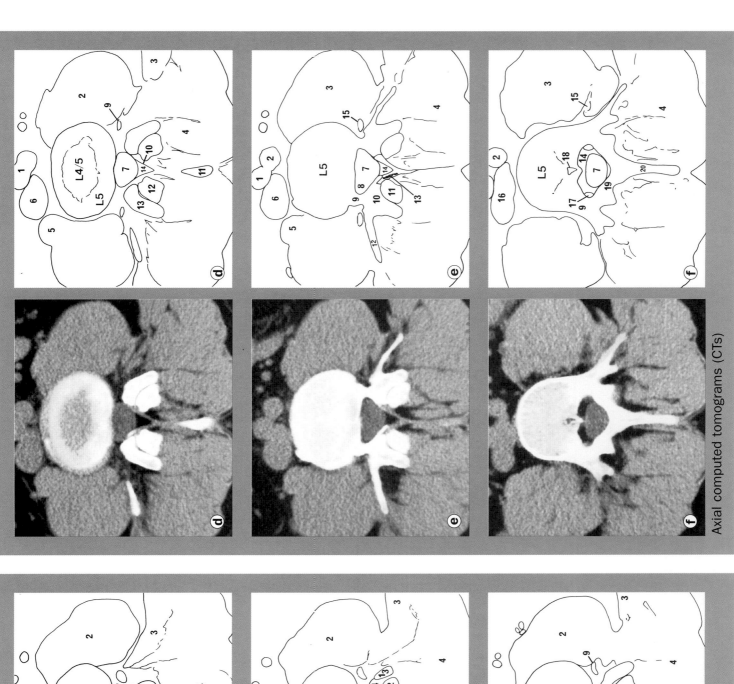

Axial computed tomograms (CTs)

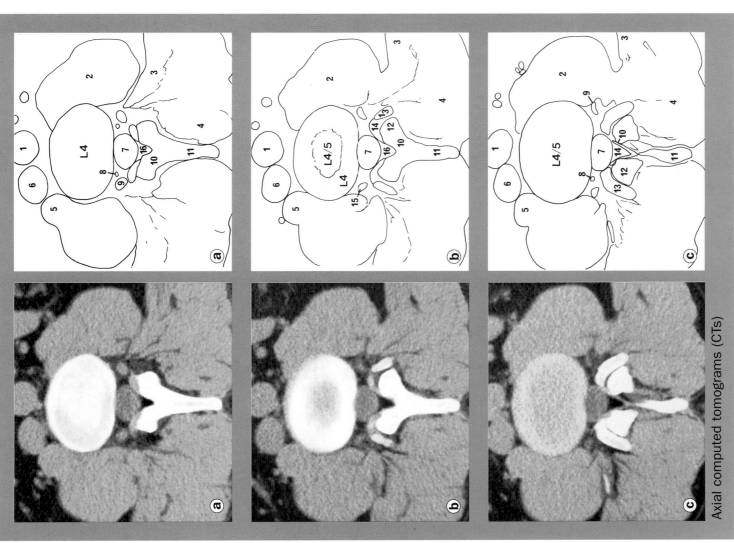

Axial computed tomograms (CTs)

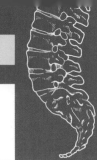

Section level

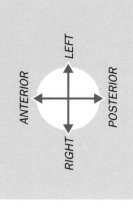

Orientation guide

ANTERIOR
LEFT
RIGHT
POSTERIOR

Images A–B
1 Aorta
2 Psoas major
3 Quadratus lumborum
4 Erector spinae
5 Psoas minor
6 Inferior vena cava
7 Dural sheath
8 Epidural vein
9 Dorsal root ganglion L4 in foramen between L4 and L5
10 Lamina L4
11 Spinous process L4
12 Inferior facet L4
13 Superior facet L5
14 Capsule L4/5 facet joint
15 L4 nerve
16 Epidural fat

Images C–D
1 Aortic bifurcation
2 Psoas major
3 Quadratus lumborum
4 Erector spinae
5 Psoas minor
6 Inferior vena cava
7 Dural sheath
8 Epidural vein
9 Ventral ramus L4
10 Flaval ligament
11 Spinous process L4
12 Inferior facet L4
13 Superior facet L5
14 Epidural fat

Images E–F
1 Right common iliac artery
2 Left common iliac artery
3 Psoas major
4 Erector spinae
5 Psoas minor
6 Inferior vena cava
7 Dural sheath
8 Pouch for L5 root
9 Pedicle L5
10 Superior facet L5
11 Inferior facet L4
12 Transverse process of L5
13 Flaval ligament
14 Epidural fat
15 Ventral ramus L4
16 Confluence of common iliac veins
17 L5 nerve root sheath
18 Basivertebral vein
19 Lamina L5
20 Spinous process L5

Notes

Images A–B
This series of six computed tomograms (a–f) demonstrates the key anatomical features of a craniocaudal segment of the lumbar spine. Although all the features can also be demonstrated by Magnetic Resonance Imaging (MRI), which is now the preferred test, Computed Tomography (CT) is perhaps easier to understand: bone appears white, soft tissues appear grey and fat black.

Image (a) traverses the slightly sclerotic endplate of L4. The L4 dorsal root ganglion (**9**) lies in the foramen, immediately caudal to the L4 pedicle.

Note how the dorsal root ganglion is clearly demarcated by normal epidural fat.

Images C–D
Image (c) traverses the L4/5 disc. Note that the posterior aspect of the disc is concave with respect to the dural sheath (**7**). A normal disc at this anatomical level either has a concave or flat interface with the sheath. A convex disc here is indicative

of an annular bulge. Note how the L4 ventral ramus (**9**) is now heading towards the psoas muscle in which the lumbar plexus is formed. The dorsal ramus is too small to be resolved by CT; it would pass just lateral to the superior facet of L5.

Image (d) shows a portion of the L5 endplate surrounding the inferior aspect of the L4/5 disc.

Images E–F
Image (e) transects the sclerotic endplate of L5. The flaval ligaments (**13**) running from the L4 to L5 laminae are well shown. Surgeons can now often operate through small openings in the flaval ligaments without the full laminectomy which used to be the standard approach for spinal surgery.

Image (f) passes through the body of the L5 vertebra – the normal bony architecture can be appreciated. The veins running through the vetebral body converge on the basivertebral vein (**18**) which has a small bony hood guarding its passage so that venous blood passes to the epidural veins see (8 image c). The right L5 root sheath (**17**) hugs the medial aspect of the pedicle (**9**).

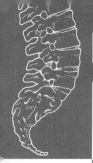

Coronal magnetic resonance image (MRI)

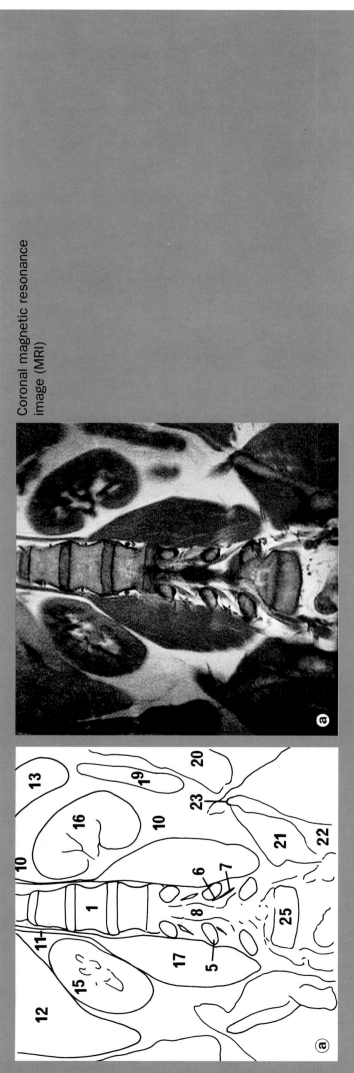

Coronal magnetic resonance image (MRI)

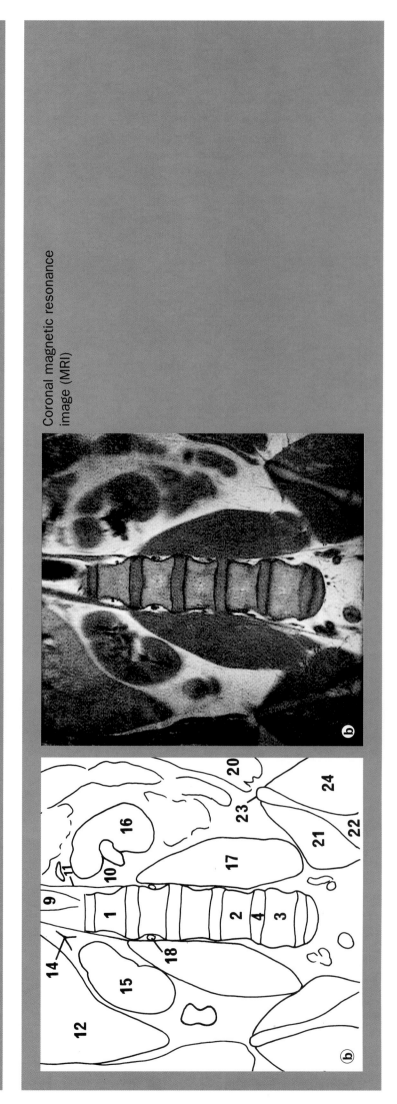

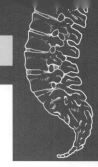

Section level

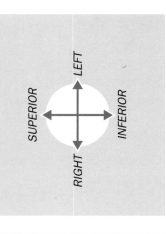

Orientation guide

SUPERIOR

LEFT

RIGHT

INFERIOR

Images A–B

1 L1 vertebral body
2 L4 vertebral body
3 L5 vertebral body
4 L4/5 intervertebral disc
5 Pedicle
6 Nerve root sheath L4
7 Dorsal root ganglion L4
8 Thecal sac
9 Aorta
10 Retroperitoneal fat
11 Crus of diaphragm
12 Liver
13 Spleen
14 Right suprarenal gland
15 Right kidney
16 Left kidney
17 Psoas
18 Lumbar vein
19 Descending colon
20 Anterior abdominal
    wall musculature
21 Iliacus
22 Ilium
23 Iliac crest
24 Gluteal muscles
25 S1 vertebral body

Notes

Images A–B

Two coronal T1 weighted images elegantly show the relationship of the lumbar spine to the psoas muscles and kidneys (within retroperitoneal fat). Note that the kidneys lie in an oblique orientation, aligned to the lateral margins of the psoas muscles; thus the upper poles lie in a more medial sagittal plane that the lower poles. Because of the lumbar lordosis, the upper poles lie in a more posterior coronal plane that the lower poles.

Because of the lumbar lordosis, the thecal sac and emerging nerve root sheaths can be seen in the L4 region while vertebral bodies are demonstrated more superiorly and inferiorly. Note the way in which each nerve root sheath hugs the medial and inferior aspect of its associated pedicle (L4 root inferomedial to the L4 pedicle). The expansion for the dorsal root ganglion can just be appreciated. The fairly constant relationship of the L4/5 disc space with the level of the superior iliac crest is well shown: this is particularly useful in patients with lumbosacral anomalies (around 25% of people).

Also apparent are the segmental lumbar veins which drain blood from the epidural veins. These run anteriorly within an important, but narrow, fat plane alongside each vertebral body.

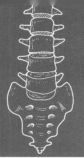

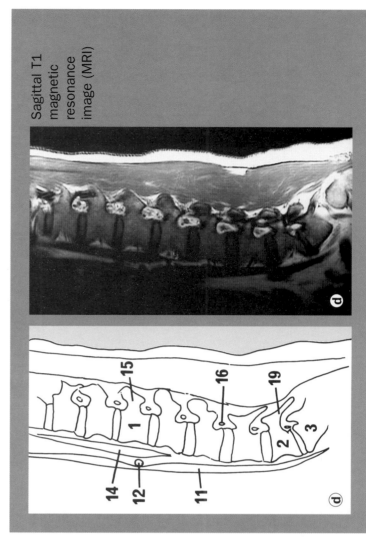

Sagittal T2 magnetic resonance image (MRI)

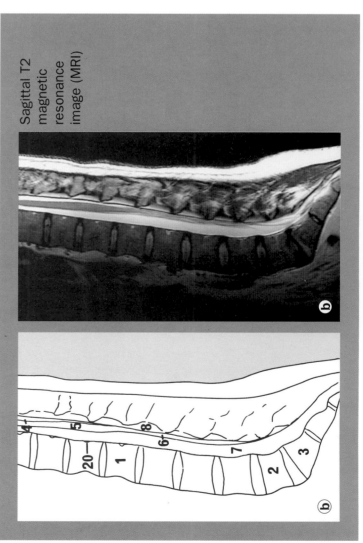

Sagittal T1 magnetic resonance image (MRI)

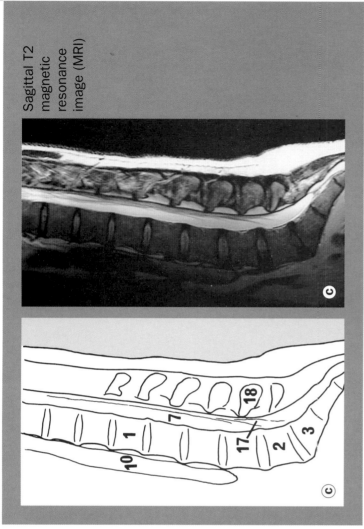

Sagittal T1 magnetic resonance image (MRI)

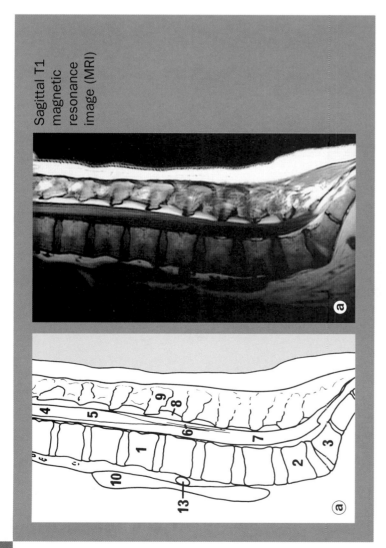

Sagittal T2 magnetic resonance image (MRI)

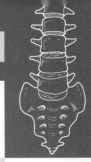

Section level

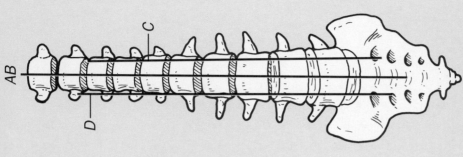

Orientation guide

POSTERIOR

SUPERIOR · INFERIOR

ANTERIOR

Images A–D

1 L1 vertebral body
2 L5 vertebral body
3 S1 vertebral body
4 Spinal cord
5 Conus medullaris
6 Cauda equina
7 Cerebrospinal fluid within thecal sac
8 Epidural fat
9 Spinous process L1
10 Aorta
11 Inferior vena cava
12 Right renal artery
13 Retroaortic left renal vein
14 Crus of diaphragm
15 Pedicle of L1 vertebra
16 L3 nerve root sheath/dorsal root ganglion
17 Nerve roots within cerebrospinal fluid
18 Spinous process L4
19 Pars interarticularis L5
20 Basivertebral vein

Notes

Images A–B

These midline sagittal MR images are of key importance in evaluating the lumbar spine (one of the commonest anatomical sites examined by MRI).

The antero-posterior diameter of the spinal canal can be readily assessed; this normally measures around 15mm from the posterior aspect of the vertebral body to the anterior aspect of the laminar arch; values under 11.5 mm indicate a degree of spinal stenosis. The height of the disc spaces can be evaluated, as can the degree of hydration within. The normal disk space yields high signal intensity on T2 weighting (image b); a degenerate disc returns low signal intensity and becomes narrower. In these images the L5/S1 disc is slightly degenerate, as judged by the slight reduction of signal. There is slight increase in fat content in the superior portion of S1 vertebral body, suggesting a long standing disc abnormality.

These sagittal images also clearly demonstrate the slight expansion of the distal cord at the T12/L1 level (the conus medullaris). The collection of nerve roots which forms the cauda equina (the horse's tail) is well seen posteriorly within the canal when the patient lies supine (as during MRI). Because normal roots move freely within the CSF, lumbar puncture is generally a very safe procedure at any level caudal to the conus medullaris.

Image C

A T2 weighted MR image about 10mm to the left of the median sagittal plane shown in the two previous (a & b) images. Here the segmental roots can be seen traversing the cerebrospinal fluid towards their respective nerve root sheaths and exit foramina. The aorta can just be seen anterior to the vertebral bodies.

Image D

A T1 weighted sagittal MR image even more lateral than the previous (c) image. However this is to the right of the midline as the right renal artery can be seen passing anterior to the diaphragmatic crus and posterior to the IVC. This plane shows the exit foramina at several segmental levels. The classical shape has been said to resemble that of the human ear. The pedicles of two adjacent vertebral bodies form the superior and inferior boundaries of the foramen. The anterior margin is formed by the vertebral body superiorly and the posterolateral portion of the intervertebral disk inferiorly. Posteriorly lie the pars interarticularis, the flaval ligament and facet joint.

Narrowing of the disc space and degenerative changes in the facet joints will reduce the capacity of the foramen; the flaval ligament gets thicker as the disk space narrows; all these changes can contribute to nerve root compression.

The nerve root sheaths, dorsal root ganglion and segmental nerve lie in the superior portion of the foramen. There are commonly two epidural veins in each foramen; a superior one between the nerve root and the body/pedicle; the second usually lies much more caudally within the foramen. Remember that in the lumbar (and thoracic and sacral) spine the segmental nerve root escapes caudal to its numbered vertebral body. For example the L5 nerve root escapes caudal to the L5 pedicle through the L5/S1 foramen. Although the L5 root can be affected by a lateral L5/S1 disc herniation or facet joint degeneration, it will much more commonly be affected by a more central herniation at the L4/5 level.

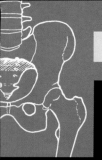

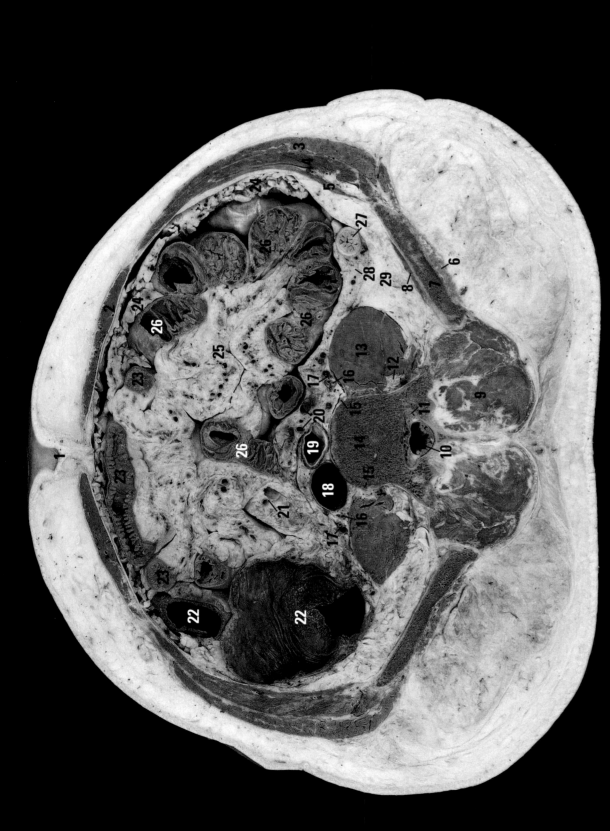

1 Umbilicus
2 Rectus abdominis
3 External oblique
4 Internal oblique
5 Transversus abdominis
6 Gluteus medius
7 Ilium
8 Iliacus
9 Erector spinae
10 Cauda equina within dural sheath

11 Dorsal root ganglion of fourth lumbar nerve
12 Ventral ramus of third lumbar nerve
13 Psoas major
14 Body of fourth lumbar vertebra
15 Lumbar sympathetic chain
16 Ureter
17 Testicular artery and vein
18 Inferior vena cava

19 Aorta
20 Inferior mesenteric artery and vein
21 Right colic artery and vein
22 Ascending colon
23 Jejunum
24 Greater omentum
25 Mesentery of small intestine
26 Ileum
27 Descending colon

28 Anterior pararenal fat of retroperitoneum
29 Posterior pararenal fat of retroperitoneum
30 Appendix vermiformis

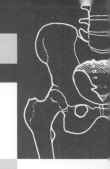

Section level

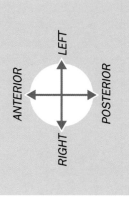

L4

Orientation guide

ANTERIOR

LEFT

POSTERIOR

RIGHT

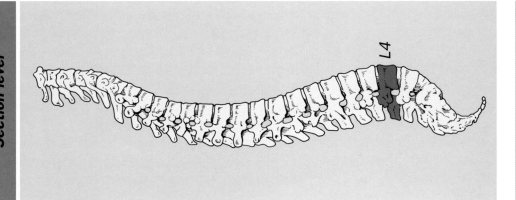

Axial computed tomogram (CT)

Notes

This section passes through the body of the fourth lumbar vertebra (**14**), the cranial portion of the iliac crests (**7**) and the umbilicus (**1**). There are quite wide individual variations in these landmarks; however the umbilicus is usually at the L3/4 intervertebral disc level and the iliac crest at the level of L4.

The inferior mesenteric artery (**20**) has just arisen from the aorta at the level of the third lumbar vertebra. More caudally, it will give rise to the superior rectal artery (see section 2, page 151). The accompanying inferior mesenteric vein (**20**) has a long ascending retroperitoneal course to enter the splenic vein.

The aorta (**19**) is commencing to bifurcate on both the section and the CT image.

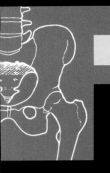

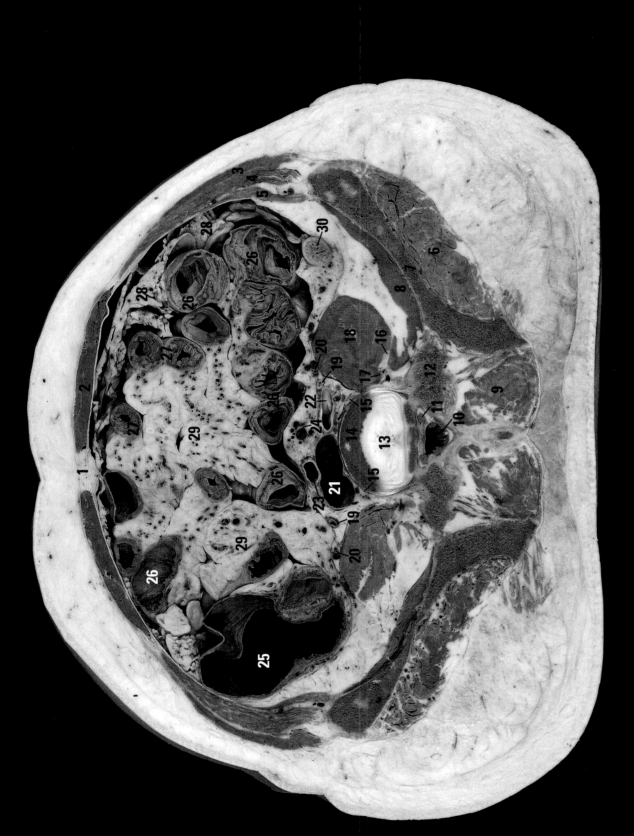

1 Linea alba
2 Rectus abdominis
3 External oblique
4 Internal oblique
5 Transversus abdominis
6 Gluteus medius
7 Ilium
8 Iliacus
9 Erector spinae

10 Cauda equina within dural sheath
11 Root of the fifth lumbar nerve
12 Transverse process of fifth lumbar vertebra
13 Part of intervertebral disc between the fourth and fifth lumbar vertebrae
14 Part of body of fourth lumbar vertebra

15 Lumbar sympathetic chain
16 Femoral nerve
17 Obturator nerve
18 Psoas major
19 Ureter
20 Testicular artery and vein
21 Inferior vena cava at origin
22 Left common iliac artery
23 Right common iliac artery

24 Superior rectal artery and vein
25 Ascending colon
26 Ileum
27 Jejunum
28 Greater omentum
29 Mesentery of small bowel
30 Descending colon

31 Appendix vermiformis

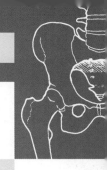

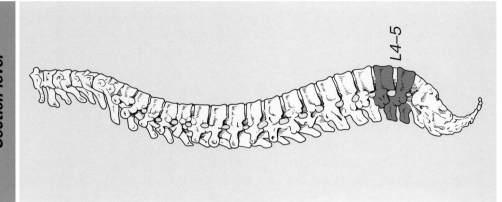

L4–5

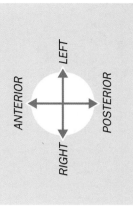

ANTERIOR

LEFT

RIGHT

POSTERIOR

Axial computed tomogram (CT)

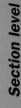

Notes

This section transects the intervertebral disc between the fourth and fifth lumbar vertebra (**13**).

The lumbar sympathetic chain (**15**) is well visualized as it lies on the fourth lumbar vertebral body (**14**); it is overlapped on the right by the inferior vena cava (**21**) and by the common iliac artery on the left (**22**). More cranially on the left it lies just lateral to the aorta, as can be seen in section 1, page 149.

The transverse processes of the fifth lumbar vertebra (**12**) are bulky and all but reach the sacrum, particularly (in this subject) on the left side. Reference to section 3, page 153,

shows that there is partial sacralisation of L5, a very common variation.

The superior rectal artery (**24**) is the continuation of the inferior mesenteric artery after this has given off its left colic branch (see section 1, page 149).

The inferior vena cava (**21**) is seen at its commencement and its oval shape in the section (more markedly oval in the CT image) is produced by the convergence of the two common iliac veins at this level.

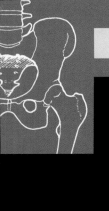

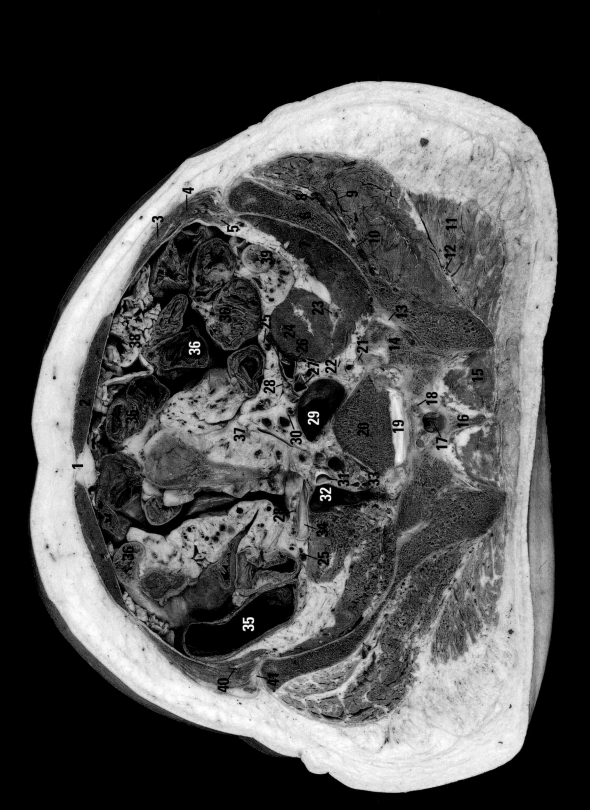

1 Linea alba
2 Rectus abdominis
3 External oblique
4 Internal oblique
5 Transversus abdominis
6 Ilium
7 Iliacus
8 Gluteus minimus
9 Gluteus medius
10 Superior gluteal artery vein
    and nerve (see also 31)
11 Gluteus maximus
12 Inferior gluteal artery
    vein and nerve

13 Sacro-iliac joint
14 Lateral mass of sacrum
15 Erector spinae
16 Spine of first segment of sacrum
17 Cauda equina within dural sheath
18 Root of first sacral nerve
19 Part of lumbosacral disc
20 Part of body of fifth lumbar
    vertebra
21 Ventral ramus of fifth lumbar
    nerve
22 Obturator nerve
23 Femoral nerve
24 Psoas major

25 Testicular artery and vein
26 Left external iliac artery
27 Left internal iliac artery
28 Ureter
29 Left common iliac vein
30 Superior rectal artery
    and vein
31 Superior gluteal artery and
    vein within pelvis
32 Right common iliac vein
33 Right internal iliac vein
34 Right common iliac artery
    at bifurcation
35 Ascending colon

36 Ileum
37 Mesentery of small bowel
38 Greater omentum
39 Descending colon
40 Iliohypogastric nerve
41 Ilio-inguinal nerve with
    deep circumflex iliac artery
    and vein
42 Left external iliac vein
43 Left internal iliac vein

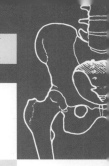

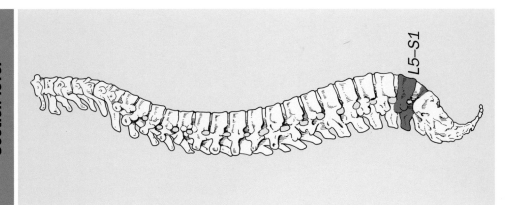

L5–S1

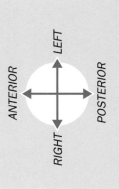

ANTERIOR
LEFT
RIGHT
POSTERIOR

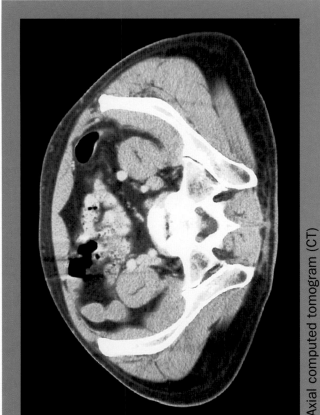

Axial computed tomogram (CT)

Notes

This section traverses the sacro-iliac joint (**13**), the lumbosacral disc (**19**) and a lower part of the body of the fifth lumbar vertebra (**20**). There is some asymmetry of the lateral mass of the sacrum (**14**) in this subject, the left side being larger. This is because there is a small articulation (which is just visible) between the left sacral mass and the 'sacralized' left L5 transverse process (see also section 2, page 151). These variations are very common.

An intravenous injection of contrast medium was given before the CT image series, hence the opacification of the blood vessels.

The superior gluteal vessels (**31**) arise from the internal iliac vessels. Together with the superior gluteal nerve (**10**), they emerge from the pelvis through the greater sciatic foramen *above* piriformis, then run between, and supply, gluteus medius (**9**) and gluteus minimus (**8**). The inferior gluteal artery, vein and nerve (**12**) emerge *below* piriformis and supply gluteus maximus (**11**).

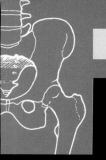

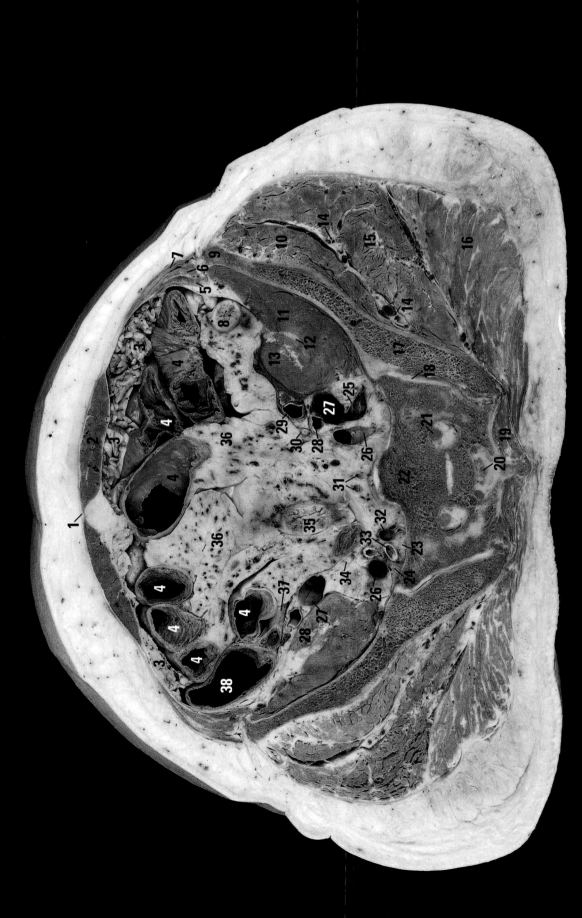

Linea alba
Rectus abdominis
Greater omentum
Ileum
Transversus abdominis
Internal oblique
External oblique aponeurosis
Descending colon
Anterior superior iliac spine
Gluteus minimus

11 Iliacus
12 Femoral nerve
13 Psoas major
14 Superior gluteal artery
   and vein
15 Gluteus medius
16 Gluteus maximus
17 Ilium
18 Sacro-iliac joint
19 Erector spinae

20 Filum terminale within
   sacral canal
21 Second sacral nerve root
22 Sacrum second segment
23 Lumbosacral trunk
24 Obturator nerve
25 Iliolumbar vein
26 Internal iliac vein
27 External iliac vein
28 Internal iliac artery

29 External iliac artery
30 Left ureter
31 Median sacral artery and vein
32 Superior gluteal vein
33 Superior gluteal artery
34 Right ureter
35 Sigmoid colon
36 Mesentery of ileum
37 Appendix vermiformis
38 Caecum

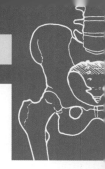

Section level

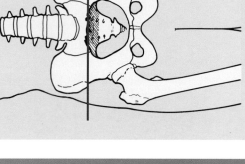
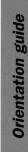
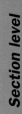

S2

Orientation guide

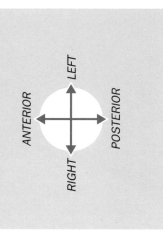

ANTERIOR

LEFT

RIGHT

POSTERIOR

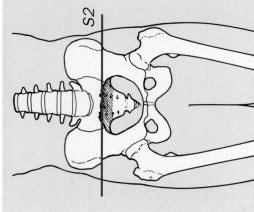

Axial computed tomogram (CT)

Notes

This section transects the second segment of the sacrum (**22**). Note that in this section the gluteal muscles on the right side are smaller and paler than on the left (**10**, **15**, **16**). This subject had suffered a cerebrovascular accident which resulted in a right-sided paresis.

The appendix vermiformis (**37**) lies posterior to the ileum (**4**) in this section – the retro-ileal position. Much more commonly

the post mortem appendix lies behind the caecum (in about 65% of cases) or descends into the pelvis (30% of cases) (see CT image, section 1, page 150 & CT image, section 2, page 152). The superior gluteal vessels in their pelvic (**32**, **33**) and gluteal (**14**) course are again clearly demonstrated (see section 3, page 153).

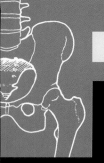

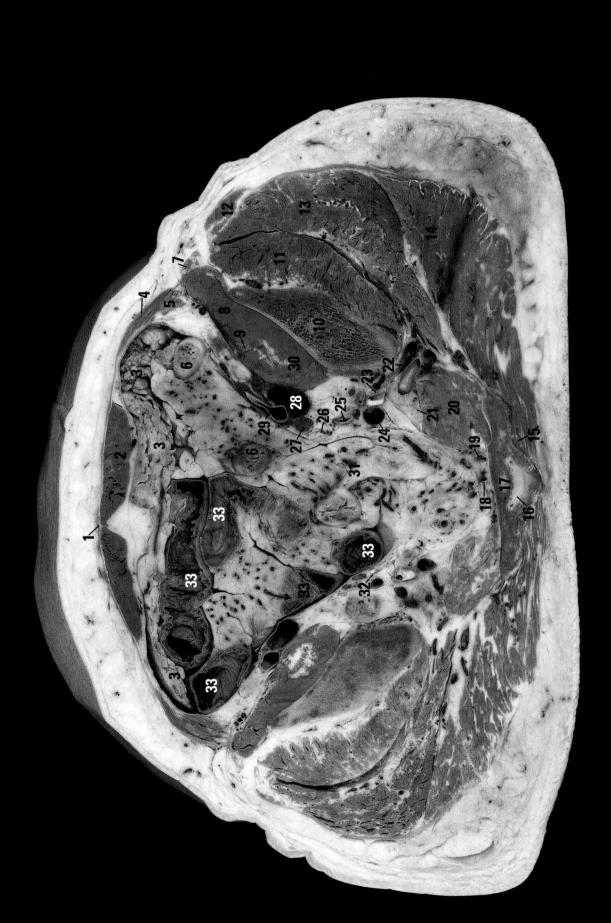

1 Linea alba
2 Rectus abdominis
3 Greater omentum
4 Internal oblique
5 Transversus abdominis
6 Sigmoid colon
7 Sartorius
8 Iliacus
9 Femoral nerve
10 Ilium

11 Gluteus minimus
12 Tensor fasciae latae
13 Gluteus medius
14 Gluteus maximus
15 Erector spinae
16 Sacral canal
17 Sacrum third segment
18 Median sacral artery and vein
19 Lateral sacral artery and vein
20 Piriformis

21 Sciatic nerve
22 Superior gluteal artery and vein
23 Obturator artery and vein
24 Internal iliac vein
25 Internal iliac artery
26 Left ureter
27 Lymph node
28 External iliac vein
29 External iliac artery

30 Psoas major
31 Sigmoid mesocolon
32 Right ureter
33 Ileum

34 Bladder
35 Vas deferens
36 Inferior epigastric artery

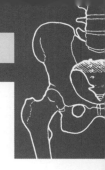

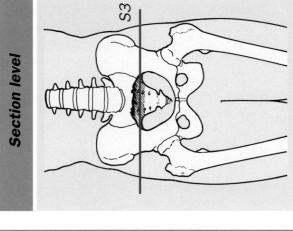

S3

ANTERIOR · LEFT · POSTERIOR · RIGHT

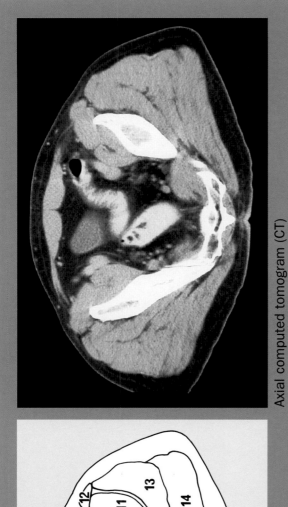

Axial computed tomogram (CT)

Notes

This section passes through the sacrum at its third segment (**17**). Piriformis (**20**) arises from the front of the sacrum by three digitations, attached to the portions of bone between the pelvic sacral foramina and also to the grooves leading laterally from these foramina. The superior gluteal vessels (**22**), together with the superior gluteal nerve, pass above piriformis through the greater sciatic foramen. In this subject, piriformis is paler and less bulky on the right side than on the left as a result of a previous cerebrovascular accident (see section 4). Piriformis is a bulky muscle which must be traversed when using the greater sciatic foramen as a route for percutaneous pelvic aspiration. On the CT image there is asymmetry of the piriformis muscles due to a degree of scoliosis. The ureter (**26**) descends into the pelvis characteristically immediately anterior to the internal iliac artery (**25**). It lies immediately deep to the pelvic peritoneum, crossed only by the vas deferens, which is seen in section 6, page 159.

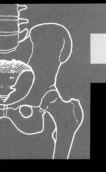

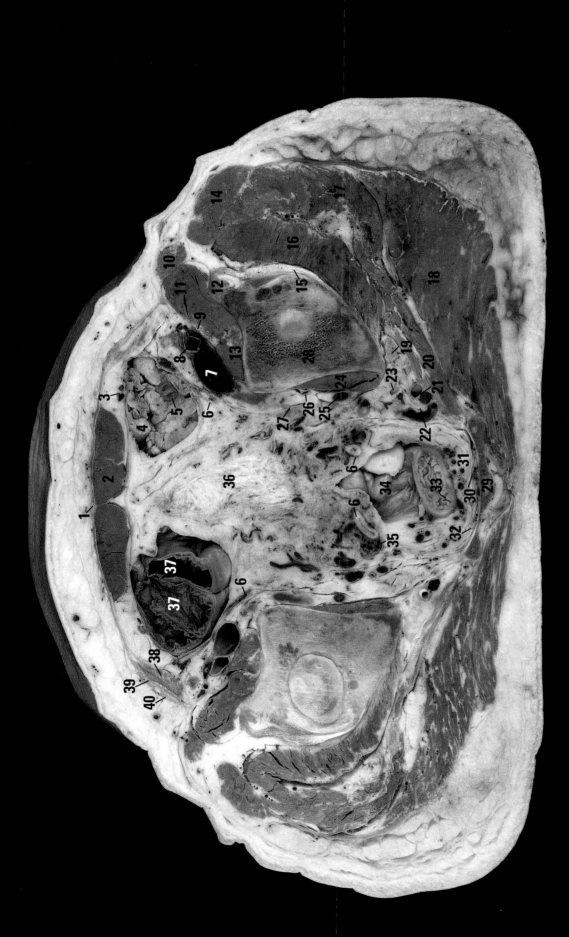

1 Linea alba
2 Rectus abdominis
3 Inferior epigastric artery
   and vein
4 Greater omentum
5 Sigmoid colon
6 Vas deferens
7 External iliac vein
8 External iliac artery
9 Femoral nerve
10 Sartorius
11 Iliacus

12 Rectus femoris straight
    head tendon
13 Psoas major and tendon
14 Tensor fasciae latae
15 Iliofemoral ligament
16 Gluteus minimus
17 Gluteus medius
18 Gluteus maximus
19 Sciatic nerve
20 Piriformis
21 Inferior gluteal artery and vein
22 Pudendal nerve

23 Internal pudendal artery
24 Obturator internus
25 Obturator vein
26 Obturator artery
27 Obturator nerve
28 Acetabulum (ilial portion)
29 Sacrum fourth segment
30 Median sacral artery and vein
31 Superior rectal artery and vein
32 Lateral sacral artery and vein
33 Rectum
34 Rectosigmoid junction

35 Seminal vesicle
36 Fundus of bladder
37 Ileum
38 Transversus abdominis
39 Internal oblique
40 External oblique

41 Perirectal fat
42 Pararectal fat (with branches of
    internal iliac artery and vein)
43 Perirectal fascia

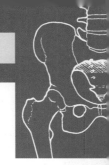

Section level

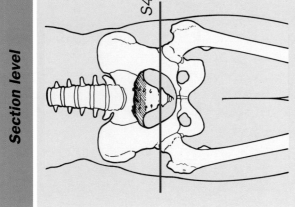

S4

Orientation guide

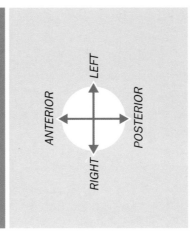

LEFT
ANTERIOR
POSTERIOR
RIGHT

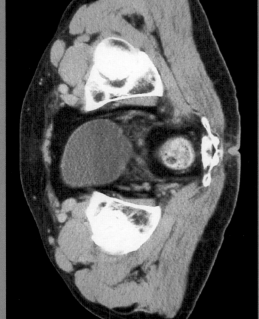

Axial computed tomogram (CT)

Notes

This section passes through the fourth segment of the sacrum (**29**), the superior portion of the acetabulum (**28**) and the fundus of the bladder (**36**).

The rectum (**33**) lies immediately in front of the sacrum, separated from it by the median sacral vessels (**30**). It commences just cranial to this line of section on the third sacral segment. The rectosigmoid junction is also seen (**34**).

The vas deferens (**6**) is the most medial structure crossing the side wall of the pelvis immediately deep to the pelvic peritoneum. More caudally it will join the seminal vesicle (**35**) to form the ejaculatory duct.

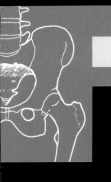

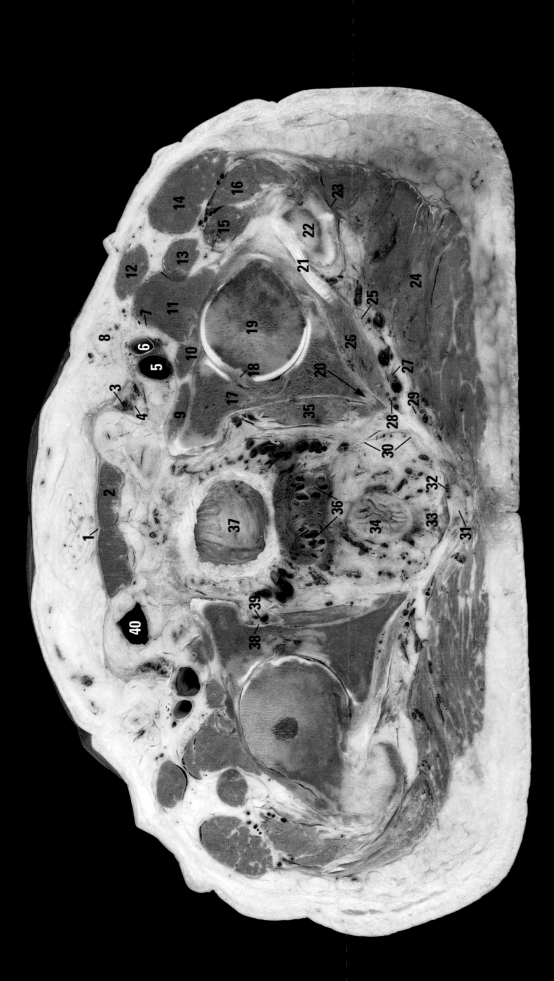

1 Linea alba
2 Rectus abdominis
3 Spermatic cord
4 Vas deferens
5 Femoral vein
6 Femoral artery
7 Femoral nerve
8 Lymph node
9 Pectineus
10 Psoas major and tendon
11 Iliacus
12 Sartorius

13 Rectus femoris
14 Tensor fasciae latae
15 Gluteus minimus
16 Gluteus medius
17 Acetabulum (pubic portion)
18 Ligamentum teres
19 Femoral head
20 Ischium leading to ischial
   spine (arrowed)
21 Obturator internus tendon
22 Greater trochanter
23 Trochanteric bursa

24 Gluteus maximus
25 Sciatic nerve
26 Gemellus superior
27 Inferior gluteal artery and vein
28 Pudendal nerve and internal
   pudendal artery and vein
29 Sacrospinous ligament
30 Perirectal fascia separating
   perirectal fat from
   pararectal fat
31 Sacrum fifth segment
32 Lateral sacral artery and vein

33 Superior rectal artery and
   vein in perirectal fat
34 Rectum
35 Obturator internus
36 Seminal vesicle
37 Bladder
38 Obturator nerve
39 Obturator artery and vein
40 Patent processus vaginalis
   (indirect inguinal hernia sac)

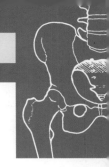

Section level

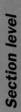

S5

Orientation guide

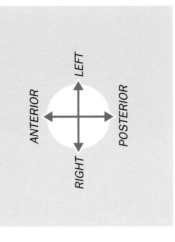

ANTERIOR

LEFT

RIGHT

POSTERIOR

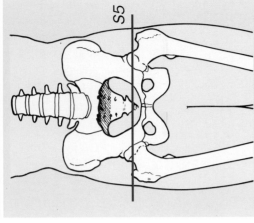

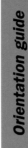

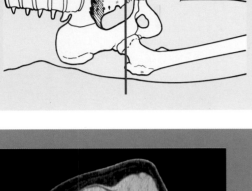

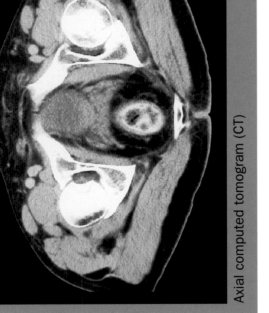

Axial computed tomogram (CT)

Notes

This section traverses the last, fifth, segment of the sacrum (**29**) the sacrospinous ligament (**31**) is transected as it passes forward to the ischial spine (**20**).

This section gives an excellent illustration of the hip joint at the level of the ligamentum teres (**18**).

The superior rectal vessels (**33**) can be seen as they lie in the loose perirectal fat, which also contains lymphatic vessels, lymph nodes and the pelvic plexuses lying on the rectal wall. The perirectal fat is separated by the perirectal fascia (**30**) from the pararectal fat.

Note that this subject has an indirect inguinal hernia sac on the right side (**40**).

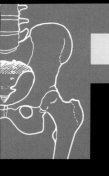

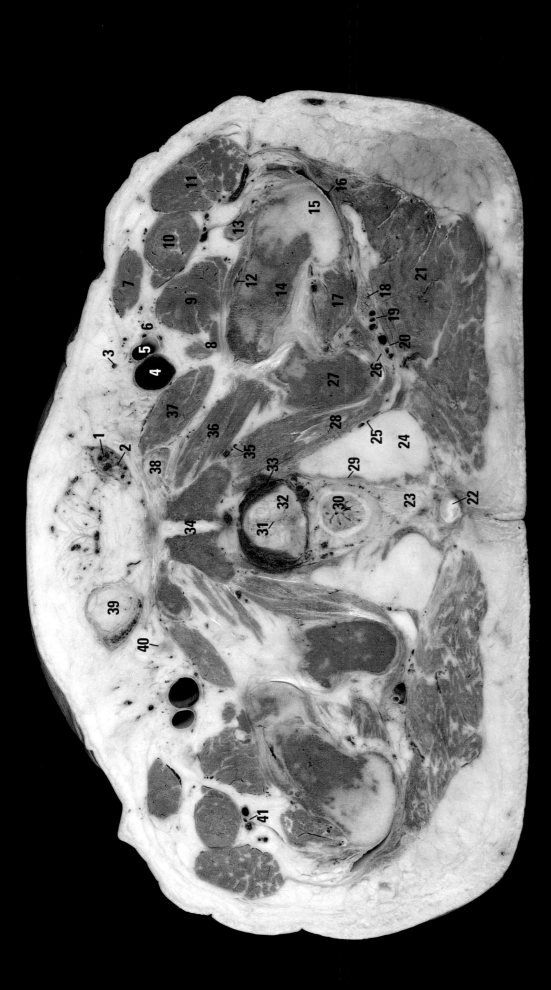

1 Spermatic cord
2 Vas deferens
3 Great saphenous vein
4 Femoral vein
5 Femoral artery
6 Femoral nerve
7 Sartorius
8 Psoas major and tendon
9 Iliacus
10 Rectus femoris
11 Tensor fasciae latae
12 Hip joint capsule

13 Vastus lateralis
14 Femoral neck
15 Greater trochanter
16 Trochanteric bursa
17 Quadratus femoris
18 Sciatic nerve
19 Inferior gluteal artery and vein
20 Internal pudendal artery and vein
   and pudendal nerve (see also 25)
21 Gluteus maximus
22 Coccyx
23 Mesorectum

24 Ischiorectal (ischioanal) fossa
25 Pudendal (Alcock's) canal
26 Obturator internus tendon
27 Ischium
28 Obturator internus
29 Levator ani (puborectalis portion)
30 Rectum
31 Prostatic urethra
32 Prostate
33 Prostatic venous plexus
34 Symphysis pubis
35 Obturator artery and vein

36 Obturator externus
37 Pectineus
38 Superior ramus of pubis
39 Extraperitoneal fat related to
   hernia sac
40 Inguinal lymph node
41 Lateral circumflex femoral artery
   and vein
42 Inferior rectal artery
43 Body of penis

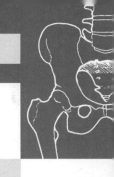

Section level

Orientation guide

ANTERIOR

LEFT

RIGHT

POSTERIOR

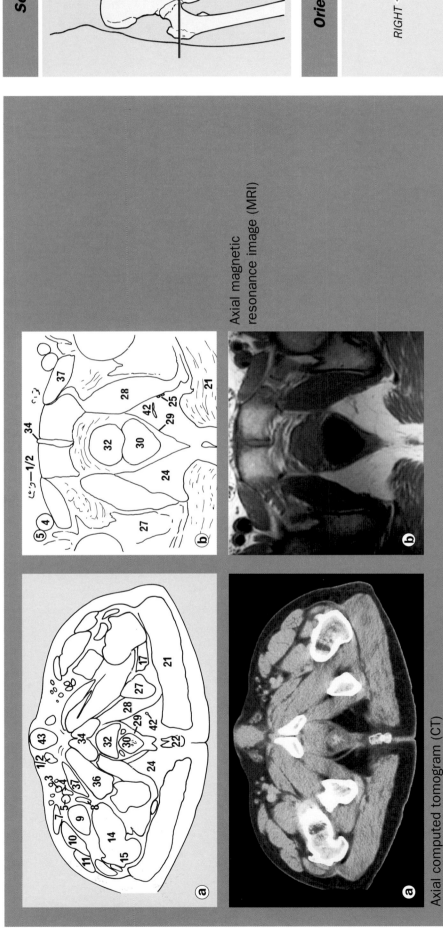

Axial magnetic
resonance image (MRI)

Axial computed tomogram (CT)

Notes

This section passes through the coccyx (**22**) and the symphysis pubis (**34**). In the standing position, the horizontal plane which passes through the coccyx corresponds to the superior margin of the symphysis.

The ischiorectal (ischioanal) fossa (**24**) is wedge shaped with its base pointing to the surface of the perineum, while its apex is the junction of obturator internus (**28**) and levator ani (**29**) covered respectively by the obturator fascia and the inferior fascia of the pelvic diaphragm. Medially it is bounded by the external anal sphincter and levator ani, laterally by

the tuberosity of the ischium and the obturator fascia and posteriorly by the lower border of gluteus maximus (**21**) and the sacrotuberous ligament. Anteriorly lies the urogenital diaphragm, but the fossa is prolonged as a narrow recess above this diaphragm, where it is limited by the fusion between the inferior fascia of the pelvic diaphragm and the superior fascia of the urogenital diaphragm.

The internal pudendal vessels and the pudendal nerve (**20**) enter the perineum through the lesser sciatic foramen and then traverse the pudendal canal of Alcock

(**25**). This canal comprises a distinct sheath of fascia fused with the lower part of the obturator fascia.

The left common femoral artery (**5**) is about to divide into the superficial femoral and profunda femoris on the section: on the CT image this has already taken place.

The spermatic cord (**1**) and vas deferens (**2**) are clearly seen on the left side. On the right these are compressed by extraperitoneal fat related to this subject's indirect inguinal hernia (**39**). This hernia is well seen in section 7, page 161.

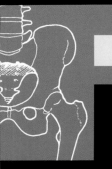

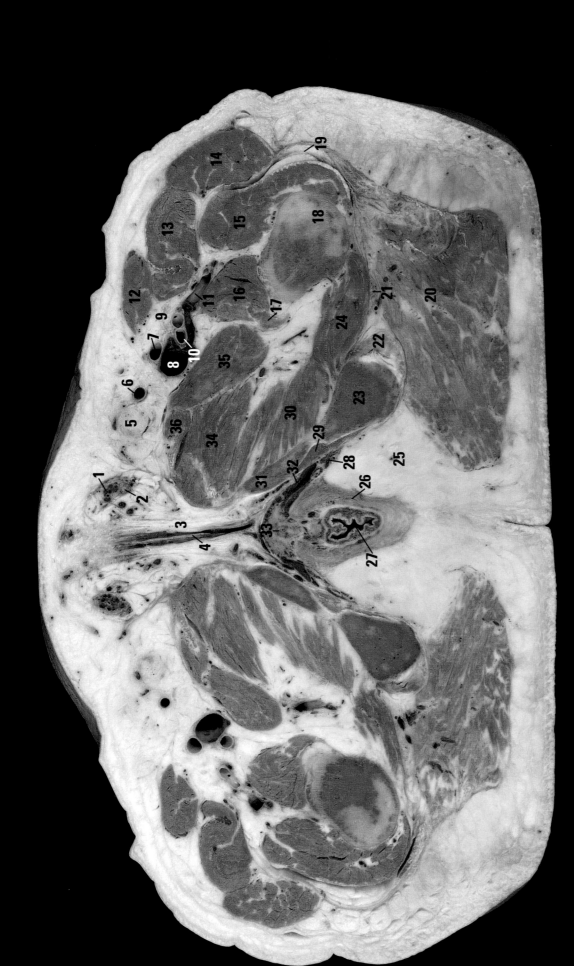

1   Spermatic cord
2   Vas deferens
3   Tunica albuginea of penis
4   Corpus cavernosum (body)
5   Inguinal lymph node
6   Great saphenous vein
7   Superficial femoral artery
8   Femoral vein
9   Femoral nerve
10 Profunda femoris artery
11 Lateral circumflex femoral vein
12 Sartorius
13 Rectus femoris
14 Tensor fasciae latae
15 Vastus lateralis
16 Iliacus
17 Tendon of psoas major
18 Greater trochanter
19 Trochanteric bursa
20 Gluteus maximus
21 Sciatic nerve
22 Biceps femoris tendon
23 Ischial tuberosity
24 Quadratus femoris
25 Ischiorectal fat
26 Levator ani
27 Anorectal junction
28 Pudendal canal
29 Obturator internus
30 Obturator externus
31 Pubis-inferior ramus
32 Corpus cavernosum (crus)
33 Urethra (in distal prostate)
34 Adductor brevis
35 Pectineus
36 Adductor longus

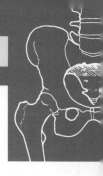

Section level

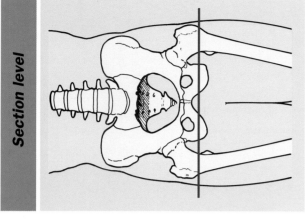
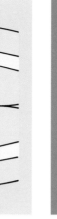

Orientation guide

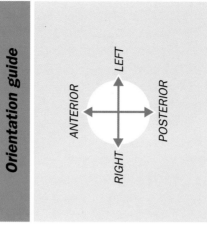

ANTERIOR

LEFT

POSTERIOR

RIGHT

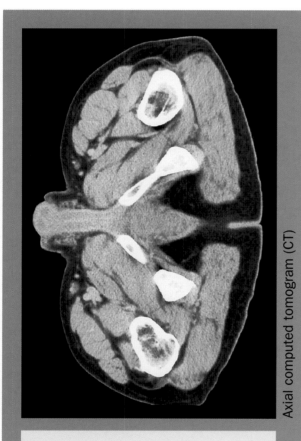

Axial computed tomogram (CT)

Notes

This section lies caudal to the coccyx and pubis but passes through the level of the ischial tuberosity (**23**). The plane of section cuts through the anorectal junction (**27**), around which lies levator ani (**26**).

The ischiorectal fossa, filled with fat (**25**), which is described in section 8, pages 163 & 164, can be seen to communicate with the fossa on the other side posterior to the anal canal. The inferior rectal artery is clearly seen in the centre of the fossa on the left side.

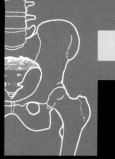

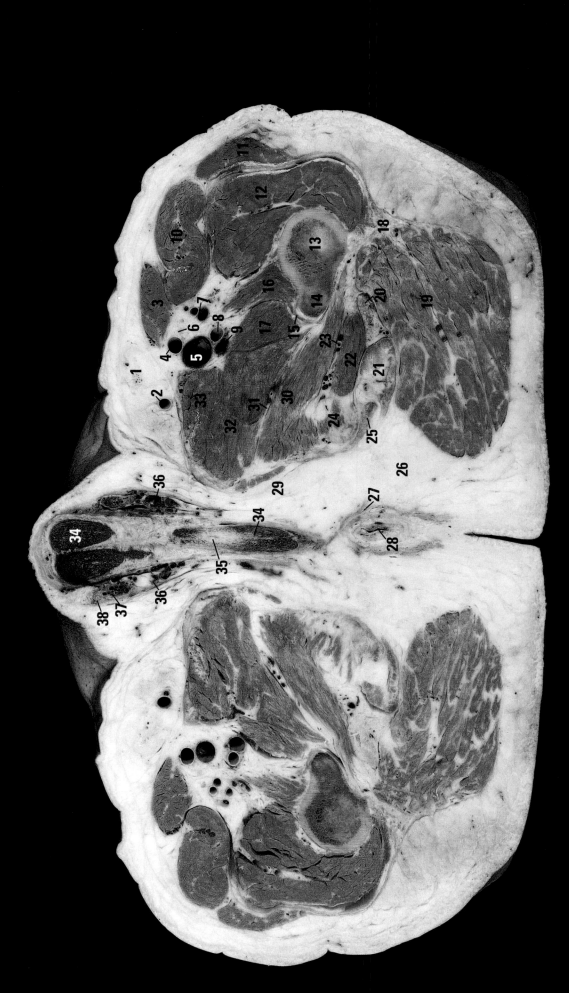

1 Inguinal lymph node
2 Great saphenous vein
3 Sartorius
4 Superficial femoral artery
5 Superficial femoral vein
6 Femoral nerve
7 Lateral circumflex femoral artery
   and vein
8 Profunda femoris artery
9 Profunda femoris vein
10 Rectus femoris
11 Tensor fasciae latae

12 Vastus lateralis
13 Femur
14 Lesser trochanter
15 Tendon of psoas major
16 Iliacus
17 Pectineus
18 Gluteus maximus tendon
19 Gluteus maximus
20 Sciatic nerve
21 Biceps femoris and
   semitendinosus tendons
22 Quadratus femoris

23 Profunda femoris artery and
   vein first perforating branches
24 Semimembranosus
25 Ischium
26 Ischiorectal fat
27 Levator ani
28 Anal canal
29 Gracilis
30 Adductor magnus
31 Obturator nerve deep branch
32 Adductor brevis
33 Adductor longus

34 Corpus cavernosum
35 Urethra
36 Pampiniform plexus
37 Spermatic cord
38 Vas deferens

39 Corpus cavernosum (crus)
40 Obturator externus

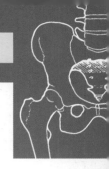

Section level

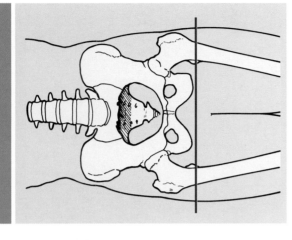

Orientation guide

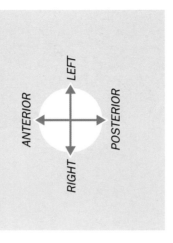

ANTERIOR

LEFT

RIGHT

POSTERIOR

Axial computed tomogram (CT)

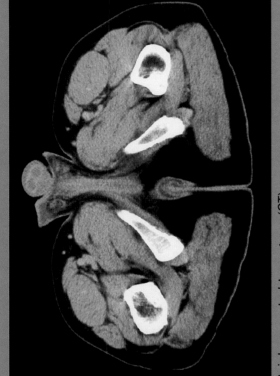

Notes

This section is completely below the pelvic girdle and transects the upper ends of the femoral shafts (**13**) at the level of the lesser trochanter (**14**). It transects the anal canal (**28**). The bulky gluteus maximus provides a good target for intramuscular injections of medications. It is worth considering the site of the sciatic nerve (**20**). Many patients have so much fat overlying the gluteal muscles that supposedly intramuscular injections are in fact placed in overlying adipose tissue!

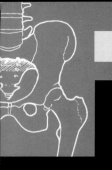

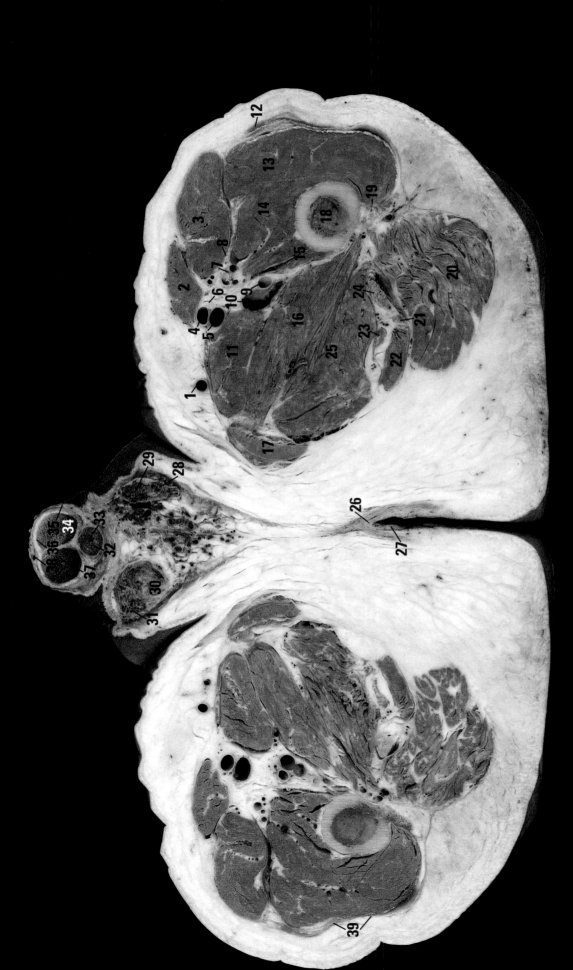

1 Great saphenous vein
2 Sartorius
3 Rectus femoris
4 Superficial femoral artery
5 Superficial femoral vein
6 Saphenous nerve
7 Lateral circumflex femoral artery and vein (inferior branch)
8 Femoral nerve (branch to quadriceps)
9 Profunda femoris artery
10 Profunda femoris vein
11 Adductor longus
12 Tensor fasciae latae
13 Vastus lateralis
14 Vastus intermedius
15 Vastus medialis
16 Adductor brevis
17 Gracilis
18 Femoral shaft
19 Gluteus maximus tendon
20 Gluteus maximus

21 Biceps femoris – tendon of long head
22 Semimembranosus
23 Semitendinosus tendon
24 Sciatic nerve
25 Adductor magnus
26 External anal sphincter
27 Anal verge
28 Vas deferens
29 Spermatic cord
30 Testis – upper pole
31 Pampiniform plexus

32 Corpus spongiosum
33 Urethra
34 Corpus cavernosum
35 Penile fascia
36 Tunica albuginea of penis
37 Deep artery of penis
38 Dorsal vein of penis
39 Investing fascia of thigh – fascia lata
40 Quadratus femoris

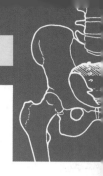

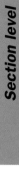

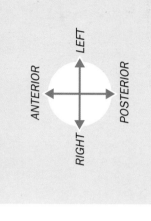

Axial computed tomogram (CT)

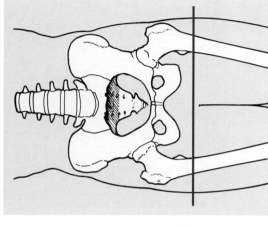

Notes

This section passes through the anal verge (**27**) surrounded by the external anal sphincter (**26**).

It demonstrates well the structure of the penis in transverse section. The penile urethra (**33**) is surrounded by the corpus spongiosum (**32**). Above and lateral to this, on either side, are the corpora cavernosa (**34**). These structures are bound together within the penile fascia (**35**). The deep artery of the penis (**37**) is a branch of the internal pudendal artery, which ends in the deep perineal pouch by dividing into the deep and the dorsal arteries of the penis and the artery to the bulb. The deep artery supplies the corpus cavernosum, the dorsal artery supplies the prepuce and glans while the artery to the bulb supplies the corpus spongiosum.

This section also demonstrates the upper pole of the testis (**30**) surrounded by its tunica albuginea, and also the vas deferens (**28**) surrounded by the pampiniform plexus (**31**).

The saphenous nerve (**6**), a branch of the femoral nerve, is here seen entering the adductor, or subsartorial, canal (Hunter's canal). This is an aponeurotic tunnel in the middle third of the thigh, formed posteriorly by adductor longus (**11**), and more distally by adductor magnus (**25**), anterolaterally by vastus medialis (**15**) and anteromedially by sartorius (**2**). Its contents are the superficial femoral artery and vein (**4**, **5**), saphenous nerve (**6**) and nerve to vastus medialis. (See also Thigh, section 3, page 197.)

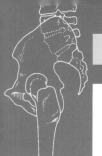

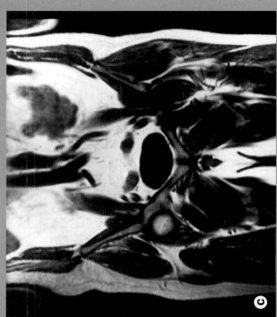

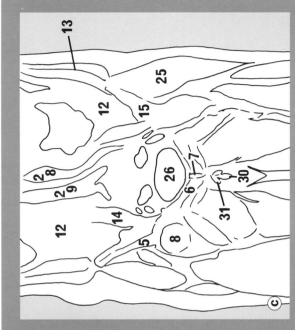

Coronal magnetic resonance image (MRI)

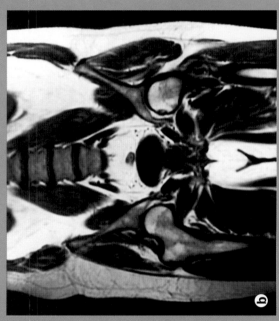

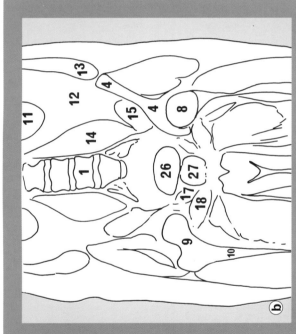

Coronal magnetic resonance image (MRI)

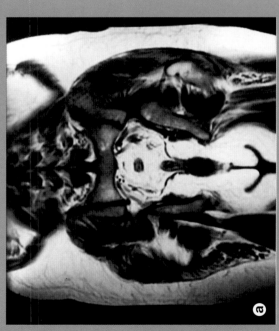

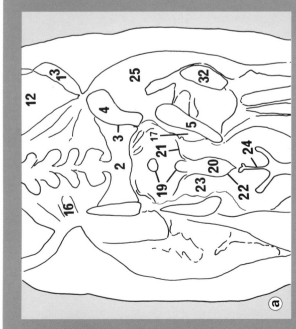

Coronal magnetic resonance image (MRI)

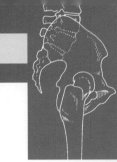

Section level

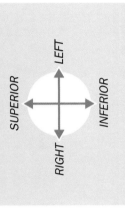

C B A

Orientation guide

SUPERIOR

LEFT

RIGHT

INFERIOR

Images A–C

1 L4 vertebral body
2 Sacrum
3 Sacro-iliac joint
4 Ilium
5 Ischium
6 Pubis
7 Pubic symphysis
8 Femoral head
9 Neck of femur
10 Shaft of femur
11 Left kidney
12 Intra-abdominal fat
13 Anterior wall musculature (transversus, internal/external obliques)
14 Psoas major
15 Iliacus

16 Quadratus lumborum
17 Obturator internus
18 Obturator externus
19 Rectum
20 Anal canal
21 Levator ani
22 Anal sphincters
23 Ischiorectal (ischioanal) fossa
24 Natal cleft
25 Gluteal muscles
26 Bladder
27 Prostate
28 Aorta
29 Inferior vena cava
30 Corpus spongiosum
31 Corpus cavernosum
32 Greater trochanter of femur

Notes

These three coronal T1 MR images provide a good overview of the relations of the structures within the male pelvis. In particular the way in which the anatomy relates to the pelvic floor is well demonstrated. So too is the way in which the anterior wall musculature merges with the bony pelvis. The copius quantity of intra-abdominal fat in men is also apparent; women have relatively much more fat in the subcutaneous tissues.

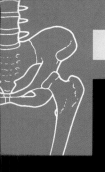

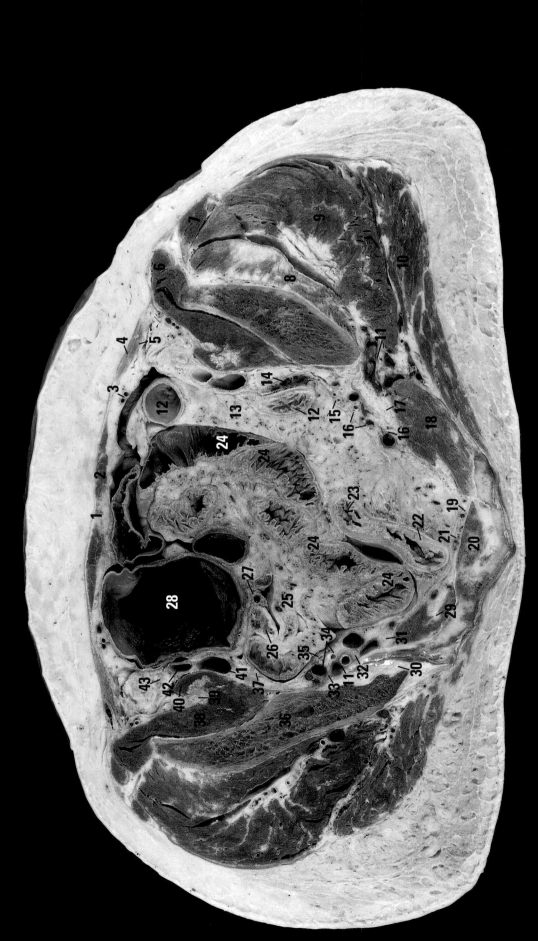

1 Linea alba
2 Rectus abdominis
3 Inferior epigastric artery and vein
4 Fused aponeurosis of external and internal oblique muscles
5 Transversus abdominis
6 Sartorius
7 Tensor fasciae latae
8 Gluteus minimus
9 Gluteus medius
10 Gluteus maximus
11 Superior gluteal artery and vein

12 Sigmoid colon
13 Sigmoid mesocolon
14 Left ovary
15 Left ureter
16 Branches of internal iliac artery and vein
17 Sciatic nerve
18 Piriformis
19 Lateral sacral artery and vein
20 Sacrum third segment
21 Median sacral artery and vein
22 Rectum
23 Rectosigmoid junction

24 Ileum
25 Mesentery of small bowel
26 Right ovary
27 Right uterine (fallopian) tube
28 Caecum
29 Ventral ramus of third sacral nerve
30 Sacro-iliac joint
31 Ventral ramus of second sacral nerve
32 Ventral ramus of first sacral nerve
33 Lumbosacral trunk

34 Uterine artery and vein
35 Right ureter
36 Ilium
37 Obturator nerve
38 Iliacus
39 Femoral nerve
40 Psoas major
41 External iliac vein
42 External iliac artery
43 Lymph node

44 Uterus (fundus)
45 Round ligament

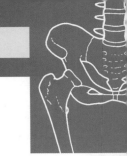

Section level

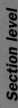

S3

Orientation guide

ANTERIOR

LEFT

POSTERIOR

RIGHT

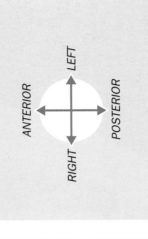

Axial computed tomogram (CT)

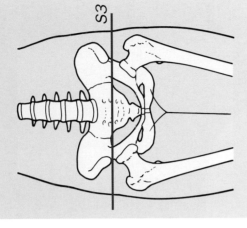

Notes

This section through the female pelvis transects the third segment of the sacrum (**20**), which defines the commencement of the rectum (**22**) at its junction with the sigmoid colon (**23**). The left ovary is seen at (**14**) and the right ovary at (**26**); in this elderly subject they are atrophic.

Along the internal iliac vessels (**16**) lies a rich lymphatic plexus, together with the internal iliac lymph nodes. These receive afferents from all the pelvic viscera, the deeper parts of the perineum and the muscles of the buttock. Their efferents pass through the common iliac nodes.

The sciatic nerve (**17**) at its origin is lying on piriformis (**18**). Its important relationships can be traced in subsequent sections as it emerges through the greater sciatic foramen below piriformis to cross, in turn, obturator internus tendon with its accompanying gemelli, quadratus femoris and, finally, adductor magnus. It is covered superficially by gluteus maximus and is crossed by the long head of biceps.

Note that a degree of scoliosis in this subject explains the asymmetry of the sciatic nerve and other structures on the two sides of this section.

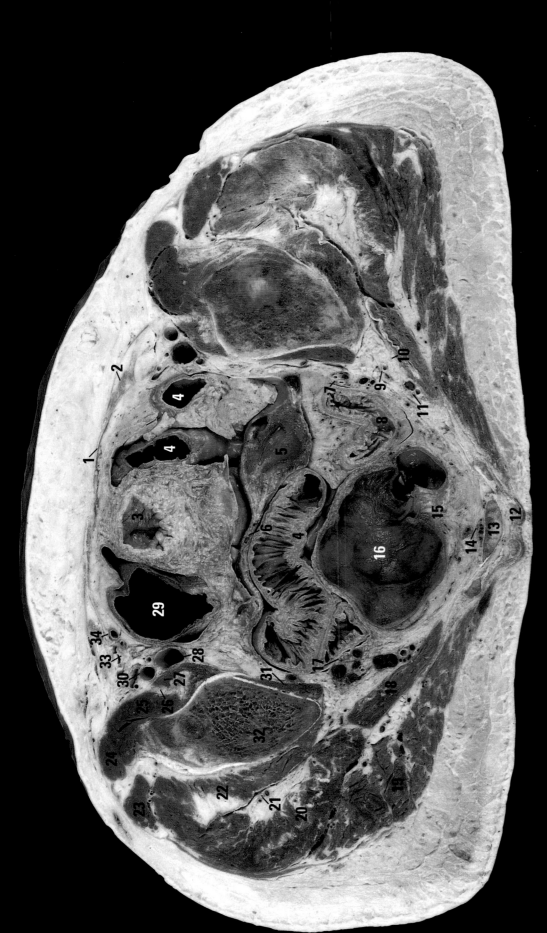

1 Rectus sheath
2 Transversus abdominis
3 Fundus of bladder
4 Ileum
5 Fundus of uterus
6 Broad ligament
7 Left ureter
8 Sigmoid colon
9 Inferior gluteal artery vein
   and nerve

10 Sciatic nerve
11 Internal pudendal artery, vein
    and pudendal nerve
12 Left sacral cornu
13 Sacrum fifth segment
14 Median sacral artery and vein
15 Mesorectum with superior
    rectal artery and vein
16 Rectum
17 Right ureter

18 Piriformis
19 Gluteus maximus
20 Gluteus medius
21 Superior gluteal artery
    and vein
22 Gluteus minimus
23 Tensor fasciae latae
24 Sartorius
25 Iliacus
26 Femoral nerve

27 Psoas major
28 External iliac vein
29 Caecum
30 External iliac artery
31 Obturator internus
32 Ilium
33 Round ligament
34 Inferior epigastric artery
    and vein

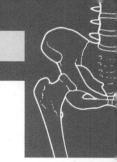

Section level

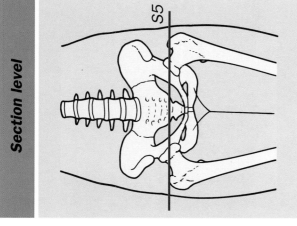
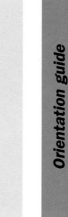

S5

Orientation guide

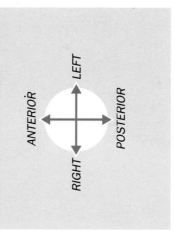

ANTERIOR

LEFT

POSTERIOR

RIGHT

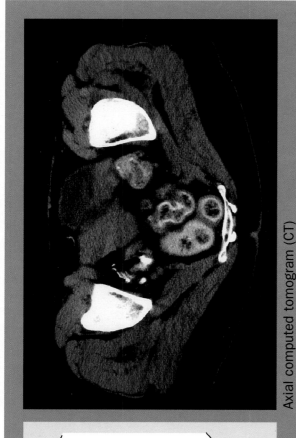

Axial computed tomogram (CT)

Notes

This section passes through the lowest, fifth, segment of the sacrum (**13**) and shaves through the fundus of the bladder (**3**) and of the uterus (**5**), together with the upper part of the broad ligament (**6**).

There is wide normal variation in the relative positions of the pelvic organs. For example, on the CT images the fundus of the uterus was first encountered on section 1, page 173. On this CT image, the body of the uterus is traversed. Conversely, the rectosigmoid junction lies at a more caudal level on the CT images than on the sections.

The rectum, from its narrow lumen at its origin, shown in the previous section, has widened into its patulous ampulla (**16**).

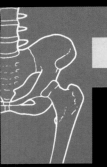

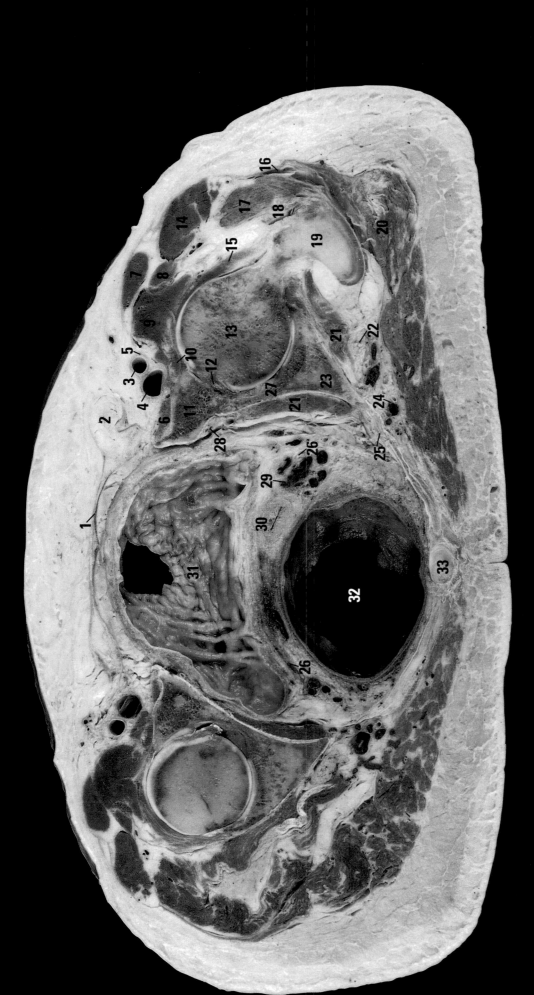

1   Inguinal ligament
2   Femoral hernia containing extraperitoneal fat
3   Femoral artery
4   Femoral vein
5   Femoral nerve
6   Pectineus
7   Sartorius
8   Rectus femoris
9   Iliacus

10   Psoas major tendon
11   Pubic component of acetabulum
12   Ligamentum teres
13   Head of femur
14   Tensor fasciae latae
15   Iliofemoral ligament
16   Iliotibial tract
17   Gluteus medius
18   Tendon of gluteus minimus
19   Greater trochanter

20   Gluteus maximus
21   Obturator internus
22   Sciatic nerve
23   Ischial spine
24   Inferior gluteal artery vein and nerve
25   Sacrospinous ligament
26   Ureter
27   Acetabulum
28   Obturator artery, vein and nerve

29   Uterine artery and vein
30   Internal os of cervix
31   Bladder
32   Ampulla of rectum
33   Coccyx

34   Ischial component of acetabulum
35   Sigmoid colon
36   Vault of vagina (with tampon)

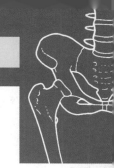

Section level

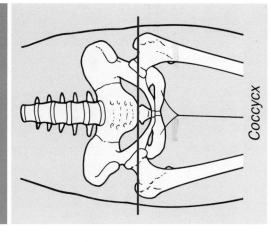

Coccyx

Orientation guide

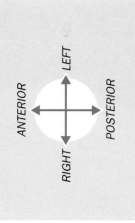

ANTERIOR

LEFT

RIGHT

POSTERIOR

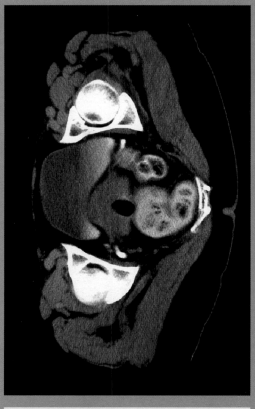

Axial computed tomogram (CT)

Notes

This section passes through the coccyx (**33**) and transects the femoral head (**13**). In this elderly subject the uterus is atrophic; note the small size of the cervix, here cut through its internal os (**30**).

Most CT units prepare all female patients undergoing pelvic CT by giving dilute iodinated contrast medium *per rectum*, as here; this renders the lumen of the rectosigmoid opaque. It is also useful if a tampon is inserted into the vagina; the air trapped by its fibres is readily recognised (**36**). This allows appreciation of the level of the vaginal vault and the external os of the cervix (**30**), even though neither structure is directly demonstrated.

The uterine artery (**29**) arises from the internal iliac artery, runs medially on levator ani towards the cervix of the uterus, and crosses above and in front of the ureter (**26**) above the lateral vaginal fornix to reach the side of the uterus, where it ascends in the broad ligament. The corresponding uterine veins (**29**), usually two in number, drain a uterine plexus along the lateral side of the uterus within the broad ligament and open into the internal iliac vein. The close relationship between the uterine vessels and the ureter is, of course, of immense importance to the gynaecological surgeon in performing a hysterectomy (see also CT image, section 4, page 180).

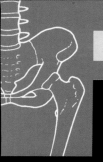

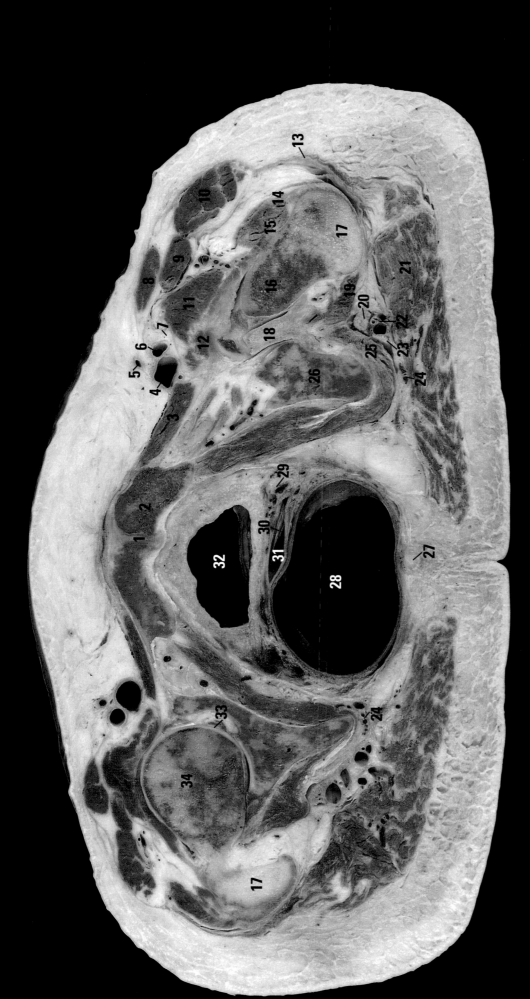

1 Pubic symphysis
2 Body of pubis
3 Pectineus
4 Femoral vein
5 Great saphenous vein
6 Femoral artery
7 Femoral nerve
8 Sartorius
9 Rectus femoris
10 Tensor fasciae latae
11 Iliacus

12 Psoas major tendon
13 Iliotibial tract
14 Gluteus medius
15 Gluteus minimus
16 Neck of femur
17 Greater trochanter
18 Ischiofemoral ligament
19 Quadratus femoris
20 Sciatic nerve
21 Gluteus maximus
22 Inferior gluteal artery and vein

23 Posterior cutaneous nerve of thigh
24 Internal pudendal artery and vein and pudendal nerve
25 Obturator internus
26 Ischium
27 Coccyx
28 Ampulla of rectum
29 Vaginal artery and vein
30 External os of cervix
31 Vagina

32 Bladder
33 Acetabulum
34 Femoral head

35 Ureter
36 Calcified pheboliths
37 Obturator artery, vein and nerve
38 Ischial spine

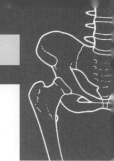

Section level

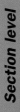

Coccycx

Orientation guide

ANTERIOR

LEFT

RIGHT

POSTERIOR

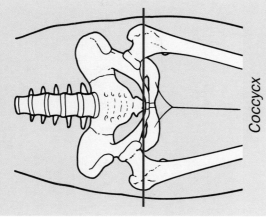

Axial computed tomogram (CT)

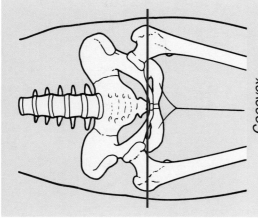

Notes

This section traverses the tip of the coccyx (**27**) and passes through the pubic symphysis in its upper part (**1**).

Note that the vagina (**31**) is transected in its upper part so that the external os of the cervix (**30**) can be seen peeping through with the posterior fornix of the vagina behind it. Alongside the vagina are the vaginal vessels (**29**). The vaginal artery usually corresponds

to the inferior vesical artery in the male and is a branch of the internal iliac artery. It is frequently double or triple. It supplies the vagina as well as the fundus of the bladder and the adjacent part of the rectum and anastomoses with branches of the uterine artery.

This section shows well the obturator internus muscle (**25**) as it sweeps around the lesser sciatic foramen with

the sciatic nerve (**20**) lying on its superficial (posterior) face covered posteriorly by gluteus maximus (**21**).

Many patients develop small outpouchings, or diverticula, in the extensive plexus of small pelvic veins. These diverticula often contain calcified thrombus to form phleboliths, as demonstrated on this CT image (**36**). On plain pelvic radiographs these may simulate ureteric calculi.

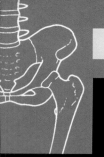

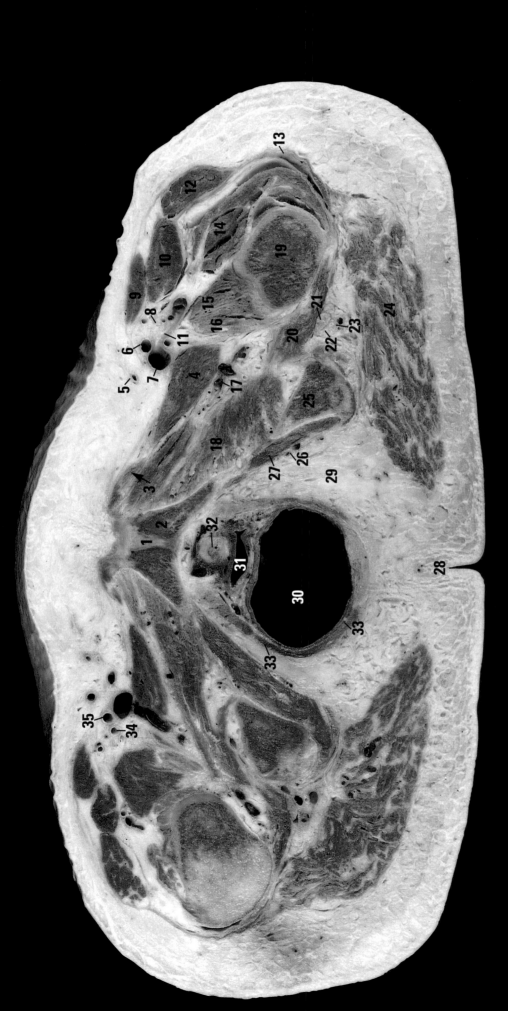

1 Symphysis pubis
2 Body of pubis
3 Adductor brevis , with adductor
   longus origin (arrowed)
4 Pectineus
5 Great saphenous vein
6 Left femoral artery
7 Femoral vein
8 Femoral nerve
9 Sartorius
10 Rectus femoris

11 Lateral circumflex
   femoral vein
12 Tensor fasciae latae
13 Iliotibial tract
14 Vastus lateralis
15 Iliacus
16 Psoas major tendon
17 Obturator artery and vein
18 Obturator externus
19 Femur
20 Quadratus femoris

21 Sciatic nerve
22 Posterior cutaneous nerve
   of thigh
23 Inferior gluteal artery and vein
24 Gluteus maximus
25 Ischial tuberosity
26 Pudendal (Alcock's) canal
   containing internal pudendal
   artery and vein and pudendal
   nerve
27 Obturator internus

28 Natal cleft
29 Ischiorectal (ischioanal) fossa
30 Rectum
31 Vagina
32 Urethra
33 Levator ani
34 Right profunda femoris artery
35 Right superficial femoral artery

36 Coccyx
37 Bladder

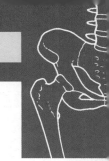

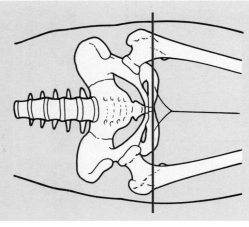

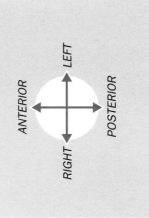

ANTERIOR

LEFT

RIGHT

POSTERIOR

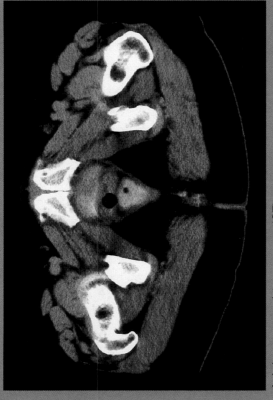

Axial computed tomogram (CT)

Notes

This section passes through the upper part of the natal cleft (**28**) and the body of the pubis (**2**).

The intimate relationship between the female urethra (**32**) and vagina (**31**) is well shown; the former is actually embedded in the anterior wall of the latter.

Unusually, the lateral circumflex femoral vein (**11**) in this subject arises from the common femoral vein (**7**); more usually, the circumflex vessels arise from the profunda femoris artery and vein. The right common femoral artery has divided into its profunda (**34**) and superficial (**35**) branches. On the left side, the femoral artery (**6**) has not yet divided.

The anatomy of the ischiorectal (ischioanal) fossa (**29**) is nicely demonstrated. It lies between levator ani (**33**) and obturator internus (**27**), on which can be seen the pudendal canal (of Alcock) (**26**) and its contents. (See also Pelvis Male, section 8, page 163).

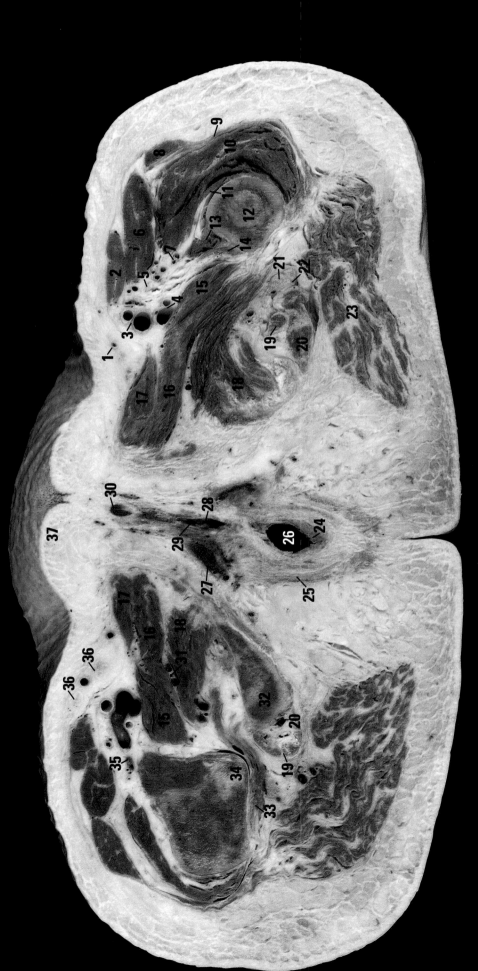

1 Great saphenous vein
2 Sartorius
3 Superficial femoral artery and vein
4 Deep femoral artery and vein
5 Femoral nerve (dividing into branches)
6 Rectus femoris
7 Lateral circumflex femoral artery and vein
8 Tensor fasciae latae
9 Iliotibial tract
10 Vastus lateralis

11 Vastus intermedius
12 Shaft of femur
13 Vastus medialis
14 Psoas major insertion to lesser trochanter with iliacus
15 Pectineus
16 Adductor brevis
17 Adductor longus
18 Adductor magnus
19 Tendon of semimembranosus
20 Origin of semitendinosus and biceps femoris muscles
21 Sciatic nerve

22 Posterior cutaneous nerve of thigh
23 Gluteus maximus
24 External anal sphincter
25 Levator ani
26 Anal canal
27 Crus of clitoris
28 Vaginal orifice
29 Urethral orifice
30 Clitoris
31 Obturator artery, vein and nerve (posterior branch)
32 Ischial tuberosity

33 Quadratus femoris
34 Lesser trochanter of femur
35 Lateral circumflex femoral vein
36 Inguinal lymph node
37 Mons pubis

38 Obturator externus
39 Ischiorectal (ischioanal) fossa

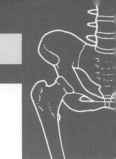

Section level

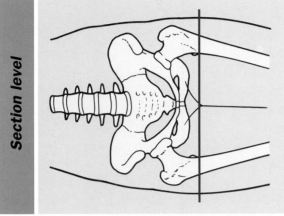

Orientation guide

ANTERIOR

LEFT

RIGHT

POSTERIOR

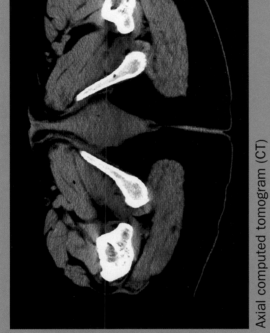

Axial computed tomogram (CT)

Notes

This section passes through the mons pubis (**37**) anteriorly and the anal canal (**26**) posteriorly. Note the close relationship between the vaginal (**28**) and urethral (**29**) orifices.

The sciatic nerve (**21**), with its accompanying posterior cutaneous nerve of the thigh (**22**) immediately superficial to it, can now be seen as it lies on quadratus femoris (**33**).

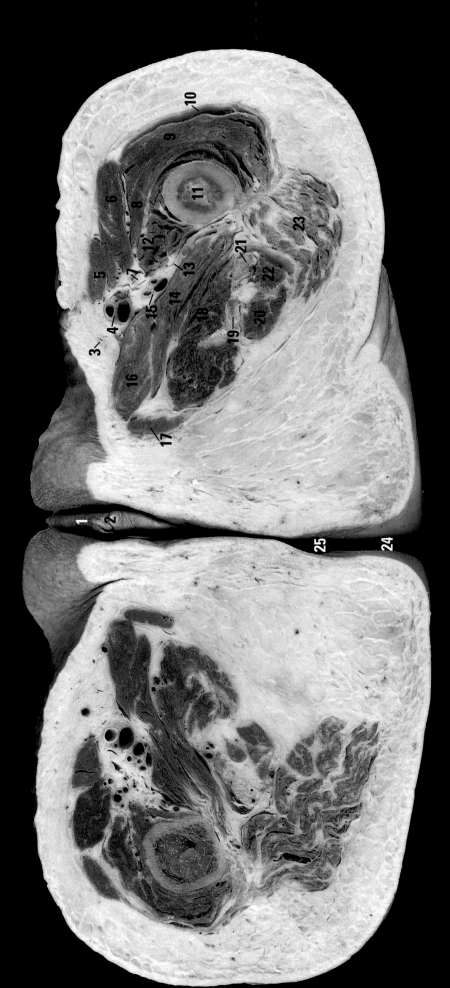

1 Prepuce of clitoris
2 Glans clitoridis
3 Great saphenous vein
4 Superficial femoral artery and
   vein
5 Sartorius
6 Rectus femoris
7 Femoral nerve (branch to
   quadratus femoris)

8 Vastus intermedius
9 Vastus lateralis
10 Iliotibial tract
11 Shaft of femur
12 Vastus medialis
13 First perforating artery and
   vein of profunda femoris
   artery and vein
14 Adductor brevis

15 Profunda femoris artery
   and vein
16 Adductor longus
17 Gracilis
18 Adductor magnus
19 Semimembranosus tendon
20 Semitendinosus
21 Sciatic nerve
22 Long head of biceps

23 Gluteus maximus
24 Natal cleft
25 Anal verge

26 Tensor fasciae latae

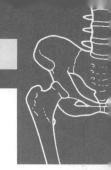

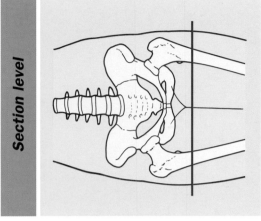

ANTERIOR

LEFT

RIGHT

POSTERIOR

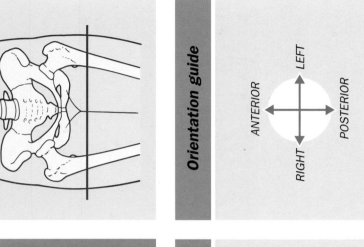

Axial computed tomogram (CT)

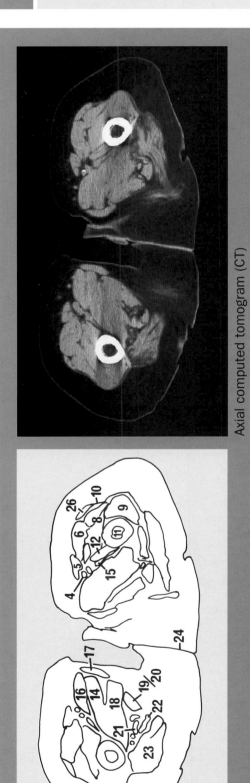

Notes

This section passes through the upper thigh but demonstrates the prepuce (**1**) and glans (**2**) of the clitoris. The anal verge (**25**) can be seen within the natal cleft (**24**). The sciatic nerve (**21**) now lies on adductor magnus (**18**) and is crossed superficially by the long head of biceps (**22**).

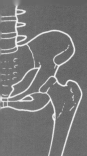

Axial magnetic
resonance image (MRI) T1

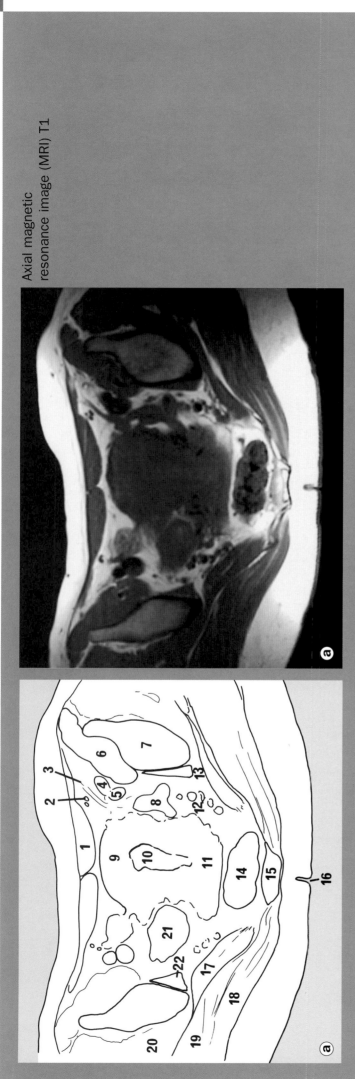

Axial magnetic
resonance image (MRI) T2

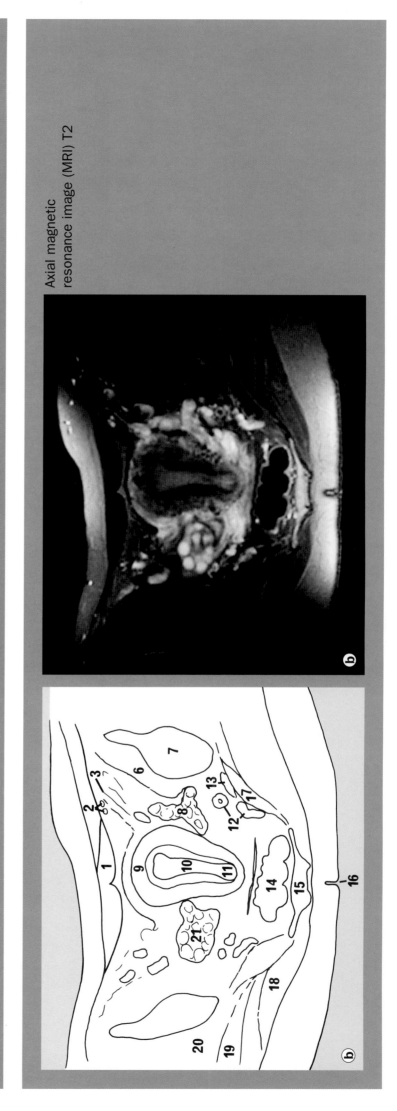

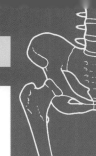

Section level

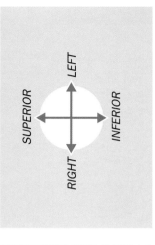

A,B

Orientation guide

SUPERIOR

LEFT

RIGHT

INFERIOR

Notes

T1 (a) and T2 (b) weighted axial MR images using a pelvic phased array coil. The design of the coil accounts for the higher signal intensity within the subcutaneous fat anteriorly and posteriorly. Note the way the T2 (image b) weighting demonstrates the internal anatomy of the uterus and the individual follicles within the ovary.

Note how there is a normal plane of fat lateral to each ovary and internal to the ilium and obturator internus. Any enlarged obturator nodes would be seen immediately posterior to the external iliac vein and would tend to disrupt the fat plane just internal to the ilium.

On the T1 weighted image the epigastric vessels return low signal intensity (signal void); on T2 weighted images they return high signal.

Note the way the round ligament passes lateral to the epigastric vessels en route to the inguinal canal.

Images A–B

1 Rectus abdominis
2 Inferior epigastric vessels
3 Round ligament
4 External iliac artery
5 External iliac vein
6 Iliopsoas
7 Ilium
8 Left ovary
9 Fundus of uterus
10 Uterine cavity
11 Cervix of uterus
12 Internal iliac vessels
13 Plane of sciatic nerve
14 Rectum
15 Sacrum
16 Natal cleft
17 Piriformis
18 Gluteus maximus
19 Gluteus medius
20 Gluteus minimus
21 Right ovary
22 Obturator internus

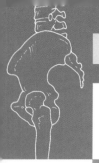

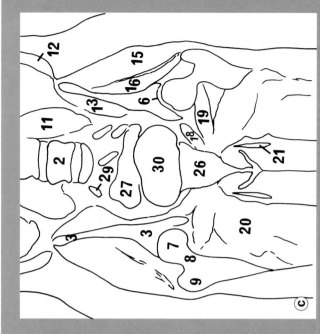

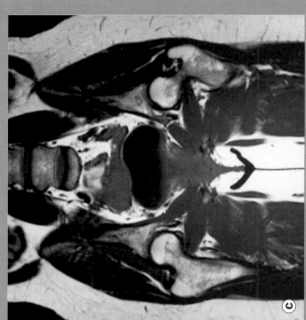

Coronal magneticresonance image (MRI)

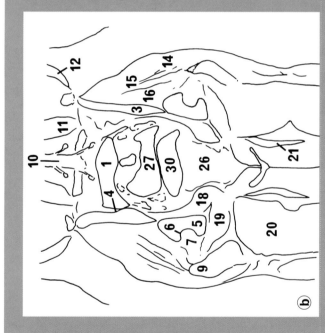

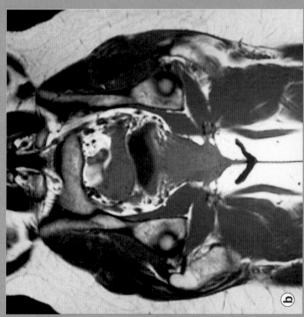

Coronal magnetic resonance image (MRI)

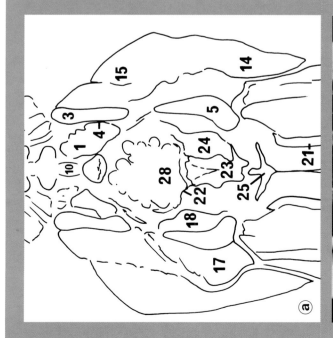

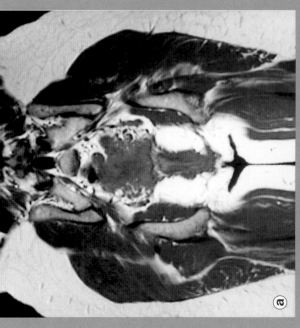

Coronal magnetic resonance image (MRI)

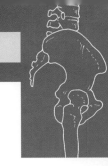

Section level

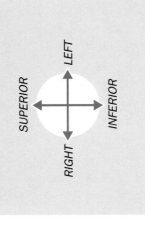

C B A

Orientation guide

SUPERIOR

RIGHT — LEFT

INFERIOR

Images A–C

1 Sacrum
2 L5 vertebral body
3 Ilium
4 Sacro-iliac joint
5 Ischium
6 Acetabulum
7 Femoral head
8 Femoral neck
9 Femur, greater trochanter
10 Thecal sac

11 Psoas major
12 Anterior abdominal wall
    musculature
13 Iliacus
14 Gluteus maximus
15 Gluteus medius
16 Gluteus minimus
17 Quadratus femoris
18 Obturator internus
19 Obturator externus
20 Adductor group of muscles

21 Gracilis
22 Levator ani
23 Anal canal
24 Ischiorectal (ischioanal)
    fossa
25 Natal cleft
26 Vagina
27 Uterus (body)
28 Uterus (cervix)
29 Common iliac vessels
30 Bladder

Notes

These coronal T1 weighted images elegantly demonstrate the way in which the anteverted uterine body rests on the bladder. It is important to realise that the support for the pelvic organs comes mainly from the tone in the pelvic musculature. The levator ani on either side are important; so too are the collective contributions of all the muscles which are attached to the inferior bony pelvis, many of which directly or indirectly converge on the region of the perineal body. All these muscles play a part in supporting the pelvic organs and ultimately preventing prolapse and incontinence. Hence the importance of pelvic floor exercises before and after pregnancy.

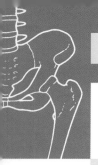

1 L5 vertebral body
2 S1 vertebral body
3 L5/S1 intervertebral disc
4 Lowest fixed point of sacrococcygeal region (here probably coccyx 1/2)
5 Rest of coccyx (mobile)
6 Pubic symphysis
7 Rectus abdominis
8 Bladder
9 Fundus of uterus
10 Myometrium of uterus
11 Junctional zone between myometrium and endometrium
12 Endometrium of uterus
13 Cavity of uterus
14 Internal os of uterus
15 External os of uterus
16 Vagina
17 Rectum

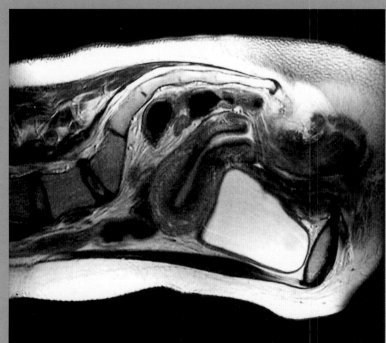

Sagittal magnetic resonance image (MRI)

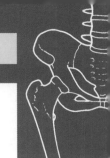

Section level

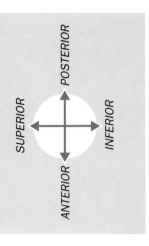

Orientation guide

POSTERIOR

SUPERIOR

INFERIOR

ANTERIOR

Notes

This midline sagittal T2 weighted MR image illustrates many of the important features of the female pelvis. The bony dimensions can be easily assessed. The anteroposterior (AP) diameter of the pelvic inlet (from the supero-posterior aspect of the pubic symphysis to the anterior aspect of the promontory on S1) is of key importance for obstetrics; this should ideally be about 12 cm – the fetal head has a diameter of about 10.5 cm. The AP diameter of the mid pelvis is usually somewhat larger; this is where rotation of the fetal head occurs during childbirth; much depends on the shape of the sacrum. The AP diameter of the pelvic outlet (from the inferior posterior aspect of the pubic symphysis to the anterior aspect of the lowest fixed point of the sacrum – usually the

sacrococcygeal junction) should be similar to that of the inlet; only rarely do the common anomalies at this site cause problems during childbirth.

The anatomy of the uterus is well shown. This anteverted uterus (the common arrangement) is clearly seen resting on a semi-distended bladder. The cavity is sharply defined by the endometrium, then by the junctional zone and the myometrium peripherally. The relationship of the internal and external ostia of the cervix to the vaginal vault is well shown, as is the close relationship of the vagina and the rectum. It is important to realise that many of these relationships vary according to the degree of distension of the urinary bladder and rectum and the strength of the pelvic floor muscles.

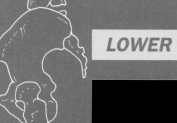

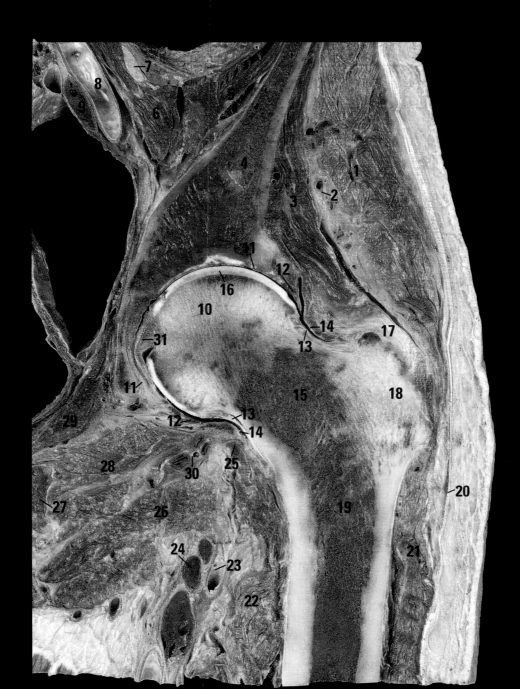

Section level

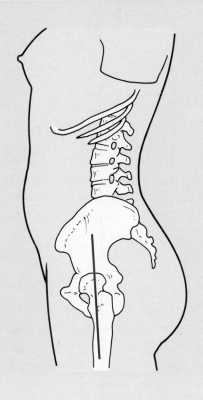

Notes

This coronal section through the hip illustrates the 'ball and socket' arrangement of the joint. This socket is much deeper and this ball much rounder than at the shoulder. Stability is an important function here. The two powerful abductors of the hip, gluteus medius (**1**) and minimus (**3**) have their own neurovascular bundle (the superior gluteal nerve, artery and vein) and these can be seen between the two sheets of muscle (**2**).

The ligament of the head of the femur (**31**), the ligamentum teres, is an important source of blood supply to the femoral head in the fetus and infant. It transmits the acetabular branch of the obturator artery. It becomes obliterated during early childhood when periosteal vessels are of key importance before vessels traverse the epiphyseal plate. The blood supply to the femoral head remains of importance throughout life: avascular necrosis due to its damage may occur in Perthes' disease, slipped femoral epiphysis and subcapital fractures of the femoral hip.

Orientation guide

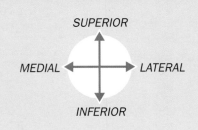

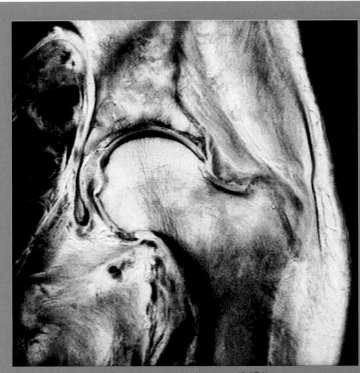

Coronal magnetic resonance image (MRI)

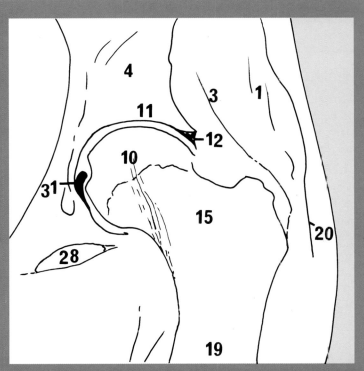

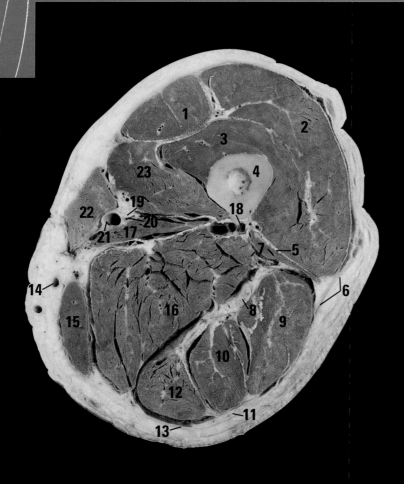

1 Rectus femoris	**12** Semimembranosus
2 Vastus lateralis	**13** Fascia lata (deep
3 Vastus intermedius	fascia of thigh)
4 Femur	**14** Great saphenous
5 Lateral intermuscu-	vein
lar septum	**15** Gracilis
6 Iliotibial tract	**16** Adductor magnus
7 Biceps femoris-	**17** Adductor logus
short head	**18** Profunda femoris
8 Sciatic nerve	artery
9 Biceps femoris-long	**19** Saphenous nerve
head	**20** Femoral vein
10 Semitendinosus	**21** Femoral artery
11 Posterior cutaneous	**22** Sartorius
nerve of thigh	**23** Vastus medialis

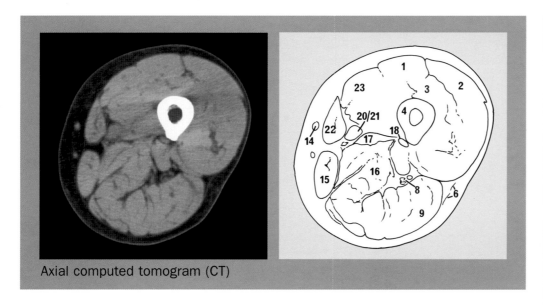

Axial computed tomogram (CT)

Orientation guide

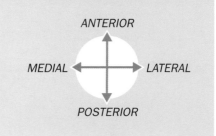

ANTERIOR

MEDIAL — LATERAL

POSTERIOR

Section level

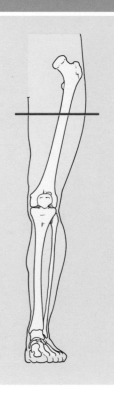

Notes

This section passes through the upper one third of the thigh and provides a useful view of the three muscular compartments of the thigh:

1 The anterior compartment – containing quadriceps femoris, made up of the vasti (**2**, **3**, **23**) and rectus femoris (**1**), supplied by the femoral nerve.

2 The adductor compartment – containing the three adductors (of which only adductor magnus (**16**) and adductor longus (**17**) are present at this level, brevis having already found insertion into the femoral shaft), together with gracilis (**15**). These muscles are supplied by the obturator nerve; adductor magnus, in addition, receives innervation from the sciatic nerve.

3 The posterior compartment – contains the hamstrings – the biceps with its long and short heads (**9** and **7** respectively), semitendinosus (**10**) and semimembranosus (**12**), all supplied by the sciatic nerve.

Sartorius (**22**) lies in a separate fascial sheath.

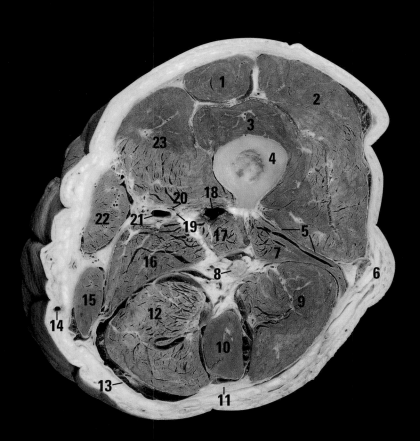

1 Rectus femoris	**14** Great saphenous vein
2 Vastus lateralis	**15** Gracilis
3 Vastus intermedius	**16** Adductor magnus medial part
4 Femur	**17** Adductor magnus lateral part
5 Lateral intermuscular septum	**18** Profunda femoris artery
6 Iliotibial tract	**19** Saphenous nerve
7 Biceps femoris-short head	**20** Superficial femoral vein
8 Sciatic nerve	**21** Superficial femoral artery
9 Biceps femoris-long head	**22** Sartorius
10 Semitendinosus	**23** Vastus medialis
11 Posterior cutaneous nerve of thigh	
12 Semimembranosus	
13 Fascia lata (deep fascia of thigh)	

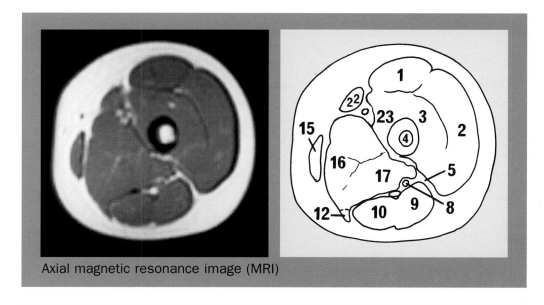

Axial magnetic resonance image (MRI)

Orientation guide

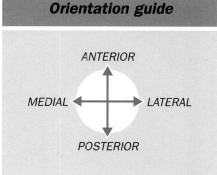

ANTERIOR

MEDIAL ←→ LATERAL

POSTERIOR

Section level

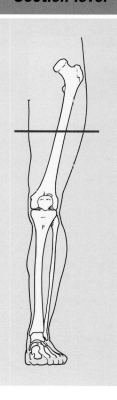

Notes

This section passes through the mid-shaft of the femur (**4**).

Note that, at this level, adductor magnus is dividing into two sections. Its lateral part (**17**), which arises from the ischial ramus, forms a broad aponeurosis which inserts along the linea aspera along the posterior border of the femoral shaft (**4**). The medial part (**16**), which arises mainly from the ischial tuberosity, descends almost vertically to a tendinous attachment to the adductor tubercle of the medial condyle of the femur. Between the two parts distally is the osseo-aponeurotic adductor hiatus, which admits the femoral vessels to the popliteal fossa.

Being a composite muscle, adductor magnus also has a composite nerve supply; the medial part is innervated by the tibial division of the sciatic nerve (**8**), the lateral part by the obturator nerve.

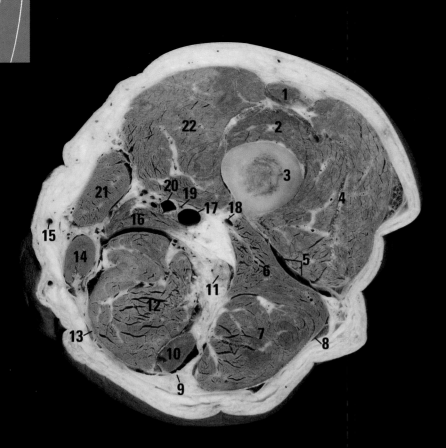

1 Rectus femoris	**13** Fascia lata (deep
2 Vastus intermedius	fascia of thigh)
3 Femur	**14** Gracilis
4 Vastus lateralis	**15** Great saphenous
5 Lateral intermuscular	vein
septum	**16** Adductor magnus
6 Biceps femoris–short	**17** Superficial femoral
head	vein
7 Biceps femoris–long	**18** Profunda femoris
head	artery and vein
8 Iliotibial tract	**19** Saphenous nerve
9 Posterior cutaneous	**20** Superficial femoral
nerve of thigh	artery
10 Semitendinosus	**21** Sartorius
11 Sciatic nerve	**22** Vastus medialis
12 Semimembranosus	

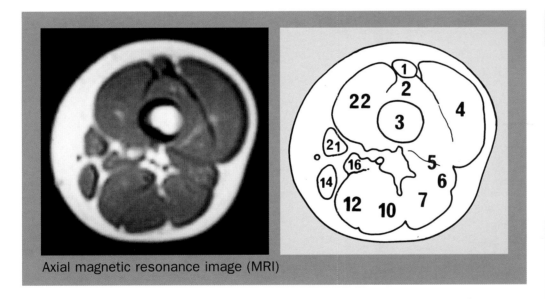

Axial magnetic resonance image (MRI)

Orientation guide

ANTERIOR

MEDIAL — LATERAL

POSTERIOR

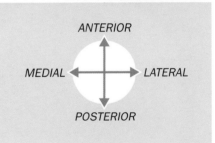

Section level

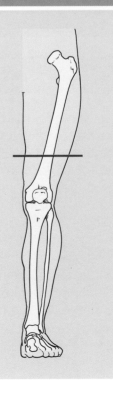

Notes

This section transects the lower third of the thigh.

This and the previous two sections demonstrate the anatomy of the adductor or subsartorial canal (Hunter's canal). This is formed as a triangular aponeurotic tunnel, which leads from the femoral triangle above to the popliteal fossa below, via the hiatus in adductor magnus. The canal lies between sartorius (**21**) anteromedially, adductor longus and, more distally, adductor magnus (**16**) posteriorly, and vastus medialis (**22**) anterolaterally. Its contents are the femoral artery (**20**) and vein (**17**), the saphenous nerve (**19**) and also the nerve to vastus medialis until this enters and supplies this muscle.

John Hunter (1728–1793) described ligation of the femoral artery within this canal in the treatment of popliteal aneurysm, and his name has been eponymously attached to the canal.

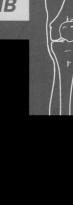

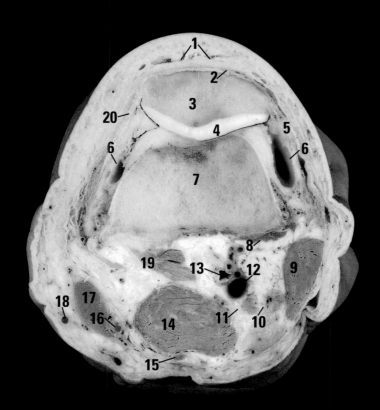

1 Prepatellar bursa	11 Tibial nerve
2 Tendon of	12 Popliteal vein
quadriceps femoris	13 Popliteal artery
3 Patella	14 Semimembranosus
4 Articular cartilage of	15 Semitendinosus
patella	16 Gracilis tendon
5 Lateral patellar	17 Sartorius
retinaculum	18 Great saphenous
6 Capsule of knee	vein
joint	19 Gastrocnemius
7 Femur	20 Tendon of vastus
8 Plantaris origin	medialis
9 Biceps femoris	
10 Common peroneal	**21 Vastus medialis**
nerve	

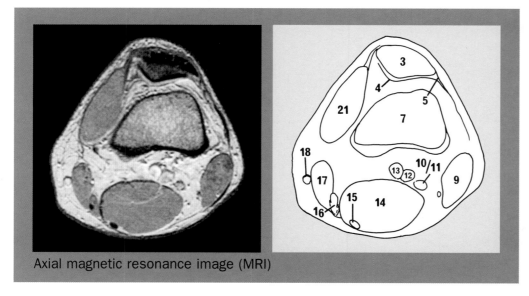

Axial magnetic resonance image (MRI)

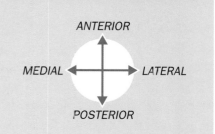

Orientation guide

ANTERIOR

MEDIAL ←→ LATERAL

POSTERIOR

Section level

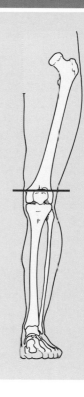

Notes

This section passes through the upper part of the patella (**3**) and the femur just as this widens into its condyles (**7**).

Note how the lateral portion of the patella (**3**) has a larger and flatter articular surface than the medial. This, together with the low insertion of vastus medialis (**20**) into the medial side of the patella, helps to prevent lateral dislocation of the patella. The exact alignment of the patellar depends on the relative contributions of the vasti muscles via their tendons (medial and lateral retinacula).

The sciatic nerve has now divided into the common peroneal nerve (**10**) and tibial nerve (**11**): the latter is usually about twice the size of the former. Division usually takes place just proximal to the knee, but the sciatic nerve may divide anywhere along its course. Indeed, its division may take place at the sciatic plexus, when the common peroneal nerve usually pierces the piriformis muscle in the greater sciatic foramen and the tibial division emerges caudal to this muscle.

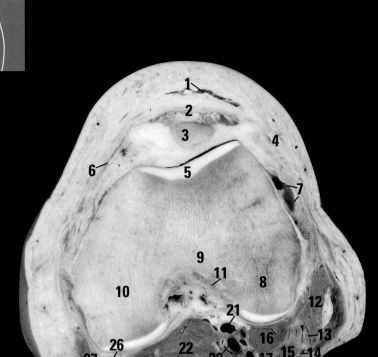

1 Prepatellar bursa	**15** Gastrocnemius- lateral head
2 Ligamentum patellae	**16** Plantaris
3 Patella	**17** Small saphenous vein – termination
4 Lateral patellar retinaculum	**18** Sural nerve
5 Articular cartilage of femur	**19** Tibial nerve
6 Medial patellar retinaculum	**20** Popliteal vein
7 Capsule of knee joint	**21** Popliteal artery
8 Lateral condyle of femur	**22** Gastrocnemius – medial head
9 Intercondylar fossa	**23** Semitendinosus tendon
10 Medial condyle of femur	**24** Semimembranosus tendon
11 Anterior cruciate ligament	**25** Great saphenous vein
12 Biceps femoris	**26** Gracilis tendon
13 Common peroneal nerve	**27** Sartorius
14 Sural communicating nerve	**28** Posterior cruciate ligament – attachment

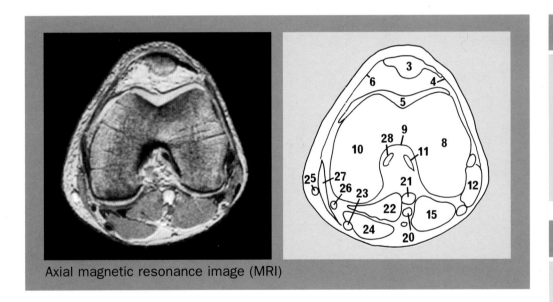

Axial magnetic resonance image (MRI)

Orientation guide

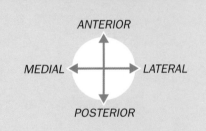

ANTERIOR

MEDIAL   LATERAL

POSTERIOR

Section level

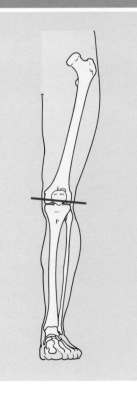

Notes

This section passes through the distal extremity of the patella (**3**) and the femoral condyles (**8**, **10**).

The anterior cruciate ligament (**11**) arises from the intercondylar fossa (**9**) of the femur laterally and slightly more proximally than the posterior cruciate ligament, whose attachment will be better seen in the next cadaveric section. The anterior cruciate ligament passes downwards and forwards laterally to the posterior cruciate ligament, to attach to the anterior intercondylar area of the tibia.

The small saphenous vein (**17**), which will be seen in later sections as it lies in the superficial fascia of the back of the calf, has here pierced the deep fascia of the popliteal fossa and is about to drain into the popliteal vein (**20**).

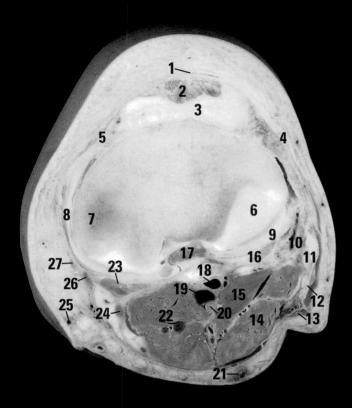

1 Infrapatellar bursa
2 Ligamentum patellae
3 Infrapatellar fat pad
4 Lateral patellar retinaculum
5 Medial patellar retinaculum
6 Sliver of cartilage over lateral condyle of tibia
7 Medial condyle of tibia
8 Medial collateral ligament
9 Lateral meniscus
10 Lateral collateral ligament
11 Tendon of biceps femoris
12 Common peroneal nerve
13 Lateral cutaneous nerve of calf
14 Gastrocnemius lateral head
15 Plantaris
16 Popliteus
17 Posterior cruciate ligament
18 Popliteal artery
19 Popliteal vein
20 Tibial nerve
21 Small saphenous vein
22 Gastrocnemius – medial head
23 Semimembranosus tendon
24 Semitendinosus tendon
25 Great saphenous vein
26 Gracilis tendon
27 Sartorius tendon

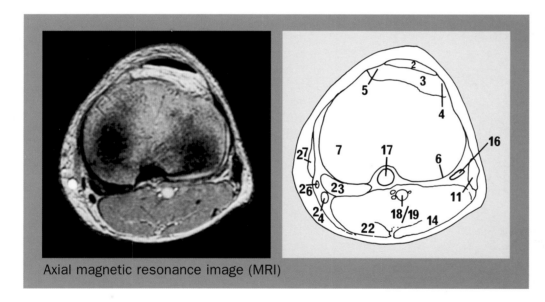

Axial magnetic resonance image (MRI)

Orientation guide

ANTERIOR
MEDIAL — LATERAL
POSTERIOR

Section level

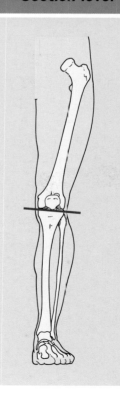

Notes

This section passes through the tibial condyles (**6**, **7**).

The posterior cruciate ligament (**17**) is here finding attachment to the posterior intercondylar area of the proximal articular surface of the tibia.

The popliteus tendon (**16**), which inserts onto the femur in a depression immediately distal to the lateral epicondyle, passes between the lateral meniscus (**9**) and the lateral collateral ligament of the knee (**10**). In contrast, the medial collateral ligament (**8**) is closely applied to the medial meniscus, which lies just proximal to this plane of section. This tethering of the medial meniscus probably accounts for the much higher incidence of tears of the medial compared with the lateral meniscus.

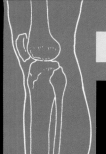

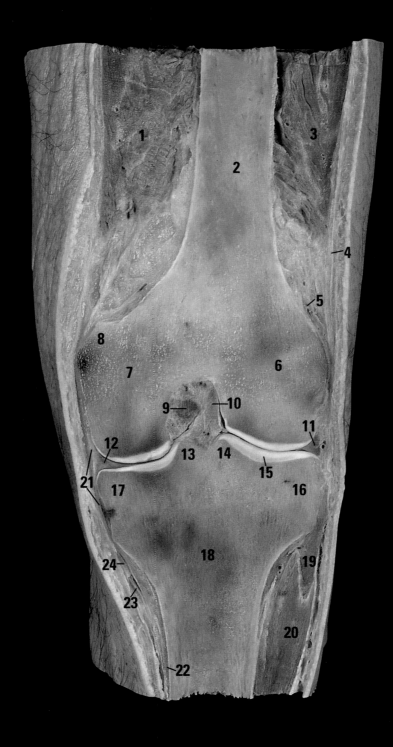

1 Vastus medialis	**15** Articular cartilage
2 Shaft of femur	**16** Lateral condyle (plateau)
3 Vastus lateralis	of tibia
4 Fascia lata	**17** Medial condyle (plateau)
5 Superior lateral genicular	of tibia
artery	**18** Tibia
6 Lateral condyle of femur	**19** Extensor digitorum longus
7 Medial condyle of femur	**20** Tibialis anterior
8 Adductor tubercle of femur	**21** Medial collateral ligament
9 Posterior cruciate ligament	**22** Popliteus (most medial fibres)
10 Anterior cruciate ligament	**23** Tendon of gracilis
11 Lateral meniscus	**24** Tendon of sartorius
12 Medial meniscus	
13 Medial intercondylar	**25** Popliteus tendon
eminence/tubercle (also	**26** Lateral collateral ligament
known as spine)	**27** Head of fibula
14 Lateral intercondylar	**28** Great saphenous vein
eminence/tubercle (also	**29** Medial gastrocnemius
known as spine)	**30** Biceps femoris

Section level

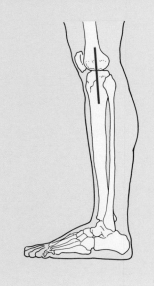

Orientation guide

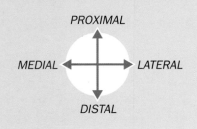

PROXIMAL

MEDIAL ←→ LATERAL

DISTAL

Notes

The posterior cruciate ligament (**9**) lies on the medial side of the anterior cruciate ligament (**10**). The former prevents posterior sliding movement of the tibia on the femur while the latter prevents anterior displacement as well as resisting torsional movement at the knee joint.

It can be seen that the menisci (**11** & **12**) do little to deepen the concavity of the knee joint on either side. However, they do act as 'shock absorbers' at the knee, for example, on jumping from a height.

Note that the medial collateral ligament is continuous with the medial meniscus whereas the lateral collateral ligament is discontinuous with the lateral meniscus. This contributes to the medial meniscus being more static and getting injured more in torsional injuries of the flexed knee; the lateral meniscus is more mobile.

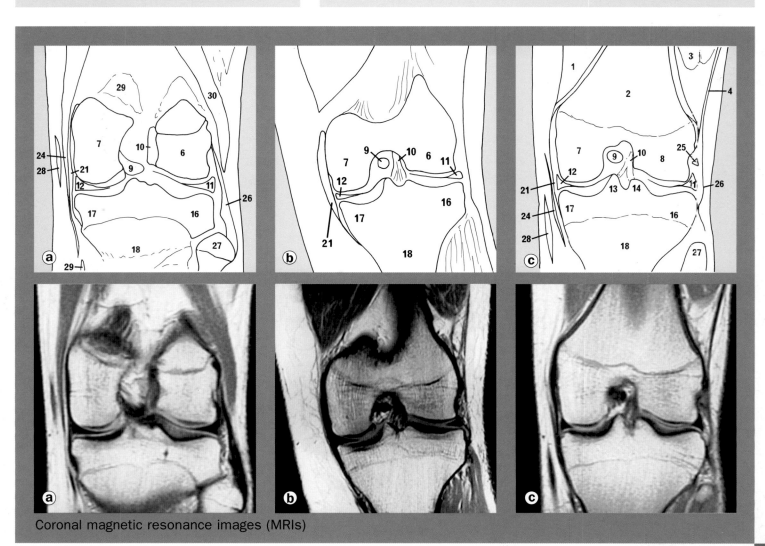

Coronal magnetic resonance images (MRIs)

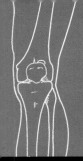

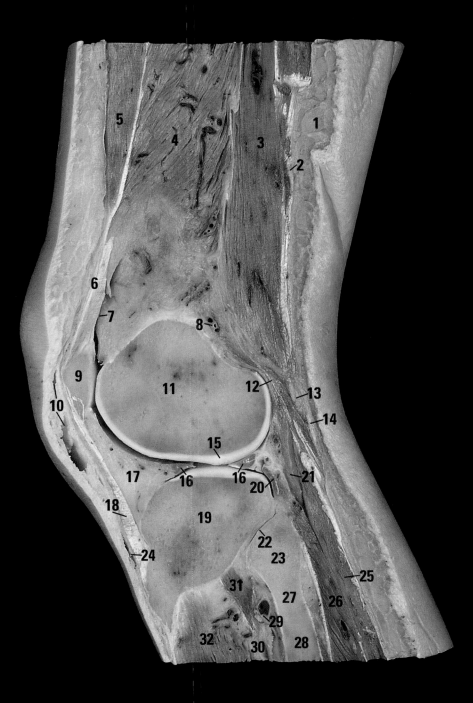

1 Superficial fascia	**17** Infrapatellar pad of fat
2 Deep fascia	extending into infrapatellar
3 Biceps femoris	fold
4 Vastus intermedius	**18** Ligamentum patellae
5 Vastus lateralis	**19** Lateral condyle (plateau) of
6 Tendon of quadriceps	tibia
femoris	**20** Tendon of popliteus
7 Suprapatellar bursa	**21** Plantaris
8 Lateral superior geniculate	**22** Superior tibiofibular joint
artery and vein	**23** Head of fibula
9 Patella	**24** Infrapatellar bursa
10 Prepatellar bursa	**25** Gastrocnemius lateral
11 Lateral condyle of femur	**26** Soleus
12 Fibrous capsule of knee	**27** Neck of fibula
joint	**28** Shaft of fibula
13 Common peroneal nerve	**29** Anterior tibial artery and
14 Lateral cutaneous nerve	vein
of calf	**30** Interosseous membrane
15 Articular cartilage	**31** Tibialis posterior
16 Lateral meniscus	**32** Tibialis anterior

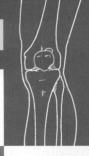

Section level

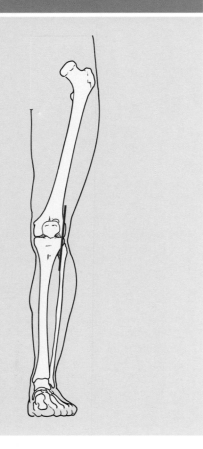

Orientation guide

PROXIMAL

ANTERIOR ← → POSTERIOR

DISTAL

Notes

The prepatellar bursa (**10**) and infrapatellar bursa (**24**) are both subcutaneous. Either may become inflamed by constant kneeling, which produces a traumatic bursitis. A prepatellar bursa comes into contact with the ground on scrubbing the floor (hence 'housemaid's knee'), while the infrapatellar bursa does so when kneeling to pray (hence 'clergyman's knee')!

The communication of the suprapatellar bursa (**7**) with the main synovial cavity of the knee is well demonstrated. It extends a handsbreadth superior to the border of the patella (**9**) and lies posterior to the quadriceps tendon (**6**). It becomes distended when there is an effusion into the knee joint.

Plantaris (**21**) is absent in about ten percent of subjects. Very rarely it has two heads.

The tendon of popliteus (**20**) is connected to the lateral meniscus (**16**) as it passes to the lateral condyle it thus helps to retract the mobile lateral meniscus during lateral rotation of the femur in flexion of the knee joint, protecting the meniscus from being crushed between the femoral and tibial condyles during this movement.

The superior tibiofibular joint (**22**) is a plane synovial joint, in contrast to the fibrous inferior tibiofibular joint.

The lateral meniscus is of even thickness throughout. Thus a lateral sagittal slice creates a 'bow-tie' appearance to this portion of the lateral meniscus.

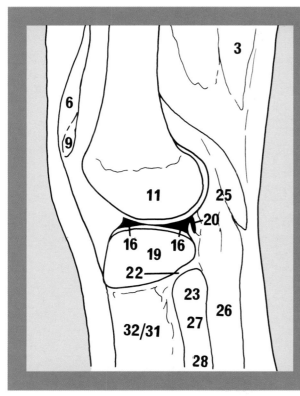

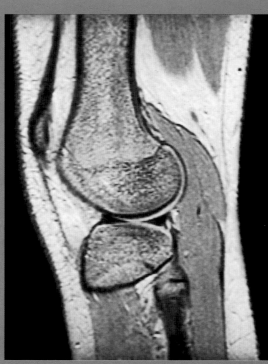

Sagittal magnetic resonance image (MRI)

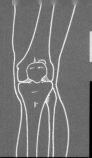

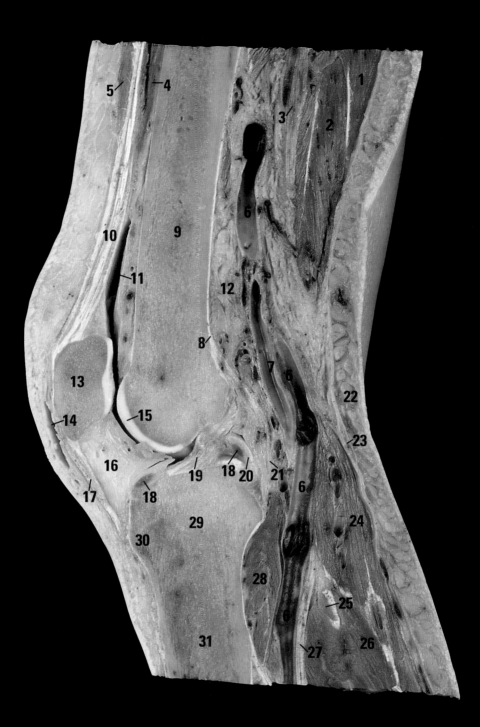

1 Semitendinosus	**17** Ligamentum patellae
2 Semimembranosus	**18** Medial meniscus
3 Sciatic nerve	**19** Anterior cruciate ligament
4 Vastus intermedius	**20** Posterior cruciate ligament
5 Rectus femoris	**21** Fibrous capsule of knee
6 Popliteal vein	joint
7 Popliteal artery	**22** Superficial fascia
8 Popliteal surface of femur	**23** Deep fascia
9 Shaft of femur	**24** Gastrocnemius
10 Tendon of quadriceps	**25** Tendon of plantaris
femoris	**26** Soleus
11 Suprapatellar bursa	**27** Tibial nerve
12 Popliteal pad of fat	**28** Popliteus
13 Patella	**29** Proximal end of tibia
14 Prepatellar bursa	**30** Tibial tuberosity
15 Articular cartilage	**31** Shaft of tibia
16 Infrapatellar pad of fat	
(Hoffa) extending into	**32** Transverse intermeniscal
infrapatellar fold	ligament

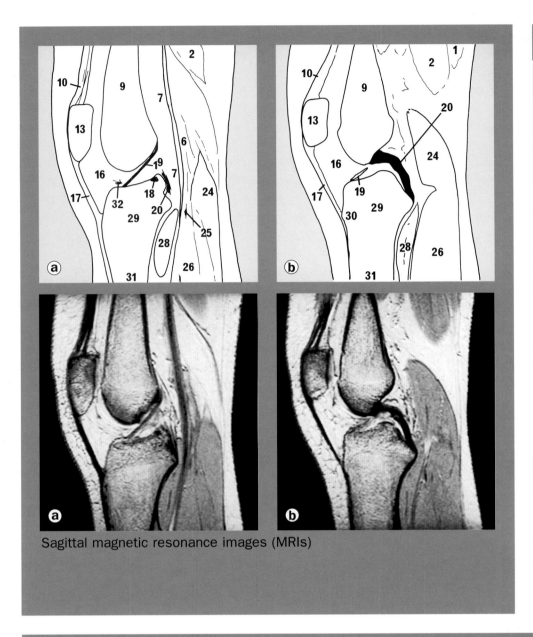

Sagittal magnetic resonance images (MRIs)

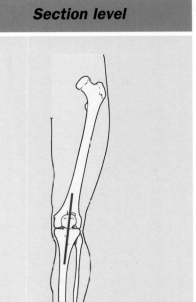

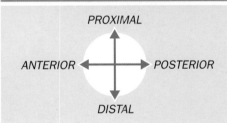

PROXIMAL

ANTERIOR ←→ POSTERIOR

DISTAL

Notes

The relationships in the popliteal fossa comprise:

The tibial nerve (**27**) most superficially, then the popliteal vein (**6**) and then, more deeply the popliteal artery (**7**). The valves in the vein are well shown.

The fossa contains a large amount of fat (**12**) as well as the rather insignificant popliteal lymph nodes, usually five or six in number. Note the composition of the floor of the politeal fossa comprises superiorly the popliteal surface of the femur (**8**), then the capsule of the knee joint (**21**) and then finally popliteus (**28**).

Both gastrocnemius (**24**) and soleus (**26**) contain large veins; an important component of the calf pump mechanism in venous return from the lower limb. Note also the density of the deep fascia (**23**), which assists the pumping action of the muscles.

Note that with the knee in the extended position the anterior cruciate ligament is taut and straight; there is less tension on the posterior cruciate which appears curved in that position. The cruciate, ligaments take their names (anterior and posterior) from the site of attachment to the tibia. The anterior cruciate passess lateral to the posterior ligament.

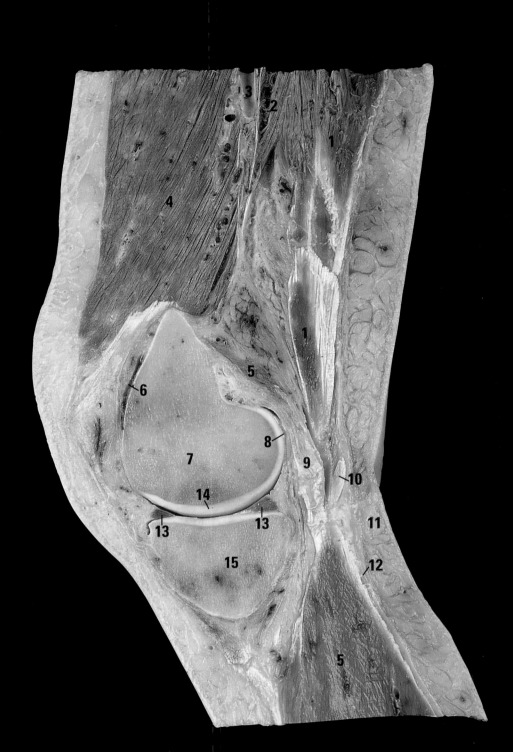

1 Semimembranosus	**9** Medial head/tendon of
2 Adductor magnus	gastrocnemius
3 Femoral artery	**10** Tendon of
4 Vastus medialis	semitendinosus
5 Medial head of	**11** Superficial fascia
gastrocnemius	**12** Deep fascia
6 Suprapatellar bursa	**13** Medial meniscus
7 Medial condyle of	**14** Articular cartilage
femur	**15** Medial condyle (plateau
8 Fibrous capsule of	of tibia)
knee joint	

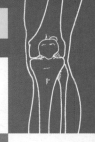

Section level

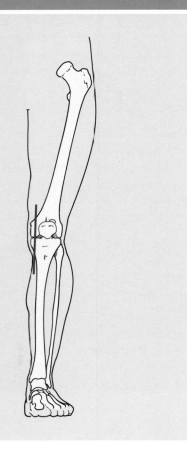

Orientation guide

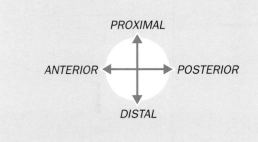

PROXIMAL

ANTERIOR ←→ POSTERIOR

DISTAL

Notes

The femoral artery (**3**) passes through the hiatus in adductor magnus (**2**) to become the popliteal artery about two-thirds of the distance along a line which joins the femoral pulse at the groin with the adductor tubercle on the medial condyle of the femur.

The posterior third of the medial meniscus is usually a little thicker than the middle and anterior thirds, in contrast to the lateral meniscus which is of constant thickness around its circumference. Furthermore the posterior third frequently undergoes myxoid change during early middle age; thus this part of the medial meniscus often appears rather heterogeneous in consistency.

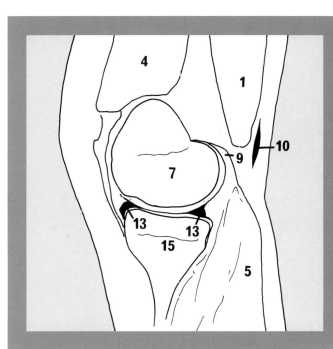

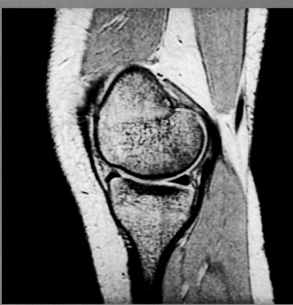

Sagittal magnetic resonance image (MRI)

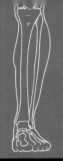

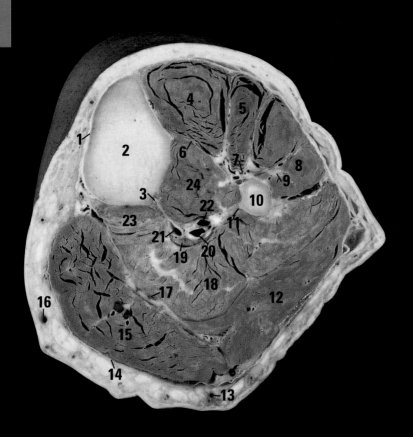

1 Subcutaneous surface of tibia
2 Tibia
3 Vertical ridge of tibia
4 Tibialis anterior
5 Extensor digitorum longus
6 Interosseous membrane
7 Anterior tibial artery and vein with deep peroneal nerve
8 Peroneus longus
9 Superficial peroneal nerve
10 Fibula
11 Medial crest of fibula
12 Gastrocnemius–lateral head
13 Small saphenous vein
14 Deep fascia of calf
15 Gastrocnemius–medial head
16 Great saphenous vein
17 Plantaris tendon
18 Soleus
19 Tibial nerve
20 Posterior tibial artery
21 Posterior tibial vein
22 Peroneal artery
23 Popliteus
24 Tibialis posterior

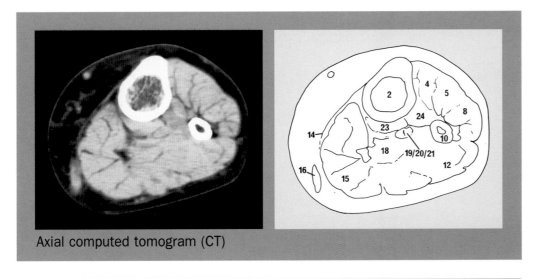

Axial computed tomogram (CT)

Orientation guide

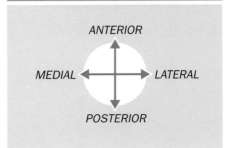

ANTERIOR

MEDIAL — LATERAL

POSTERIOR

Section level

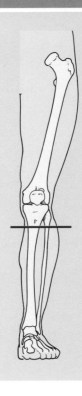

Notes

This section traverses the proximal end of the tibial shaft (**2**) and the shaft of the fibula (**10**) immediately distal to the neck of the fibula.

At this level the common peroneal nerve, which sweeps round the neck of the fibula deep to peroneus longus (**8**), has divided into its superficial peroneal (**9**) and deep peroneal (**7**) branches. The superficial peroneal nerve lies deep to peroneus longus. The deep peroneal nerve passes obliquely forwards deep to extensor digitorum longus (**5**) to descend with the anterior tibial vessels (**7**).

The tendon of plantaris (**17**) lies in a well defined tissue plane between soleus (**18**) and gastrocnemius (**12**, **15**). Fluid enters this plane following rupture of a semimembranosus bursa (Baker's cyst).

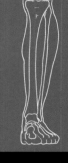

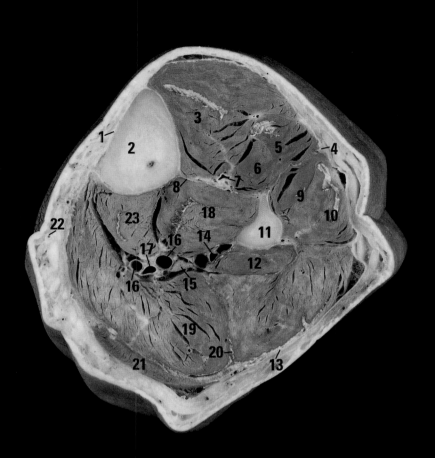

1 Subcutaneous border of tibia
2 Tibia
3 Tibialis anterior
4 Superficial peroneal nerve
5 Extensor digitorum longus
6 Extensor hallucis longus
7 Anterior tibial artery and vein with deep peroneal nerve
8 Interosseous membrane
9 Peroneus brevis
10 Peroneus longus
11 Fibula
12 Flexor hallucis longus
13 Deep fascia of calf
14 Peroneal artery with venae comitantes
15 Tibial nerve
16 Venae comitantes of posterior tibial artery
17 Posterior tibial artery
18 Tibialis posterior
19 Soleus
20 Plantaris tendon
21 Gastrocnemius
22 Great saphenous vein
23 Flexor digitorum longus

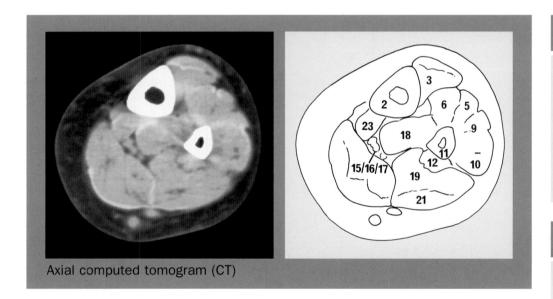

Axial computed tomogram (CT)

Orientation guide

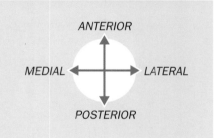

ANTERIOR

MEDIAL ←→ LATERAL

POSTERIOR

Section level

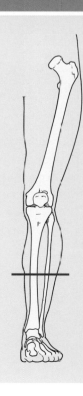

Notes

This section traverses the mid calf.

Note that the whole of the anteromedial aspect of the shaft of the tibia (**1**) is subcutaneous, covered only by skin, superficial fascia and periosteum, and crossed, in its lower part, only by the great saphenous vein (**22**) and saphenous nerve.

The neurovascular bundle of the anterior tibial vessels and deep peroneal nerve (**7**), having descended first between extensor digitorum longus (**5**) and tibialis anterior (**3**), now runs between the latter and extensor hallucis longus (**6**) as this takes origin from the anterior aspect of the fibular shaft (**11**).

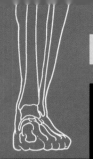

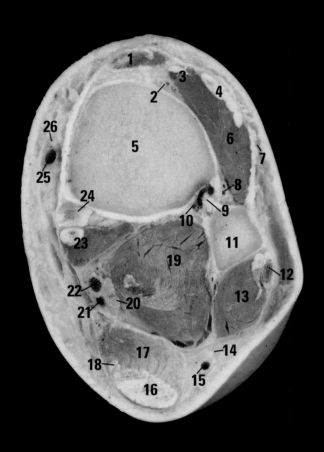

1 Tibialis anterior tendon	11 Fibula
2 Anterior tibial artery with venae comitantes and deep peroneal nerve	12 Peroneus longus tendon
	13 Peroneus brevis
	14 Sural nerve
3 Extensor hallucis longus and tendon	15 Small saphenous vein
4 Extensor digitorum longus tendon	16 Tendo calcaneus (Achilles tendon)
5 Tibia	17 Soleus
6 Peroneus tertius	18 Plantaris tendon
7 Superficial peroneal nerve	19 Flexor hallucis longus
	20 Tibial nerve
8 Perforating branch of peroneal artery	21 Posterior tibial vein
	22 Posterior tibial artery
9 Inferior tibiofibular joint (interosseous ligament)	23 Flexor digitorum longus and tendon
	24 Tibialis posterior tendon
10 Peroneal artery	25 Great saphenous vein
	26 Saphenous nerve

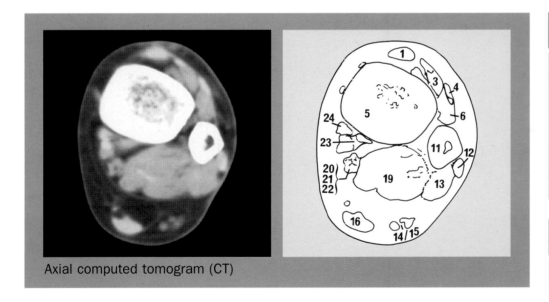

Axial computed tomogram (CT)

Orientation guide
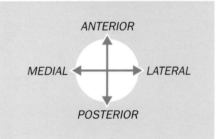
ANTERIOR / MEDIAL / LATERAL / POSTERIOR

Section level
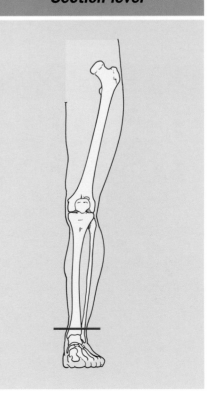

Notes

This section passes immediately above the ankle joint at the level of the inferior tibiofibular joint (**9**). This is the only fibrous joint, apart from the skull sutures, and represents, in fact, the thickened distal extremity of the interosseous membrane. (See also section 2, page 212.)

At this level, gastroncnemius has already become tendinous (**16**), although soleus (**17**) still displays muscle fibres. A little more distally this too will become tendinous and fuse into the tendo calcaneus (tendo Achilles).

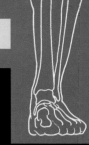

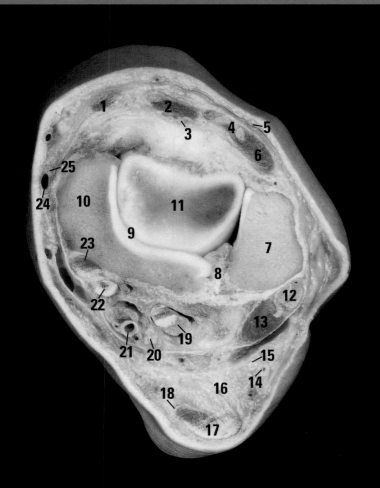

1 Tibialis anterior tendon	13 Peroneus brevis
2 Extensor hallucis longus and tendon	14 Small saphenous vein
3 Anterior tibial artery and venae comitantes with deep peroneal nerve	15 Sural nerve
	16 Fat
	17 Tendo calcaneus
	18 Plantaris tendon
4 Extensor digitorum tendon	19 Flexor hallucis longus tendon
5 Superficial peroneal nerve	20 Tibial nerve
6 Peroneus tertius and tendon	21 Posterior tibial artery with venae comitantes
7 Lateral malleolus	22 Flexor digitorum longus tendon
8 Inferior tibiofibular joint	23 Tibialis posterior tendon
9 Ankle joint	24 Great saphenous vein
10 Medial malleolus	25 Saphenous nerve
11 Talus	
12 Peroneus longus tendon	

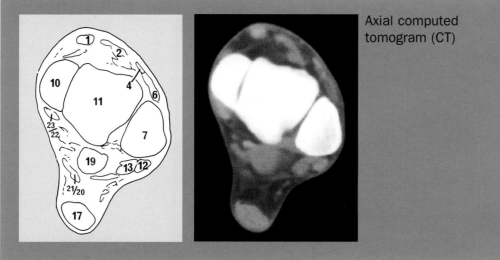

Axial computed tomogram (CT)

Orientation guide

ANTERIOR

MEDIAL ←→ LATERAL

POSTERIOR

Section level

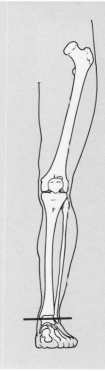

Notes

This section passes through the ankle joint (**9**) and the inferior tibiofibular joint (**8**).

Note that this section illustrates the fibrous nature of the inferior tibiofibular joint.

Peroneus brevis (**12**) and peroneus longus (**13**) pass behind the lateral malleolus (**7**) of the fibula and will groove the bone a little more distally to form the malleolar fossa.

This section demonstrates the order of structures which pass behind the medial malleolus (**10**). These are, from the medial to the lateral side, the tendon of tibialis posterior (**23**), the tendon of flexor digitorum longus (**22**), the posterior tibial artery with its venae comitantes (**21**), the tibial nerve (**20**) and, most laterally, the tendon of flexor hallucis longus (**19**).

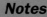

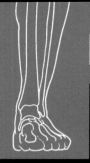

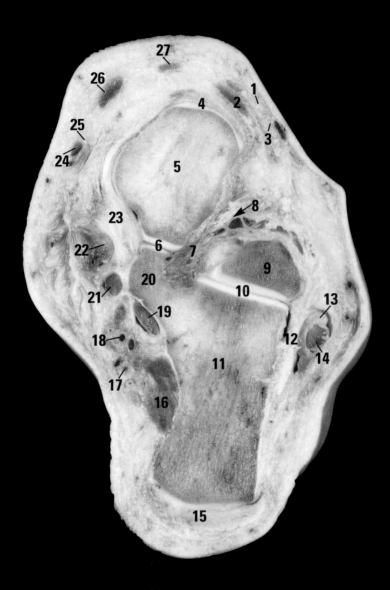

1 Extensor digitorum longus tendon
2 Extensor digitorum brevis
3 Peroneus tertius tendon
4 Talocalcaneonavicular joint (anterior talonavicular part)
5 Head of talus
6 Talocalcaneonavicular joint (posterior part)
7 Interosseous talocalcanean ligament
8 Sulcus tali (arrowed)
9 Lateral process of talus
10 Talocalcanean (subtalar) joint
11 Calcaneus
12 Capsule of talocalcanean joint
13 Peroneus brevis tendon
14 Peroneus longus tendon
15 Tendo Achilles
16 Flexor accessorius

17 Lateral plantar neurovascular bundle
18 Medial plantar neurovascular bundle
19 Flexor hallucis longus tendon
20 Sustentaculum tali
21 Flexor digitorum longus tendon
22 Tibialis posterior tendon
23 Deltoid ligament of ankle
24 Great saphenous vein
25 Saphenous nerve
26 Tibialis anterior tendon
27 Extensor hallucis longus tendon

28 Tibia
29 Medial Malleolus
30 Abductor hallucis
31 Abductor digiti minimi

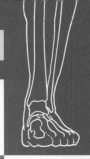

Section level

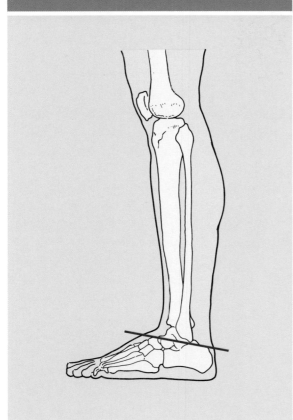

Orientation guide

ANTERIOR

MEDIAL ← → LATERAL

POSTERIOR

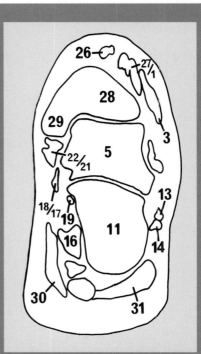

Computed tomogram (CT)

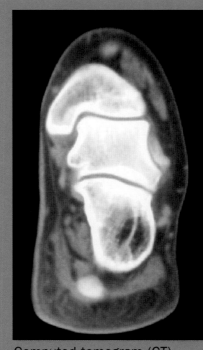

Notes

This section passes through the head (**5**) and lateral process (**9**) of the talus and the calcaneus (**11**). The CT image is in a more coronal plane, hence the tibia (**28**) is seen with its articulation with the talus (**5**).

The tendon of flexor hallucis longus (**19**) passes behind the sustentaculum tali (**20**) and, more distally, grooves its inferior aspect. The sulcus tali (**8**), with its corresponding sulcus calcanei, forms the sinus tarsi and contains the strong interosseous talocalcanean ligament.

The talocalcanean joint (**10**), also termed the subtalar joint, lies between the convex posterior facet on the upper surface of the calcaneus and the concave posterior facet on the inferior surface of the

talus. The talocalcaneonavicular joint is complex. It is formed by the rounded head of the talus (**5**) which fits into the concavity on the posterior aspect of the navicular, the upper surface of the plantar calcaneon-avicular ligament (the spring ligament), which runs between the sustentaculum tali and the inferior aspect of the navicular, and the anterior and middle facets for the talus on the calcaneus. The anterior and posterior portions of this joint are shown at (**4**) and (**6**).

A considerable degree of inversion and eversion of the foot takes place at the talocalcanean and talocalcaneonavicular joints.

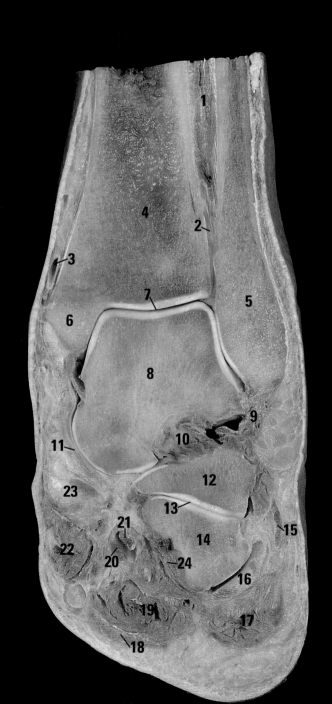

Section level

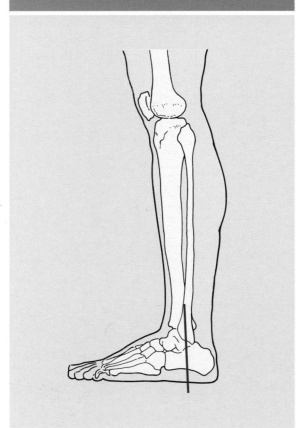

Orientation guide

PROXIMAL

MEDIAL ←→ LATERAL

DISTAL

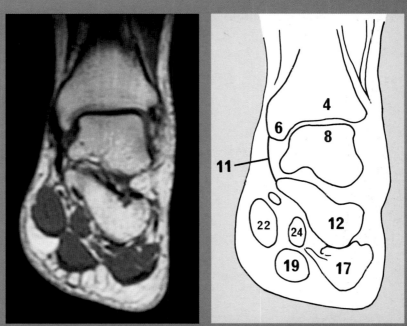

Coronal magnetic resonance image (MRI)

Notes

By convention, the articulation between the lower end of the fibula and the tibia is described as the inferior tibiofibular joint (**2**) and it is stated to be the only fibrous joint apart from those pertaining to the skull. In effect this 'joint' represents the considerable thickening of the lowermost part of the interosseous membrane between the shafts of these two bones.

The mortice joint of the ankle (**7**) is well demonstrated. The lateral collateral ligament (**9**), especially its anterior talofibular component, is commonly injured.

The plantar aponeurosis (**18**) is thick and tough. It closely adheres to flexor digitorum brevis (**19**).

The hyaline cartilage and subchondral bone of the talar dome (**8**) is commonly damaged by relatively minor trauma. Loose fragments may break off and cause symptoms. Cystic degenerative change may follow in later life.

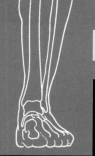

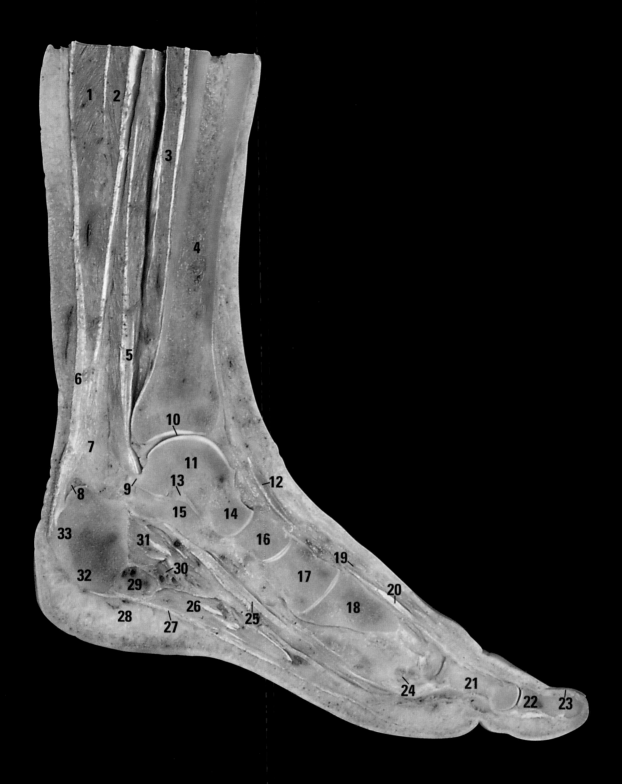

1 Gastrocnemius	13 Interosseous talocalcanean	26 Abductor hallucis
2 Soleus	ligament	27 Plantar aponeurosis
3 Flexor digitorum longus	14 Head of talus	28 Dense subcutaneous fibro
4 Tibia	15 Sustentaculum tali	fatty tissue
5 Tendon of flexor hallucis longus	16 Navicular	29 Abductor digiti minimi
(posterior relation to ankle joint	17 Medial cuneiform	30 Lateral plantar artery, vein
– see also 25)	18 First metatarsal bone	and nerve
6 Tendo calcaneus (Achilles	19 Tributary of great	31 Flexor accessorius
tendon)	saphenous vein	32 Medial process of tuberosity
7 Fat deep to tendo calcaneus	20 Extensor hallucis longus	of calcaneus
8 Bursa deep to tendo calcaneous	21 Proximal phalanx of hallux	33 Calcaneus
9 Medial tubercle of posterior	22 distal phalanx of hallux	34 Plantar calcaneonavicular
process of talus	23 Nail bed	(spring) ligament
10 Ankle joint	24 Sesamoid bone	35 Tendon of tibialis posterior
11 Body of talus	25 Tendon of flexor hallucis longus	
12 Tendon of tibialis anterior	(in foot – also see 5)	

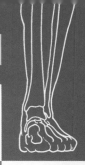

Section level

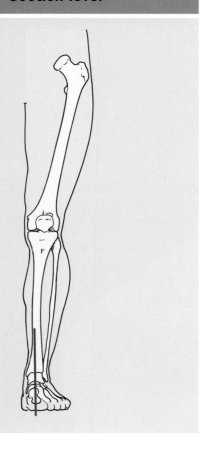

Orientation guide

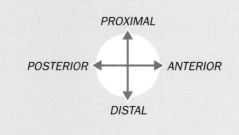

PROXIMAL

POSTERIOR ←——→ ANTERIOR

DISTAL

Notes

Flexor hallucis longus (**5**) is the immediate posterior relation of the ankle joint. It grooves the posterior aspect of the lower extremity of the tibia (**4**) then, distal to the capsule of the ankle joint (**10**) it grooves the posterior process of the talus between its medial (**9**) and lateral tubercle. The tendon (**25**) then grooves a third bone, as it passes beneath the sustentaculum tali of the calcaneus (**15**). Suprisingly the flexor hallucis longus at this point is lateral to the flexor digitorum longus; they cross in the foot.

This section shows clearly the role of the plantar calcaneonavicular (or spring) ligament (**34**) as this passes from the sustentaculum tali (**15**) to the navicular (**16**). It supports the head of the talus (**14**).

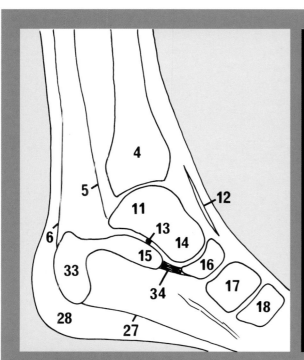

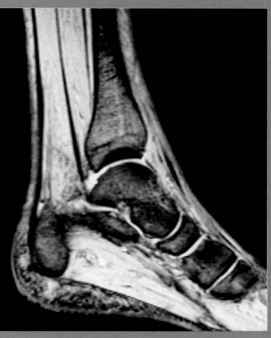

Sagittal magnetic resonance image (MRI)

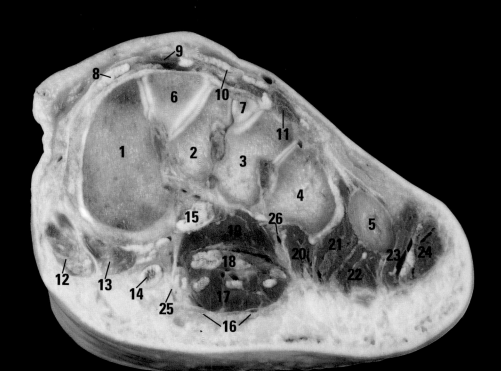

Section level

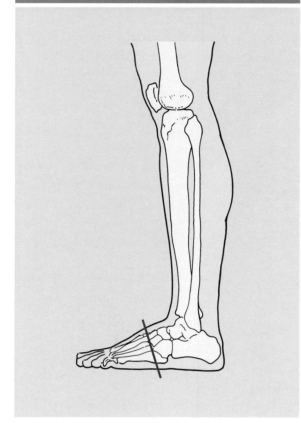

Notes

This section of the lower limb passes through the forefoot and the bases of the metatarsal bones. It demonstrates the appearance of the transverse arch of the foot.

The tendon of peroneus longus (**15**), having grooved the inferior aspect of the cuboid, passes forward and medially to insert into the inferolateral aspect of the medial cuneiform (**6**) and the base of the first metatarsal (**1**). The sling-like action of this tendon helps maintain the transverse arch.

Orientation guide

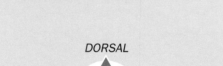
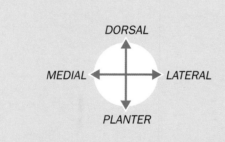

DORSAL

MEDIAL   LATERAL

PLANTER

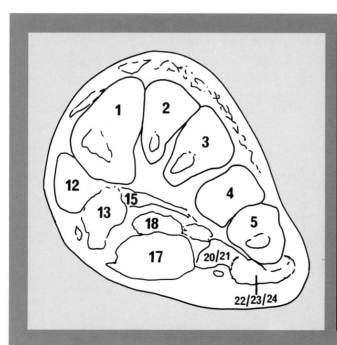

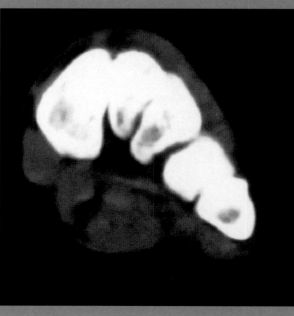

Coronal computed tomogram (CT)

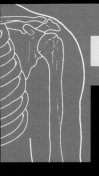

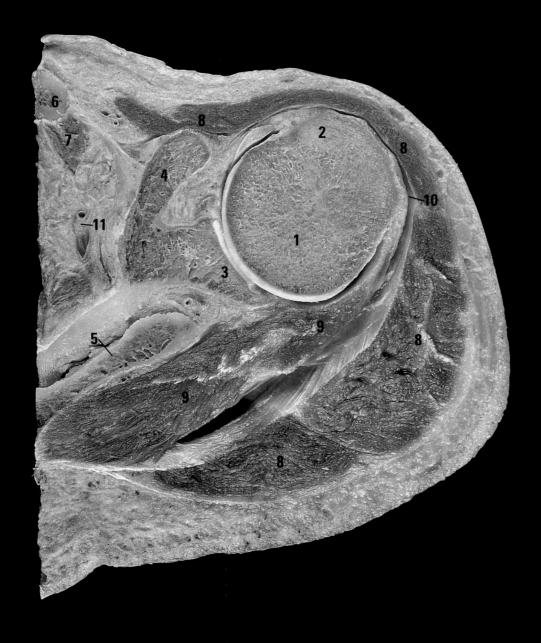

1 Head of humerus
2 Greater tubercle
   of humerus
3 Glenoid fossa of
   scapula
4 Coracoid process
   of scapula
5 Spine of scapula
6 Clavicle
7 Subclavius
8 Deltoid
9 Infraspinatus
10 Subdeltoid bursa
11 Suprascapular artery
   and vein

12 Labrum of glenoid
13 Subscapularis tendon
14 Middle glenohumeral
   ligament
15 Long head of biceps
   tendon in bicipital
   groove (intertubercular
   groove)
16 Attachment of
   coraco-acrominal and
   coraco-humeral
   ligaments
17 Lesser tubercle of
   humerus
18 Transverse humeral
   ligament

Section level

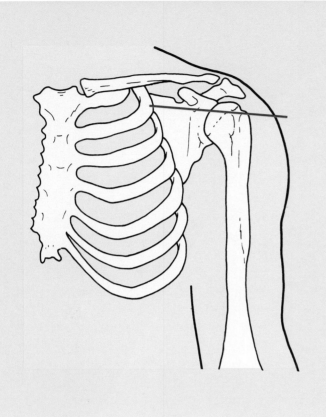

Orientation guide

ANTERIOR

MEDIAL ←→ LATERAL

POSTERIOR

Notes

The greater tubercle of the humerus (**2**) is the most lateral bony landmark around the shoulder. The subacromial bursa passes below the acromion and above supraspinatus to continue into the subdeltoid bursa (**10**) between the upper shaft of the humerus and the deltoid muscle (**8**).

Infraspinatus (**9**), together with supraspinatus, teres minor and subscapularis, forms a protective rotator cuff around the shoulder joint, which, as can be seen in this section, has little stability afforded either by its bony configuration or capsular strength.

The shallow glenoid is in sharp contrast to the deep acetabulum in the hip; stability has been sacrificed for mobility to allow a greater range of movement.

The orientation and shape of the coracoid process is an important feature; the coraco-acromial ligament can impinge on the rotator cuff.

The tendon of subscapularis mainly attaches to the lesser tubercle but some slips attach to the floor of the intertubercular sulcus. Furthermore the transverse humeral ligament, which retains the long head of biceps tendon, could be regarded as fibres from the subscapularis attachment on the lesser tubercle extending on towards the greater tubercle.

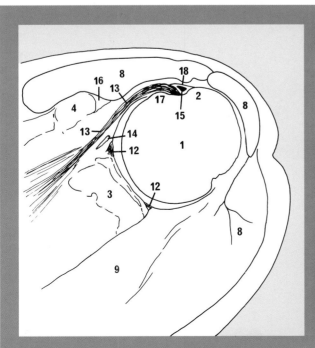

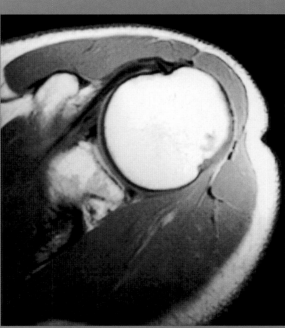

Axial magnetic resonance image (MRI)

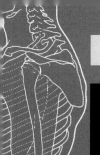

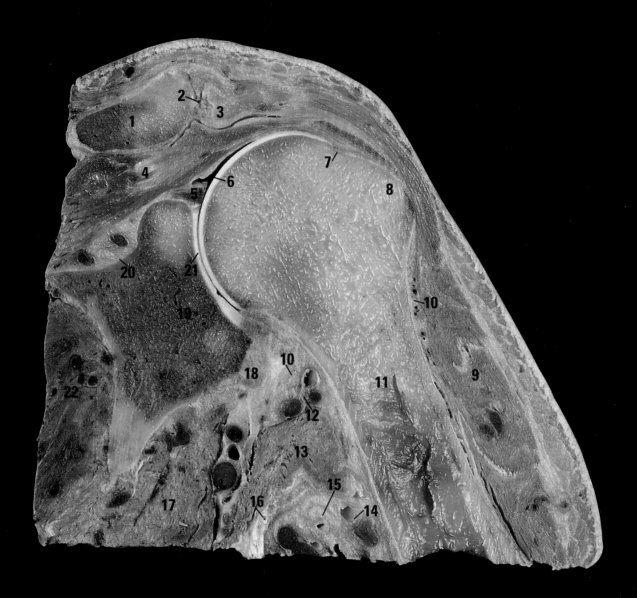

1 Clavicle	**13** Latissimus dorsi
2 Acromioclavicular joint	**14** Brachial artery and vein
3 Acromion of scapula	**15** Nerves of brachial
4 Supraspinatus	plexus
5 Glenoid labrum	**16** Tendon of teres major
6 Shoulder joint cavity	**17** Teres minor
7 Anatomical neck of	**18** Long head of triceps
humerus	**19** Head of scapula
8 Greater tubercle of	**20** Neck of scapula
humerus	**21** Glenoid fossa of
9 Deltoid	scapula
10 Axillary nerve	**22** Subscapularis
accompanied by	
posterior circumflex	**23** Long head of biceps
humeral artery and vein	tendon
11 Shaft of humerus	**24** Surgical neck of
12 Medial circumflex	humerus
artery and vein	

Section level

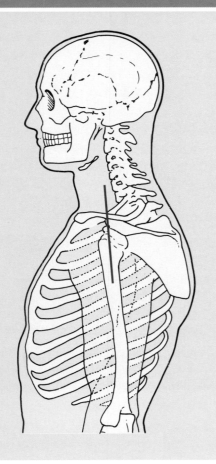

Notes

The important relationship of the supraspinatus tendon (**4**) to the acromion process (**3**) and clavicle (**1**) is well demonstrated. This muscle initiates abduction of the shoulder, which is then powerfully continued by deltoid (**9**). Degenerative changes in the acromio-clavicular joint frequently cause impingement on the musculotendinous junction of supraspinatus; tendonitis and a tear in the rotator cuff may follow.

Note the close relationship of the axillary nerve (**10**), together with its accompanying vessels, the posterior circumflex humeral artery and vein, to the surgical neck of the humerus (**24**). Fractures commonly occur in the region of the surgical neck; the axillary nerve may be affected.

This MR image is in a somewhat coronal oblique plane in order to demonstrate the supraspinatus muscle, tendon and insertion as a continuum

Orientation guide

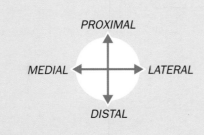

PROXIMAL

MEDIAL ← → LATERAL

DISTAL

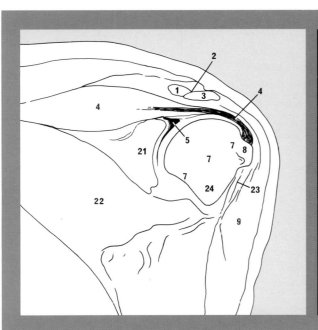

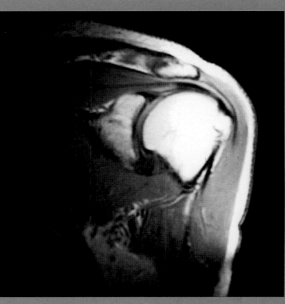

Coronal magnetic resonance image (MRI)

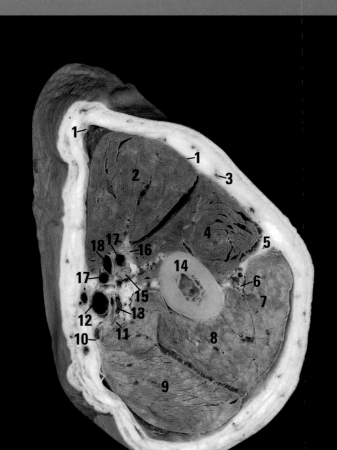

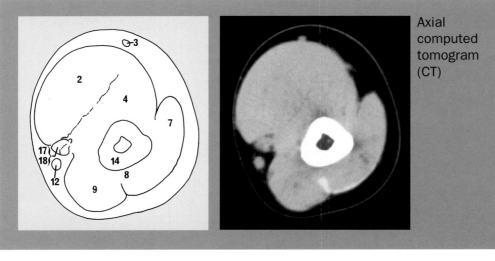

1 Deep fascia of arm	**10** Medial intermuscular
2 Biceps	septum
3 Cephalic vein	**11** Ulnar nerve
4 Brachialis	**12** Basilic vein
5 Lateral intermuscular	**13** Superior ulnar collateral
septum	artery and vein
6 Radial nerve with	**14** Humerus shaft
profunda brachii artery	**15** Median nerve
and vein	**16** Musculocutaneous nerve
7 Triceps – lateral head	**17** Venae comitantes of
8 Triceps – medial head	brachial artery
9 Triceps – long head	**18** Brachial artery

Axial computed tomogram (CT)

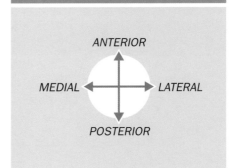

Orientation guide

ANTERIOR

MEDIAL ←→ LATERAL

POSTERIOR

Section level

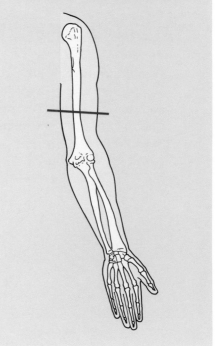

Notes

This section passes through the mid-shaft of the humerus (**14**). It gives a clear view of the fascial arrangements of the upper arm; the investing sheath of the deep fascia (**1**) with its lateral (**5**) and medial (**10**) intermuscular septa which attach to the humeral shaft. These septa divide the extensor group of muscles, comprising the three heads of triceps (**7**, **8**, **9**), from the anterior flexor group. The medial septum is pierced by the ulnar nerve (**11**) and its accompanying vessels (**13**), the lateral by the radial nerve with its accompanying profunda brachii artery and vein (**6**).

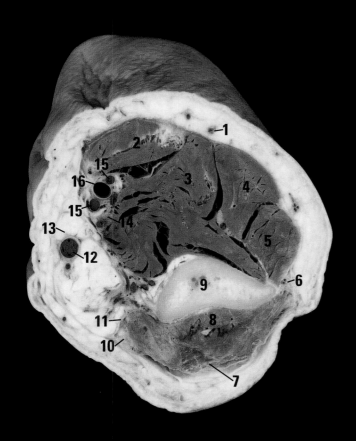

1 Cephalic vein
2 Biceps
3 Brachialis
4 Brachioradialis
5 Extensor carpi radialis long
6 Lateral intermuscular septum
7 Triceps tendon
8 Triceps
9 Humerus
10 Ulnar nerve
11 Medial intermuscular septum
12 Basilic vein
13 Medial cutaneous nerve of forearm
14 Median nerve
15 Venae comitantes of brachial artery
16 Brachial artery

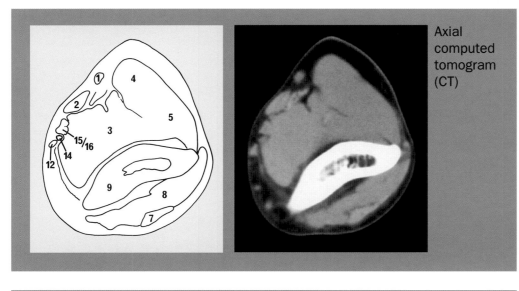

Axial computed tomogram (CT)

Orientation guide

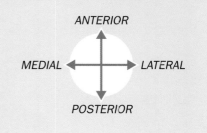

ANTERIOR

MEDIAL — LATERAL

POSTERIOR

Section level

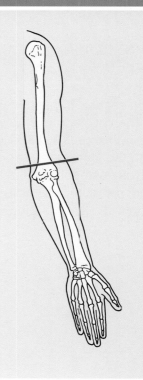

Notes

This section transects the distal end of the humeral shaft as it expands to form its medial and lateral supracondylar ridges.

The origin of extensor carpi radialis longus (**5**) is from the upper part of the lateral ridge and this muscle arises superior to, and separate from, the remaining extensor muscles of the forearm, which originate from a common origin from the lateral epicondyle of the humerus.

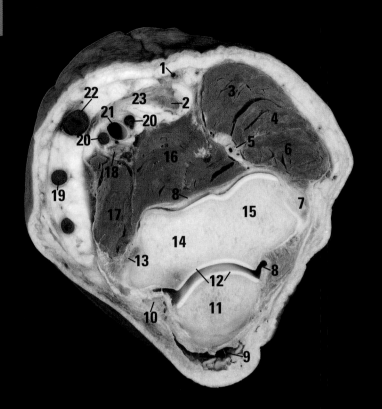

1 Cephalic vein
2 Biceps tendon
3 Brachioradialis
4 Extensor carpi radialis longus
5 Radial nerve with profunda brachii artery and vein
6 Common extensor origin
7 Lateral collateral ligament of elbow
8 Joint capsule of elbow
9 Olecranon bursa
10 Ulnar nerve
11 Olecranon process of ulna
12 Articular cartilage
13 Medial collateral ligament of elbow
14 Trochlea of humerus
15 Capitulum of humerus
16 Brachialis
17 Common flexor origin
18 Median nerve
19 Basilic vein
20 Venae comitantes of brachial artery
21 Brachial artery
22 Median cubital vein
23 Bicipital aponeurosis

24 Anconeus

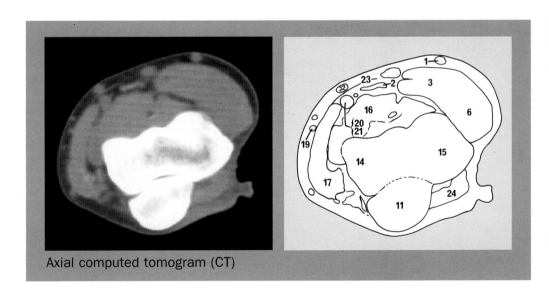

Axial computed tomogram (CT)

Orientation guide

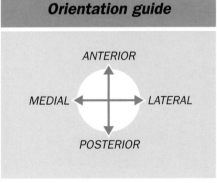

ANTERIOR

MEDIAL — LATERAL

POSTERIOR

Section level

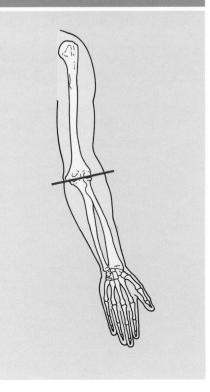

Notes

This section transects the elbow joint.

The cartilage (**12**) covering the articular surfaces of the lower end of the humerus (**14**, **15**) and the olecranon process of the ulna (**11**), together with the joint cavity and collateral ligaments (**8**) are readily appreciated.

The posterior surface of the olecranon process of the ulna is separated from the skin by a bursa (**9**). This is a common site for bursitis ('Student's elbow' or 'Miner's elbow').

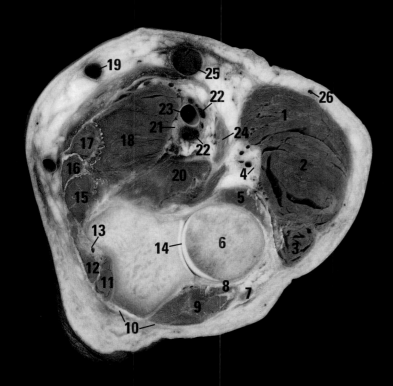

1	Brachioradialis	**12**	Flexor carpi ulnaris
2	Extensor carpi radialis longus	**13**	Ulnar nerve with posterior recurrent ulnar artery and vein
3	Extensor carpi radialis brevis	**14**	Radial notch of ulna
4	Radial nerve with radial recurrent artery	**15**	Flexor digitorum superficialis
5	Supinator	**16**	Palmaris longus
6	Head of radius	**17**	Flexor carpi radialis
7	Common extensor origin	**18**	Pronator teres
		19	Basilic vein
8	Annular ligament of superior radio-ulnar joint	**20**	Brachialis
		21	Median nerve
9	Anconeus	**22**	Venae comitantes of brachial artery
10	Deep fascia of the forearm	**23**	Brachial artery
		24	Tendon of biceps
11	Flexor digitorum profundus	**25**	Median cubital vein
		26	Cephalic vein

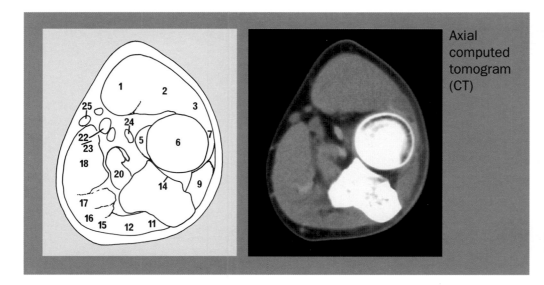

Axial computed tomogram (CT)

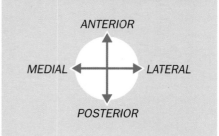

Orientation guide

ANTERIOR

MEDIAL ←→ LATERAL

POSTERIOR

Section level

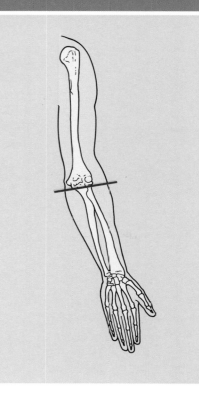

Notes

This section passes through the superior radio-ulnar joint between the head of the radius (**6**) and the radial notch of the ulnar (**14**). The annular ligament (**8**), which maintains the congruity of this pivot joint, is well shown. In this CT image the hand is in the neutral position alongside the body.

The median cubital vein (**25**) passes obliquely across the front of the elbow between the cephalic vein (**26**) and the basilic vein (**19**). It is separated from the underlying brachial artery (**23**) by a condensation of the deep fascia (**10**) termed the bicipital aponeurosis. Occasionally in high division of the brachial artery, an abnormal ulnar artery may lie immediately below the median cubital vein in the superficial fascia. This vein is therefore safer avoided for intravenous injections to protect against inadvertent intra-arterial injection.

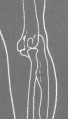

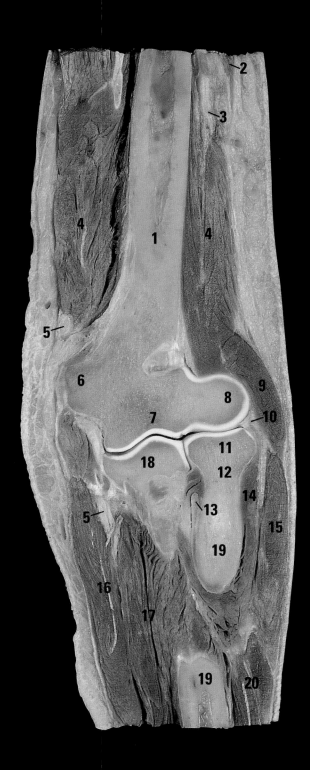

1 Shaft of humerus
2 Lateral head of triceps
3 Radial nerve
4 Medial head of triceps
5 Ulnar nerve
6 Medial epicondyle of

15 Extensor carpi radialis
   longus
16 Flexor carpi ulnaris
17 Flexor digitorum
   profundus
18 Coronoid process of ulna

Section level

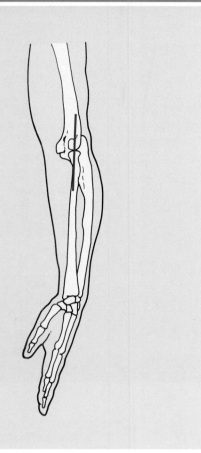

Notes

The ulnar nerve (**5**) passes posterior to the medial epicondyle of the humerus (**6**), where it may be palpated. It may be injured at this site in fractures or dislocations around the elbow or stretched in valgus deformity of this joint.

The tendon of biceps (**13**) inserts into the posterior lip of the tuberosity of the radius. It is a powerful supinator of the radio-ulnar joints as well as flexor of the elbow joint.

The brachial vessels are in close anterior proximity to the elbow joint; the artery may be compromised in supracondylar fractures which are relatively common in children.

The epicondyles have developed to provide attachment of the common extensor (lateral epicondyle) and common flexor (medial epicondyle) muscle groups.

Inflammation of the extensor origin on the lateral epicondyle (**22**) is known as 'tennis elbow'.

Orientation guide

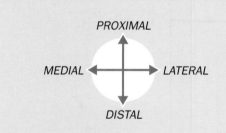

PROXIMAL

MEDIAL — LATERAL

DISTAL

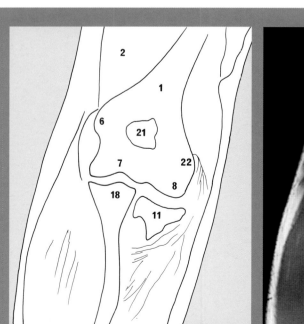

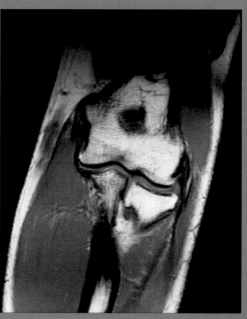

Coronal magnetic resonance image (MRI)

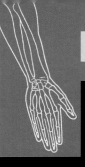

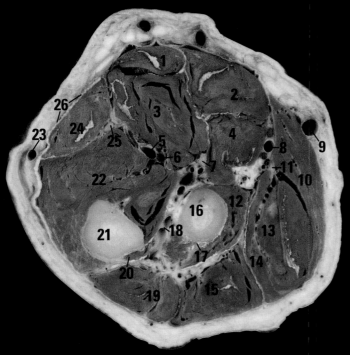

1 Palmaris longus
2 Flexor carpi radialis
3 Flexor digitorum superficialis
4 Pronator teres – humeral head
5 Ulnar artery
6 Ulnar vein
7 Median nerve with anterior interosseous artery and vein
8 Radial artery with venae comitantes
9 Cephalic vein
10 Brachioradialis
11 Radial nerve
12 Supinator
13 Extensor carpi radialis longus
14 Extensor carpi radialis brevis
15 Extensor digitorum
16 Radius
17 Posterior interosseous nerve
18 Posterior interosseous artery and vein
19 Extensor carpi ulnaris
20 Anconeus
21 Ulna
22 Flexor digitorum profundus
23 Basilic vein
24 Flexor carpi ulnaris
25 Ulnar nerve
26 Deep fascia of forearm

27 Pronator teres (ulnar head)

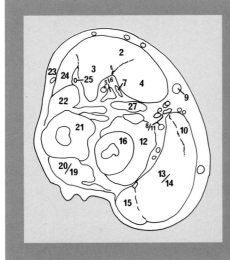

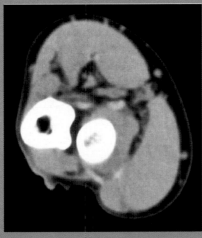

Axial computed tomogram (CT)

Orientation guide

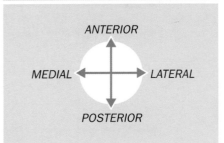

ANTERIOR

MEDIAL ←→ LATERAL

POSTERIOR

Section level

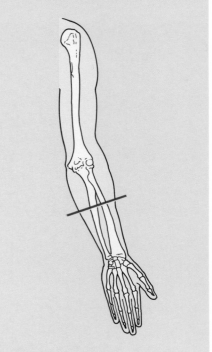

Notes

This section passes through the mid forearm. In both the section and CT image the forearm is viewed in the supinated position.

Note how the median nerve (**7**) characteristically hugs the deep aspect of flexor digitorum superficialis (**3**). The ulnar nerve (**25**) lies sandwiched between flexor carpi ulnaris (**24**) and flexor digitorum profundus (**22**) and the radial nerve (**11**) lies beneath brachioradialis (**10**).

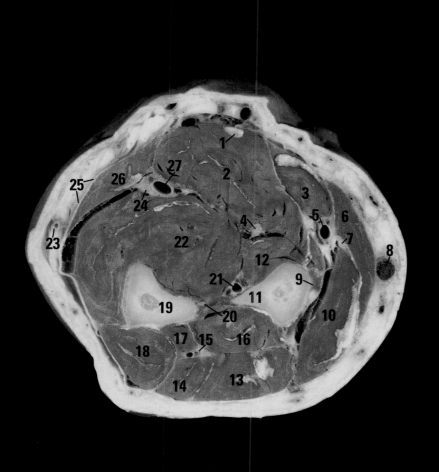

1 Palmaris longus tendon
2 Flexor digitorum superficialis
3 Flexor carpi radialis
4 Median nerve
5 Radial artery
6 Brachioradialis
7 Radial nerve
8 Cephalic vein
9 Pronator teres tendon
10 Extensor carpi radialis longus and brevis
11 Radius
12 Flexor pollicis longus
13 Extensor digitorum
14 Extensor digiti minimi
15 Posterior interosseous nerve with artery and vein
16 Abductor pollicis longus
17 Extensor pollicis longus
18 Extensor carpi ulnaris
19 Ulna
20 Interosseous membrane
21 Anterior interosseous artery, vein and nerve
22 Flexor digitorum profundus
23 Basilic vein
24 Ulnar nerve
25 Deep fascia of forearm
26 Flexor carpi ulnaris
27 Ulnar artery with venae comitantes

28 Superficial flexor group of muscles
29 Extensor group of muscles

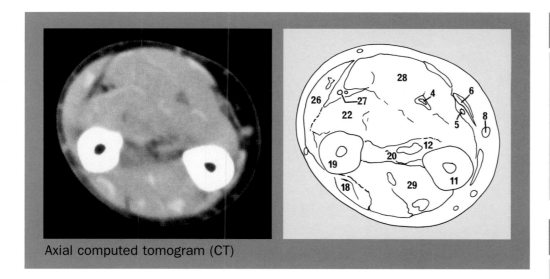

Axial computed tomogram (CT)

Orientation guide

ANTERIOR
MEDIAL — LATERAL
POSTERIOR

Section level

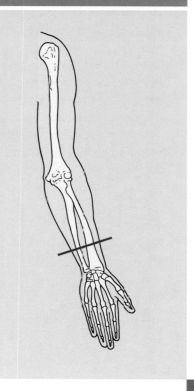

Notes

This section transects the supinated forearm at the junction of its upper two thirds and lower one-third.

Note that the very extensive origin of flexor digitorum profundus (**22**) is clearly demonstrated by this section. It arises from both the anterior and medial surfaces of the upper three quarters of the ulna (**19**), from the ulnar half of the interosseous membrane (**20**) and also from the superior three quarters of the posterior border of the ulna by an aponeurosis which is in common with that of flexor carpi ulnaris (**26**) and extensor carpi ulnaris (**18**).

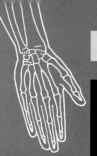

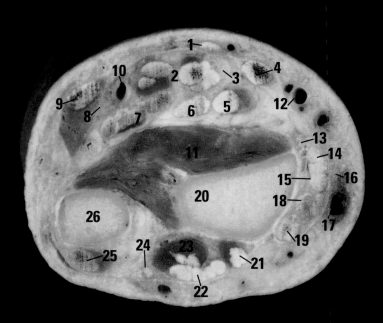

1	Palmaris longus tendon	**14**	Abductor pollicis longus tendon
2	Flexor digitorum superficialis tendons	**15**	Extensor pollicis brevis tendon
3	Median nerve	**16**	Radial nerve
4	Flexor carpi radialis tendon	**17**	Cephalic vein
5	Flexor pollicis longus tendon	**18**	Extensor carpi radialis longus tendon
6	Flexor digitorum profundus tendon to index finger	**19**	Extensor carpi radialis brevis tendon
7	Flexor digitorum profundus tendon to remaining fingers	**20**	Radius
		21	Extensor pollicis longus tendon
8	Ulnar nerve	**22**	Extensor digitorum tendon
9	Flexor carpi ulnaris tendon	**23**	Extensor indicis
10	Ulnar artery	**24**	Extensor digiti minimi tendon
11	Pronator quadratus	**25**	Extensor carpi ulnaris tendon
12	Radial artery	**26**	Ulna
13	Brachioradialis insertion		

27 Superficial vein

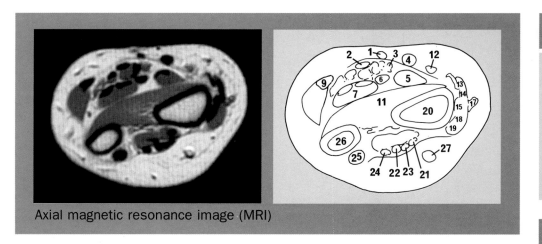

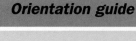

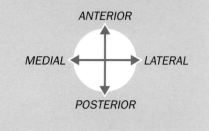

Axial magnetic resonance image (MRI)

Orientation guide

ANTERIOR

MEDIAL ←→ LATERAL

POSTERIOR

Section level

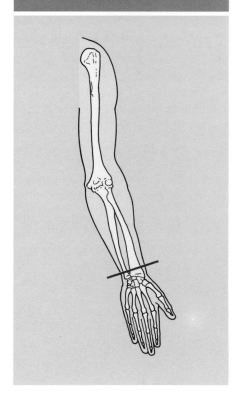

Notes

This section transects the forearm immediately proximal to the wrist joint.

The arrangement of the extensor tendons on the posterior and radial aspects of the wrist can be clearly appreciated. Note that extensor carpi ulnaris tendon (**25**) grooves the dorsal aspect of the distal ulna (**26**).

At this level, flexor digitorum profundus has given off a separate tendon to the index finger (**6**) while those for the remaining three fingers are still closely applied to each other (**7**).

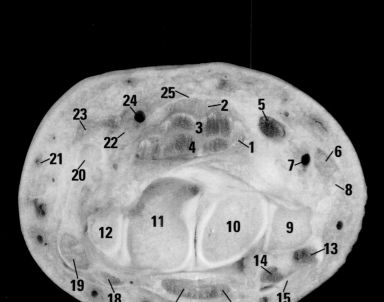

1 Flexor pollicis longus tendon
2 Median nerve
3 Flexor digitorum superficialis tendons
4 Flexor digitorum profundus tendons
5 Flexor carpi radialis tendon
6 Abductor pollicis longus tendon
7 Radial artery
8 Extensor pollicis brevis tendon
9 Styloid process of radius
10 Scaphoid
11 Lunate
12 Triquetral
13 Extensor carpi radialis longus tendon
14 Extensor carpi radialis brevis tendon

15 Extensor pollicis longus tendon
16 Extensor indicis tendon
17 Extensor digitorum tendon
18 Extensor digiti minimi tendon
19 Extensor carpi ulnaris tendon
20 Pisiform
21 Basilic vein
22 Ulnar nerve
23 Flexor carpi ulnaris tendon
24 Ulnar artery
25 Flexor retinaculum

26 Capitate
27 Hamate
28 Trapezoid
29 Trapezium

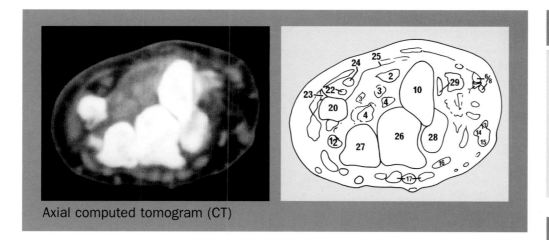

Axial computed tomogram (CT)

Orientation guide

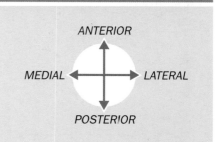

ANTERIOR

MEDIAL ←—→ LATERAL

POSTERIOR

Section level

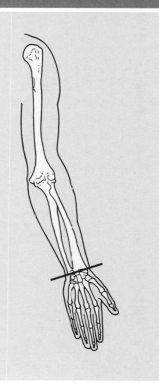

Notes

This section passes through the proximal row of carpal bones and the radial styloid process. The CT image is at a more distal level.

The radius (**9**) extends more distally than the ulna; thus abduction of the wrist is more limited than adduction.

The pisiform bone (**20**) can be considered as a sesamoid within the termination of the tendon of flexor carpi ulnaris (**23**), which anchors via the pisohamate ligament to the hook of the hamate and via the pisometacarpal ligament to the base of the fifth metacarpal bone.

The flexor retinaculum (**25**) is a tough fibrous band across the front of the carpus, which converts its concavity into the carpal tunnel, transmitting the flexor tendons of the digits together with the median nerve (**2**). Its attachments can be seen in this section and in section 3; medially to the pisiform (**20**) and to the hook of the hamate (**27**), laterally as two laminae, the more superficial one being attached to the tubercles of the scaphoid (**10**) and the trapezium (**29**) and the deep lamina to the medial lip of the groove on the latter.

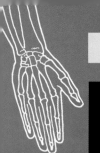

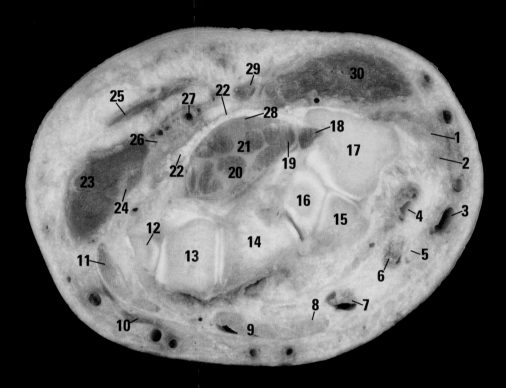

1	Abductor pollicis longus tendon	**17**	Trapezium
2	Extensor pollicis brevis tendon	**18**	Flexor carpi radialis tendon
3	Cephalic vein	**19**	Flexor pollicis longus tendon
4	Radial artery	**20**	Flexor digitorum profundus tendons
5	Extensor pollicis longus tendon	**21**	Flexor digitorum superficialis tendons
6	Extensor carpi radialis longus tendon	**22**	Flexor retinaculum
7	Extensor carpi radialis brevis tendon	**23**	Muscles of hypothenar eminence
8	Extensor indicis tendon	**24**	Pisometacarpal ligament
9	Extensor digitorum tendons	**25**	Palmaris brevis
10	Extensor digiti minimi tendon	**26**	Ulnar nerve
11	Extensor carpi ulnaris tendon	**27**	Ulnar artery
12	Triquetral	**28**	Median nerve
13	Hamate	**29**	Palmaris longus tendon
14	Capitate	**30**	Muscles of thenar eminence
15	Trapezoid		
16	Scaphoid		

31	Base of thumb metacarpal

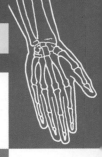

Section level

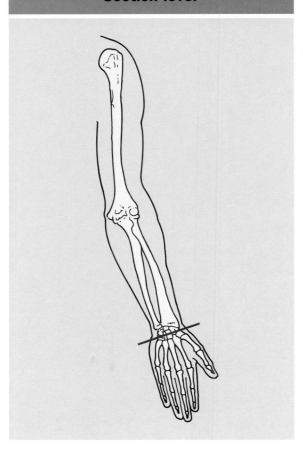

Orientation guide

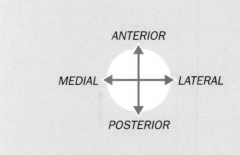

ANTERIOR

MEDIAL ← → LATERAL

POSTERIOR

Notes

This section passes through the distal part of the carpus. The bony arch is well seen.

The flexor retinaculum (**22**) has already been described (see section 2). Here its distal attachment to the trapezium (**17**) and the hook of the hamate (**13**) can be seen. Note the tendon of flexor carpi radialis (**18**) lying in the tunnel formed by the groove on the trapezium and the two laminae of the lateral attachment of the retinaculum.

Swelling or deformity within the carpal tunnel compresses the median nerve (**28**) and produces the carpal tunnel syndrome.

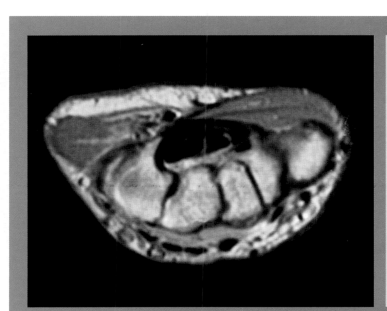

Axial magnetic resonance image (MRI)

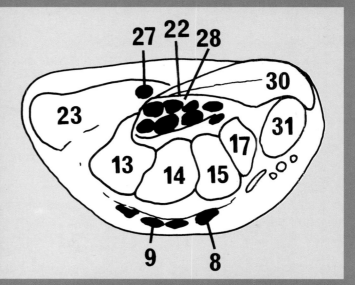

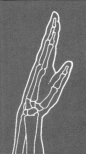

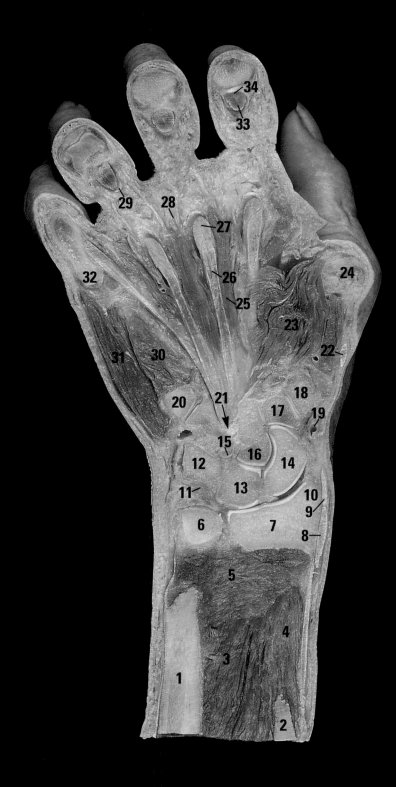

1 Shaft of ulna	**16** Capitate	**28** Common digital artery, vein and nerve
2 Shaft of radius	**17** Trapezoid	**29** Digital fibrous sheath of ring finger
3 Flexor digitorum profundus (see also 33)	**18** Trapezium	**30** Flexor digiti minimi
4 Flexor pollicis longus	**19** Radial artery in anatomical snuffbox	**31** Abductor digiti minimi
5 Pronator quadratus	**20** Base of metacarpal of little finger bone	**32** Base of proximal phalanx of little finger
6 Head of ulna	**21** Distal opening of carpal tunnel (arrowed)	**33** Tendon of flexor digitorum profundus of index finger (see also 3)
7 Distal end of radius	**22** Extensor pollicis longus	**34** Tendon of flexor digitorum superficialis of index finger
8 Abductor pollicis longus	**23** Abductor pollicis	
9 Extensor pollicis brevis	**24** Head of first metacarpal	
10 Radial styloid process	**25** Second lumbrical	
11 Articular disc (Triangular fibrocartilaginous complex TFCC)	**26** Tendon of flexor digitorum profundus	**35** Ulnar styloid
12 Triquetral	**27** Tendon of flexor digitorum superficialis	**36** Base of index metacarpal bone
13 Lunate		
14 Scaphoid		
15 Hamate		

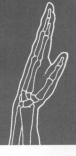

Section level

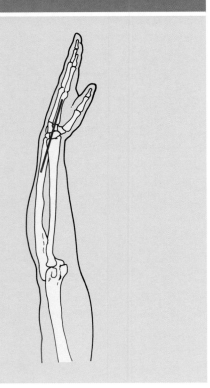

Orientation guide

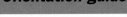
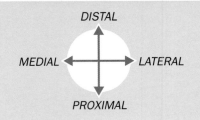

DISTAL

MEDIAL ←→ LATERAL

PROXIMAL

Notes

Note that in the anatomical position of the wrist joint the scaphoid (**14**) and lunate (**13**) are in contact with the distal end of the radius (**7**). The triquetral (**12**) only articulates against the articular disc (**11**) when the hand is adducted. The triquetral is therefore virtually never injured in falls on the hand.

The pulse of the radial artery (**19**) can be palpated in the anatomical snuff box as the artery lies against the underlying scaphoid (**14**).

The distal end of ulna is fractionally shorter than that of the radius. Thus an articular disc (the triangular fibro-cartilaginous complex – TFCC) runs from the ulnar styloid to the radius to complete the proximal part of the ellipsoid wrist joint. An articular disc implies two types of movement; the radius supinates and pronates around the ulna proximal to the disc. Minor variance in ulnar length probably contributes to damge to the TFCC in later life.

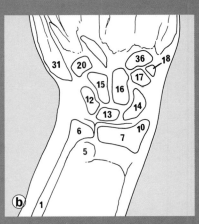

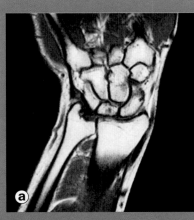

Coronal magnetic resonance image (MRI)

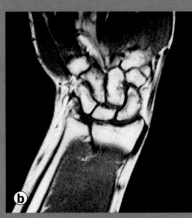

Coronal magnetic resonance image (MRI)

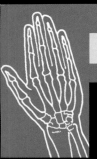

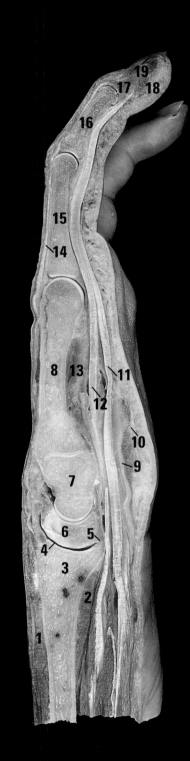

1 Extensor digitorum
2 Pronator quadratus
3 Distal end of radius
4 Wrist joint
5 Capsule of wrist joint
6 Lunate
7 Capitate
8 Metacarpal bone of
  middle finger
9 Flexor retinaculum
10 Palmar aponeurosis
11 Tendon of flexor
  digitorum superficialis

12 Tendon of flexor
  digitorum profundus
13 Adductor pollicis
14 Extensor expansion
15 Proximal phalanx of
  middle finger
16 Middle phalanx of
  middle finger
17 Distal Phalanx of middle
  finger
18 Pulp space of distal
  phalanx
19 Nail bed

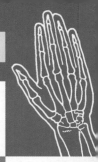

Section level

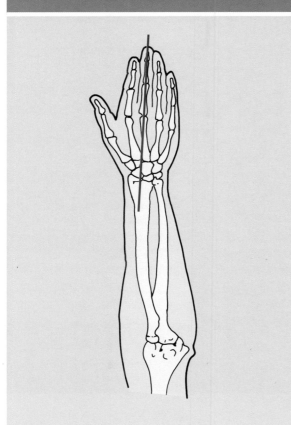

Orientation guide

DISTAL

DORSAL ←→ PALMAR

PROXIMAL

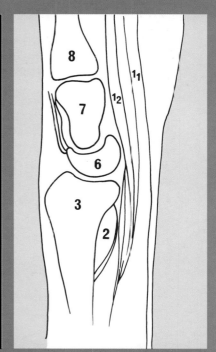

Sagittal magnetic resonance image (MRI)

Notes

The 'half moon' of the lunate (**6**) is well demonstrated in this sagittal section. This characteristic appearance enables it to be identified readily in a lateral radiograph of the hand. Lateral radiographs are needed to assess lunate or perilunate dislocations which are often missed on AP radiographs. Note the continuous alignment of radius, lunate, capitate and metacarpal bones.

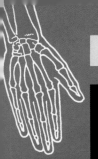

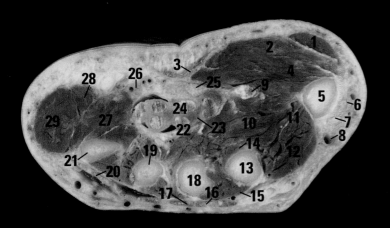

1	Abductor pollicis brevis	**17**	Extensor digitorum tendon
2	Flexor pollicis brevis	**18**	Third metacarpal
3	Palmar aponeurosis	**19**	Fourth metacarpal
4	Oponens pollicis brevis	**20**	Extensor digiti minimi tendon
5	First metacarpal	**21**	Fifth metacarpal
6	Extensor pollicis brevis tendon	**22**	Flexor digitorum profundus tendons
7	Extensor pollicis longus tendon	**23**	Lumbrical
8	Cephalic vein	**24**	Flexor digitorum superficialis tendons
9	Flexor pollicis longus tendon	**25**	Median nerve
10	Adductor pollicis	**26**	Ulnar artery and nerve
11	Radial artery	**27**	Opponens digiti minimi
12	First dorsal interosseous	**28**	Flexor digiti minimi
13	Second metacarpal	**29**	Abductor digiti minimi
14	Second palmar interosseous		
15	Second dorsal interosseous	**30**	Muscles of thenar eminence
16	Extensor indicis tendon	**31**	Muscles of hypothenar eminence

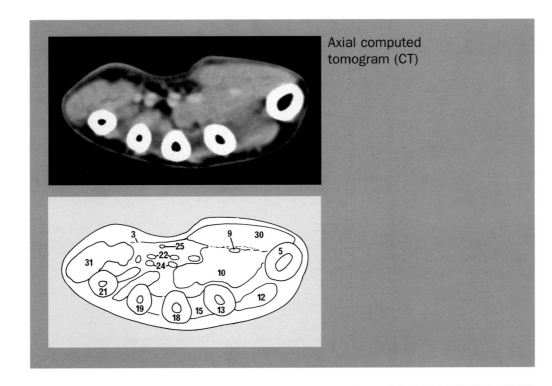

Axial computed tomogram (CT)

Orientation guide

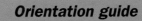

ANTERIOR

MEDIAL — LATERAL

POSTERIOR

Section level

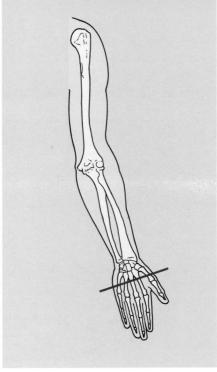

Notes

This section passes through the proximal shafts of the metacarpals.

The dense central part of the palmar aponeurosis (**3**) is triangular, its apex being continuous with the distal margin of the flexor retinaculum (see Wrist section 2 page, 234 and section 3, page 235). The expanded tendon of palmaris longus (see Wrist section 3, page 235), is attached to it. It is strongly bound to the overlying skin by dense fibroareolar tissue. Compare this with the loose superficial fascia over the extensor aspect of the hand. Oedema of the hand thus occurs mainly on its dorsal aspect. The lateral and medial extensions of the palmar aponeurosis are the thin superficial coverings of the thenar and hypothenar muscles respectively.

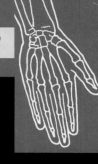

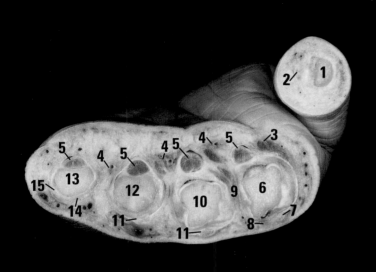

1 Proximal phalanx of thumb
2 Flexor pollicis longus tendon
3 First lumbrical
4 Neurovascular bundle
5 Flexor tendons within sheath
6 Second metacarpal head
7 Extensor digitorum tendon to index finger
8 Extensor indicis tendon
9 Interosseous muscles
10 Third metacarpal head
11 Extensor digitorum tendon
12 Fourth metacarpal head
13 Fifth metacarpal head
14 Extensor digitorum tendon to little finger
15 Extensor indicis tendon

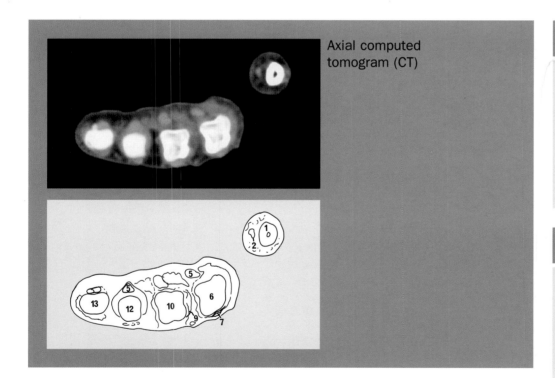

Axial computed tomogram (CT)

Orientation guide

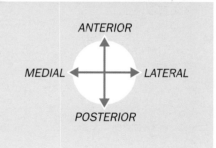

ANTERIOR

MEDIAL ← → LATERAL

POSTERIOR

Section level

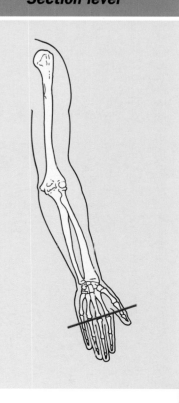

Notes

This section passes through the heads of the metacarpals of the fingers and through the proximal phalanx of the thumb (**1**).

In the distal part of the palm, the digital arteries pass deeply between the divisions of the digital nerves so that, on the sides of the digits, the neurovascular bundle (**4**) has the digital nerve lying anterior to the digital artery and vein. The bundles lie adjacent to the tendon sheaths anterior to the metacarpal heads and this relationship is also maintained in the fingers. Thus an incision along the anterior border of the bone will avoid these important structures.

244